BARNEY FLEMING, PhD, ATP

Pressure Ulcer Research

D. Bader · C. Bouten · D. Colin · C. Oomens (Eds.)

Dan Bader · Carlijn Bouten
Denis Colin · Cees Oomens

Pressure Ulcer Research

Current and Future Perspectives

With 76 Figures and 23 Tables

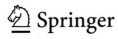 Springer

DAN L. BADER, PhD, DSc
Queen Mary University of London
Mile End Road
London E1 4NS
United Kingdom

CARLIJN V.C. BOUTEN, PhD
Eindhoven University of Technology
Biomedical Engineering Department
Den Dolech 2, P/O Box 513
5600 MB Eindhoven
The Netherlands

DENIS COLIN, MD
Medical Director
Centre de l'Arche
72650 Saint Saturnin
Le Mans, France

CEES W.J. OOMENS, PhD
Eindhoven University of Technology
Biomedical Engineering Department
Den Dolech 2, P/O Box 513
5600 MB Eindhoven
The Netherlands

ISBN-10 3-540-25030-1 Springer Berlin Heidelberg New York
ISBN-13 978-3-540-25030-2 Springer Berlin Heidelberg New York

Library of Congress Control Number: 2005928443

Springer is a part of Springer Science+Business Media

springeronline.com

© Springer-Verlag Berlin · Heidelberg 2005
Printed in Germany

Editor: Gabriele Schröder, Springer-Verlag
Desk Editor: Stephanie Benko, Springer-Verlag
Production: Pro Edit GmbH, Elke Beul-Göhringer, Heidelberg, Germany
Typesetting: K+V Fotosatz GmbH, Beerfelden
Cover design: Estudio Calamar, F. Steinen-Broo, Pau/Girona, Spain

24/3151/beu-göh – 5 4 3 2 1 0 – Printed on acid-free paper

...In the morning she was asked how she had slept. "Oh, very badly!" said she. "I have scarcely closed my eyes all night. Heaven only knows what was in the bed, but I was lying on something hard, so that I am black and blue all over my body. It's horrible!" Now they knew she was really a princess because she had felt the pea right through the twenty mattresses and the twenty eider-down beds...
(Hans Christian Andersen:
The Princess & The Pea)

We dedicate this book to all the princesses and princes in the world

Preface

Although the clinical condition of pressure ulcers has existed since time immemorial, with evidence of its occurrence in ancient Egypt, there has been a paucity of tomes devoted to the subject. Of the few which have highlighted the scientific aspects of the topic, two edited books, "Bed Sore Biomechanics" [1] and "Pressure Sores – Clinical Practice and Scientific Approach" [2] were published around 30 and 15 years ago, respectively. It is interesting to note that the name of the condition has changed during this period, from bed sores to pressure sores to pressure ulcers. The current term has been widely adopted worldwide by various organisations, such as the National Pressure Ulcer Advisory Panel (NPUAP) in the USA, the EPUAP in Europe and the Japanese Pressure Ulcer Society. Each body is committed to prevention and treatment strategies, but despite their efforts incidence figures remain unacceptably high. So what was our motivation for the current book? Well, we have already invested many years, with only minor success, in trying to alleviate this horrendous condition, which Pam Hibbs regularly described as "the hidden epidemic beneath the sheets". However, as in most walks of life, politics and monetary considerations have reared their heads. As an example, a financial audit in 1997 in the Netherlands encompassing all clinical conditions revealed that the prevention and treatment of pressure ulcers represented the fourth largest financial burden on the Dutch health service. This stimulated a wealth of activity in the Biomedical Engineering Department at the Technological University of Eindhoven, which brought us, the editors, together. In addition, the medico-legal implications of ulcer development have stimulated the interests of financial managers, who run hospitals and homes, and the associated medical insurance companies. Further considerations involve conditions that previously were life threatening but now are manageable with the advances in medical technologies. This has resulted in an ever-ageing population in many countries. It is only right for every individual to demand an improved healthspan to match this increased lifespan. Again, technology can provide solutions, and, as researchers, we firmly believe that much can be gained from applying many of the new sciences, ranging from genomics over cellular and tissue engineering to medical imaging and computational modelling. These tools can be used to provide a clearer understanding of the mechanisms associated with the aetiology of pressure ulcers, extending beyond the conventional wisdom of the effects of pressure ischaemia alone. Ultimately, they will also be used to identify the risk levels of individuals and provide appropriate support systems. This was the motivation for us to bring together a number of multidisciplinary world experts, who have contributed generously to this volume.

The Editors

References

1. Kenedi RM, Cowden JM, Scales JT (eds) (1976) Bed sore biomechanics. Macmillan, London
2. Bader DL (ed) (1990) Pressure sores: clinical practice and scientific approach. Macmillan, London

Contents

List of Contributors

DAN BADER
Department of Engineering
& IRC in Biomedical Materials
Queen Mary University of London
Mile End Road
London, E1 4NS
UK

NANCY BERGSTROM
Center on Aging
6901 Bertner Avenue, 625
Houston, TX 77030,
USA

KATH BOGIE
Rehabilitation Engineering Center
Cleveland FES Center
Hamann Building, Room 601
MetroHealth Medical Center
2500 MetroHealth Drive
Cleveland, OH 44109-1998
USA

CARLIJN BOUTEN
Biomedical Engineering Department
Eindhoven University of Technology
P/O Box 513
5600 MB Eindhoven
The Netherlands

DEBBIE BRONNEBERG
Eindhoven University of Technology
P/O Box 513
5600 MB Eindhoven
The Netherlands

DENIS COLIN
Rehabilitation Hospital
Centre de l'Arche
72650 Saint Saturnin
France

MARTIN FERGUSON-PELL
Centre for Disability Research
and Innovation
Institute of Orthopaedics
& Musculo-Skeletal Science
University College London
RNOH Trust
Brockley Hill, Stanmore
Middlesex, HA7 4LP
UK

DEBBY GAWLITTA
Biomedical Engineering Department
Eindhoven University of Technology
P/O Box 513
5600 MB Eindhoven
The Netherlands

JEEN HAALBOOM
Universitair Medisch Centrum Utrecht
Interne Geneeskunde
P.O. Box 85500
3508 GA Utrecht
The Netherlands

SATSUE HAGISAWA
Department of Nursing
Kumamoto Health Science University
Izumi 325
Kumamoto 861-5598
Japan

MARIA HOPMAN
Radboud University Nijmegen
Medical Centre
Department of Physiology
Nijmegen
The Netherlands

TIM JAMES
Department of Clinical Biochemistry
Oxford Radcliffe Hospital
Headington
Oxford, OX3 1XX
UK

THOMAS JANSSEN
Faculty of Human Movement Sciences
Vrije Universiteit
Van der Boechorststraat 9
1081 BT Amsterdam
The Netherlands

SARAH KNIGHT
Spinal Research Centre
Royal National Orthopaedic Hospital
Brockley Hill
Stanmore, Middlesex, HA7 4LP
UK

COURTNEY LYDER
School of Nursing
University of Virginia
McLeod Hall
Charlottesville, VA 22908
USA

CHARLES MICHEL
Imperial College London
South Kensington Campus
London, SW7 2AZ
UK

KLAAS NICOLAY
Department of Biomedical Technology
Eindhoven University of Technology
P/O Box 513
5600 MB Eindhoven
The Netherlands

CEES OOMENS
Biomedical Engineering Department
Eindhoven University of Technology
P/O Box 513
5600 MB Eindhoven
The Netherlands

ADRIAN POLLIACK
Department of Clinical Biochemistry
Oxford Radcliffe Hospital
Headington
Oxford, OX3 1XX
UK

JEANINE PROMPERS
Department of Biomedical Technology
Eindhoven University of Technology
P/O Box 513
5600 MB Eindhoven
The Netherlands

JOAN SANDERS
Bioengineering, 357962
University of Washington
Seattle, WA 98195
USA

TATSUO SHIMADA
School of Nursing
Oita University
Hasama 1-1, Oita 879-5593
Japan

CHRISTOF SMIT
Rehabilitation Center Amsterdam
Overtoom 283
1054 HW Amsterdam
The Netherlands

ANKE STEKELENBURG
Biomedical Engineering
Eindhoven University of Technology
P/O Box 513
5600 MB Eindhoven
The Netherlands

GUSTAV STRIJKERS
Department of Biomedical Technology
Eindhoven University of Technology
P/O Box 513
5600 MB Eindhoven
The Netherlands

IAN SWAIN
Department of Medical Physics
& Biomedical Engineering
Salisbury District Hospital
Salisbury Wiltshire, SP2 8BJ
UK

RICHARD TAYLOR
Department of Clinical Biochemistry
Oxford Radcliffe Hospital
Headington
Oxford, OX3 9DU
UK

PANKAJ VADGAMA
IRC in Biomedical Materials
Queen Mary University of London
Mile End Road
London, E1 4NS
UK

WEN WANG
Medical Engineering Division
Department of Engineering
Queen Mary University of London
Mile End Road
London E1 4NS
UK

YAK-NAM WANG
Department of Bioengineering
357962, Harris 309
University of Washington
Seattle, WA 98195
USA

The Aetiopathology of Pressure Ulcers: A Hierarchical Approach [1]

CARLIJN BOUTEN, CEES OOMENS, DENIS COLIN, DAN BADER

Introduction

Pressure ulcers are localized areas of tissue breakdown in skin and/or underlying tissues [1]. They can occur in all situations where subjects are subjected to sustained mechanical loads, but are particularly common in those who are bedridden, wheelchair bound or wearing a prosthesis or orthosis. The ulcers are painful, difficult to treat, and represent a burden to the community in terms of healthcare and finances. Consequently, they may affect the quality of life of many young and elderly individuals. To date, attempts to prevent pressure ulcers have not led to a significant reduction of the problem. As is detailed in Chaps. 2 and 3, prevalence figures remain unacceptably high, ranging between 8 and 23% depending on the severity of wounds included and the subject group under investigation [2–4]. It is widely established that this is, at least partly, due to the limited fundamental knowledge related to the aetiology of the clinical condition. Thus, the design and application of preventive aids and risk assessment techniques are so far dominated by subjective measures or, at best, based on a relatively small amount of data focusing on skin tissues.

A striking example is the traditionally quoted value for capillary closure pressure of 32 mmHg (4.3 kPa) that is still frequently used as a threshold for tissue damage [5]. Interface pressures at the contact area between skin and supporting surfaces (such as mattresses or cushions) in excess of this value are assumed to produce a degree of ischaemia which, if applied for a sufficient period of time, may lead to tissue breakdown [6–8]. Leaving aside the discussion of whether ischaemia is the principal factor for tissue breakdown in pressure ulcers, capillary closure depends on local pressure gradients across the vessel wall and not just on interface pressures at the skin level. Hence interface pressures well above capillary pressures can be supported by the soft tissues before blood flow is seriously impaired [9]. An interesting observation reported by Husain [10] in 1953 was that localized interface pressures obliterated more vessels in the skin and subcutaneous tissue than in the muscle, while the latter was severely damaged and

---

[1] The content of this chapter is based on the authors' paper: "The aetiology of pressure sores: skin deep or muscle bound?" (Arch Phys Med Rehab 84:616–619; 2003) [39].

the skin and subcutis were not. Later studies also demonstrated that muscle tissue is more susceptible to mechanical loading than skin [6, 11, 12]. Notwithstanding these facts the primary focus in pressure ulcer prevention and treatment has traditionally been on skin, and the risks of tissue degeneration in other tissues is generally neglected. This is to a large extent due to the availability and possibilities of existing methodologies and technologies, which limited the aetiological knowledge progression of pressure ulcer development to the skin.

In order to be able to reduce the prevalence of pressure ulcers it is essential to improve and expand our knowledge of the aetiopathogenesis in terms of both basic science and clinical application. In terms of the former we propose a more rigorous analysis of existing data, followed by a hierarchical research approach in which the effects of mechanical loading are studied at different tissue levels and at the level of different functional units of soft tissues. Tissue levels refer to superficial (skin) and/or deep tissue layers (muscle, subcutaneous fat), whereas tissue units involve the cells and extracellular matrix composing the tissue as well as the vessels providing for fluid transport inside the tissue. The separate tissues and tissue units and their relevance in pressure ulcer development are reviewed in detail in various chapters of this book. An integrated approach, combining the presented knowledge and proposed (new) research technologies, should lead to a thorough understanding of the aetiopathology and subsequent prevention and treatment of pressure ulcers.

Deep Versus Superficial Ulcers

As a guide to pressure ulcer prevention, research has focused on determining the minimal degree of loading that will consistently lead to persistent tissue damage. Typically, such physical conditions are derived from animal experiments [6, 8, 13, 14] with some degree of variable control, and, more rarely, from human studies, the most prominent of which is nearly 30 years old but still regularly quoted [15]. In the animal studies soft tissues are loaded externally via prescribed pressures or shear stresses applied to the skin, whereas the onset of tissue breakdown is generally observed from histological examinations after predetermined periods of time, as is detailed in Chaps. 12 and 15. Despite large variations in absolute measures these studies all demonstrate an inverse relationship between the magnitude and duration of loading, indicating that the higher loads require less time to initiate tissue breakdown. More importantly, they suggest that pressure ulcers can develop either superficially or from within the deep tissue depending on the nature of the surface loading. The superficial type forms in the skin with maceration and detachment of superficial skin layers and is predominantly caused by shear stresses within the skin layers. If allowed to progress the damage may form an ulcer, which is easily detected [13, 16]. Deep ulcers, on the other hand, arise in deep muscle layers covering bony prominences and are mainly caused by sustained compression of the tissue [6, 8, 10, 12, 17]. These ulcers are very harmful, developing at a faster rate than superficial ulcers and yielding more extensive ulceration. The damage progresses towards the surface, so that considerable necrosis of muscle, fascia and subcutaneous tissue may occur even at a stage when the skin shows only minor signs of tissue breakdown. Hence the initial pathological changes which lead to the most severe ulcers are in the deep tissues and therefore are difficult to identify with techniques currently available. Although this is recognized in clinical practice, where tactile examinations are prescribed to examine the tissue for deep pressure ulcers [19–21], this fact is frequently overlooked by objective risk assessment techniques, clinical classification schemes and techniques for prevention, such as those reviewed in Chap. 4, most of which focus on the skin and ignore the underlying tissues. Although these approaches have relevance in clinical practice because the skin is easily accessible, it should be realized that by the time a deep pressure ulcer becomes visible clinical intervention is too late and the prognosis is variable.

Pathways of Tissue Breakdown

Although it is well acknowledged that pressure ulcers are primarily caused by sustained mechanical loading of the soft tissues of the body, prevention of the ulcers by reducing the degree of loading alone remains difficult. This is mainly due to the fact that the underlying pathways whereby mechanical loading leads to tissue breakdown are poorly understood. It is not clear how global, external loading conditions are transferred to local stresses and strains inside the tissues and how these internal conditions may ultimately lead to tissue breakdown at a cellular level.

Considerable efforts have been made to determine the most effective way of measuring and reducing surface pressures at skin level [22, 23], as is also reviewed in Chap. 5. However, surface pressures are not representative of the internal mechanical conditions inside the tissue, which are most relevant for tissue breakdown. This is especially the case when tissue geometry and composition are complex and surface pressures result in highly inhomogeneous internal mechanical conditions, as is the case adjacent to bony prominences, like the trochanter, the sacrum, the heel or the ischial tuberosities. Nonetheless, in order to study the response of various tissue layers to mechanical loading the local mechanical environment within these layers needs to be known. The transition from global external loads to local internal stresses and strains requires the use of computer models [24, 25] (Chaps. 9 and 10) typically unfamiliar to experimentalists and clinical and nursing staff. Although not yet clinically validated these models may provide better insights into the mechanical conditions of separate tissue layers, extending from skin to muscle tissue. As an example, Fig. 1.1 shows a simplified computer model of the mechanical response of the separate soft tissue layers in the human buttock during sitting on a foam cushion. The ischial tuberosity is simulated by an undeformable bony indenter, whereas representative visco-elastic mechanical properties are incorporated for the individual tissue layers and the cushion material [26]. Using the finite element approach, detailed information on the magnitude and location of internal stresses and strains as a result of external loading can be obtained. Figure 1.1 clearly shows the inhomogeneous mechanical condition of the various tissue layers and areas of large tissue strains in the deeper fat and muscle layers. Combining such models with experimental data on the load-bearing capacity of the individual tissue layers will provide predictive measures of when and where tissue damage is likely to occur. This is, however, not straightforward, since the load-bearing capacity of the biological tissues is influenced by many systemic and local factors, such as temperature, nutritional status and disease.

Although computer models will provide insight into the internal mechanical conditions relevant for tissue damage, experimental research is required to validate material properties and to explain how these conditions eventually lead to tissue breakdown. There is surprisingly little consensus about the pathophysiological response to mechanical loading that triggers soft tissue breakdown. Theories involve localized ischaemia [6–8, 13], impaired interstitial fluid flow and lymphatic drainage [23, 27, 28], reperfusion injury [29, 30] and sustained deformation of cells [14, 31]. Traditionally, these theories have been proposed following experimental observations limited to the depth of skin layers determined by the physical characteristics derived from such measurement techniques as that involving blood flow and oxygen tension. However, with the development of new techniques, including magnetic resonance imaging (MRI; Chap. 18), it is cer-

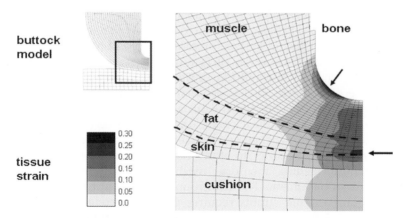

Fig. 1.1. Simplified computer model of deformed buttock (*top left*) of an 80-kg male subject demonstrating the differential response of the separate soft tissue layers (*right*) during sitting on a foam cushion. Because of assumed symmetry only half a buttock is used for calculations. Values indicate tissue strains, representing distortional energy. Note the areas of high strain in the subcutaneous fat and deep muscle layers (*arrows*) (adapted from [39])

tainly possible to relate mechanical loading to pathophysiological phenomena within deeper tissues [32, 33].

Theories focusing on ischaemia and impaired lymphatic drainage have been studied in vivo and generally confirm that sustained tissue loading will influence tissue perfusion and/or lymph flow, thereby affecting the transport of nutrients to and metabolic waste products away from cells within the tissue. Although this is appropriate for muscle tissue, which is metabolically more active than skin, these theories can only partly explain the onset of pressure ulcers and have not been fully verified. The same argument also applies to reperfusion injury mediated through oxygen free radicals. This theory states that it is the restoration of blood flow after load removal, rather than impaired blood flow during loading per se, which exacerbates the compromise to the tissue viability. Although described for other post-ischaemic pathologies, such as cardiac infarction, the specific role of reperfusion injury in the causation of pressure ulcers is still the subject of extensive study (Chap. 12). However, if reperfusion injury is indeed an important factor in promoting pressure ulcers, many traditional clinical practices involving patient-turning and pressure-relieving systems need to be carefully evaluated.

Existing histopathological data [14, 34] suggest a cellular origin of pressure ulcer development and it has been hypothesized that cellular damage is caused by sustained cell deformation. Indeed, cell deformation triggers a variety of effects, such as volume changes and cytoskeletal reorganization, which may be involved in early tissue breakdown. As it is impossible to examine the cellular response to loading in vivo independently of other factors, in-vitro models of cultured cells or engineered tissues under compressive or shear loading have been employed [35, 36]. Recent studies, described in Chaps. 15 and 16, demonstrate that such models are useful in studying the damaging effects of well-controlled compressive loading regimens in terms of cell damage or death. Although in-vitro models may prove to be an important tool in defining thresholds for cellular breakdown they are, as yet, difficult to relate to patient studies.

Overall the existing theories focus on the different functional units of soft tissue, involving the cells, the interstitial space with extracellular matrix, and blood and lymph vessels. These units are affected by mechanical loading to varying degrees and hence have different relevance for tissue breakdown. Most probably each of them contributes to the causation of pressure ulcers, although their individual and combined role in tissue breakdown will undoubtedly vary depending on the nature of the mechanical insult and patient characteristics such as illness or age [37], which affect soft tissue properties and hence the vulnerability to tissue breakdown.

Hierarchical Approach

To investigate the differential response of the various tissue functional units to mechanical loading and their relative contributions to the development of pressure ulcers a hybrid methodology involving a combination of computational and experimental studies must be adopted. The experimental studies should aim at elucidating the relationships between mechanical loading, the pathophysiological response to loading and tissue breakdown in testing hypotheses on the aetiopathogenesis of pressure ulcers. The computational models should be designed to predict the association between external and internal mechanical conditions within soft tissues and their functional units. This methodology must incorporate all soft tissue layers involved in pressure ulcers, extending from superficial stratum corneum of the epidermis to dermal layers, to subcutaneous fat, fascia, and deep muscle layers. Moreover, a hierarchical approach is proposed, in which the effects of loading are studied in different, yet complementary, model systems with increasing complexity and length scale and incorporating one or more functional tissue units. Thus, in-vitro models, ranging from the single cell (micrometer scale) to cell-matrix constructs (millimeter scale) and individual tissue layers (millimeter-centimeter scale) might be used to study the relationship between cell deformation and cell damage [38], as well as the influence of the surrounding extracellular matrix and three-dimensional tissue architecture on this relationship. The role of tissue (re)perfusion and lymph flow as well as the interaction between tissue layers in bulk tissue might further be assessed using in-vivo studies with animal models or human subjects. The different length scales of these models can be coupled by multi-scale computer calculations that enable the prediction of the internal microscopic mechanical environment within a given model from global, macroscopic loading conditions, such as interface pressures (and vice versa). In this way relationships between, for instance, cell deformation and cell damage [36] can be extrapolated to the level of bulk tissue to give clinically relevant predictions on tissue breakdown.

After setting the scene of pressure ulcer-related medical perspectives, costs and medico-legal aspects in Sect. 1, the proposed hierarchical approach is reflected in the chapters of Sects. 2 and 3. This approach can strongly benefit from new technologies, such as cell and tissue engineering and vital imaging techniques including MRI or vital microscopy, which are reviewed in Sect. 4. Cell and tissue engineering strategies enable the fabrication of in-vitro model systems with well-defined, controllable properties, which are designed to test specific hypotheses independently of predisposing factors associated with the onset of pressure ulcers. Vital imaging techniques permit monitoring of the pathophysiological response to loading in real time with none of the ethical considerations associated with the histological examination of loaded tissue in animal studies. Moreover, these techniques offer the potential of both examining the effects of mechanical loading in human subjects and, ultimately, serving as predictive tools for the screening of tissues for superficial or deep pressure ulcers in a clinical setting.

Despite the considerable amount of existing clinical experience, it is our opinion that the proposed hierarchical approach will improve fundamental knowledge about the aetiopathology of pressure ulcers, which can serve as a sound basis for effective clinical identification and prevention. The hierarchy of model systems can be used to establish well-defined thresholds for tissue damage, which can provide new guidelines for pressure ulcer prevention and to redirect available pressure-relieving strategies. In addition, the established thresholds can be related to biochemical markers for the identification of early, reversible tissue damage. Adequate guidelines for damage prevention and early identification of damage will lead to a reduction of medical costs and time of hospitalisation, as well as a more efficient and economic use of available support systems.

References

1. American Pressure Ulcer Advisory Panel (1998) Pressure ulcers prevalence, cost and risk assessment: consensus development conference statement. Decubitus 2:24–8
2. Dealey C (1991) The size of the pressure sore problem in a teaching hospital. J Adv Nurs 16:663–70
3. Meehan M (1990) Multisite pressure ulcer prevalence study. Decubitus 3:14–17
4. Haalboom JRE (1997) Decubitus anno 1997. Ned Tijdschr Geneesk 141:35 (in Dutch)
5. Landis EM (1930) Micro-injection studies of capillary blood pressure in human skin. Heart 15:209–228
6. Daniel RK, Priest DL, Wheatley DC (1982) Etiologic factors in pressure sores: an experimental model. Arch Phys Med Rehab 62:492–498
7. Bar CA (1988) The response of tissues to applied pressure. University of Wales College of Medicine, Cardiff, UK
8. Kosiak M (1961) Etiology of decubitus ulcers. Arch Phys Med Rehab 42:19–29
9. Bader DL (1990) The recovery characteristics of soft tissues following repeated loading. J Rehabil Res Dev 27:141–150
10. Husain T (1953) Experimental study of some pressure effects on tissue, with reference to the bed sore problem. Path Bact 66:347–363
11. Nola GT, Vistnes LM (1980) Differential response of skin and muscle in the experimental production of pressure sores. Plast Reconstr Surg 66:728–733
12. Salcido R, Donofrio JC, Fisher SB, LeGrand EK, Dickey K, Carney JM (1994) Histopathology of pressure ulcers as a result of sequential computer-controlled pressure sessions in a fuzzy rat model. Adv Wound Care 7:23–40
13. Dinsdale SM (1974) Decubitus ulcers: Role of pressure and friction in causation. Arch Phys Med Rehab 55:147–152
14. Bouten CVC, Bosboom EMH, Oomens CWJ (1999) The aetiology of pressure sores: A tissue and cell mechanics approach. In: Van der Woude LHV, Hopman MTE, Van Kemenade CH (eds) Biomedical aspects of manual wheelchair propulsion. IOS Press, Amsterdam, pp 52–62

15. Reswick J, Rogers J (1976) Experience at Rancho Los Amigos Hospital with devices and techniques to prevent pressure sores. In: Kennedy RM, Cowden JM, Scales JT (eds) Bedsore biomechanics. University Park Press, Baltimore, pp 301–310
16. Reuler IB, Coonery TJ (1981) The pressure sore: pathophysiology and principles of management. Ann Intern Med 94:661–666
17. Groth KE (1942) Klinische Beobachtungen und experimentelle Studien über die Entstehung des Dekubitus. Acta Chir Scand 87 [Suppl 76]:1–209 (in German)
18. Bliss MR (1992) Acute pressure area care: Sir James Paget's legacy. Lancet 339:221–223
19. Bergstrom N (1992) A research agenda for pressure ulcer prevention. Decubitus 5:22–30
20. Garber SL, Rintala DH, Rossi CD, Hart KA, Fuhrer MJ (1996) Reported pressure ulcer prevention and management techniques by persons with spinal cord injury. Arch Phys Med Rehabil 8:744–749
21. AHCPR (1994) Treatment of pressure ulcers. Clinical practice guideline no. 15. US Dept. of Human Services, PHS
22. Silver-Thorn MB, Steege JW, Childress DS (1996) A review of prosthetic interface stress investigations. J Rehab Res Dev 33:253–266
23. Barbenel JC (1991) Pressure management. Prosth Orth Int 15:225–231
24. Oomens CWJ, Van Campen DH (1987) A mixture approach to the mechanics of skin. J Biomech 9:877–885
25. Zhang JD, Mak AFT, Huang LD (1997) A large deformation biomechanical model for pressure ulcers. J Biomech Eng 119:406–408
26. Oomens CWJ, Bressers OFJT, Bosboom EMH, Bouten CVC, Bader DL (2003) Can loaded interface characteristics influence strain distributions in muscle adjacent to bony prominences. Comp Meth Biomech Biomed Eng 6:171–180
27. Miller GE, Seale J (1981) Lymphatic clearance during compressive loading. Lymphology 14:161–166
28. Reddy NP, Patel H, Krouskop TA (1981) Interstitial fluid flow as a factor in decubitus ulcer formation. J Biomech 14:879–881
29. Herrman EC, Knapp CF, Donofrio JC, Salcido R (1999) Skin perfusion responses to surface pressureinduced ischemia: Implication for the developing pressure ulcer. J Rehab Res Develop 36:109–120
30. Peirce SM, Skalak TC, Rodeheaver GT (2000) Ischemia-reperfusion injury in chronic pressure ulcer formation: a skin model in the rat. Wound Repair Regeneration 8:68–76
31. Ryan TJ (1990) Cellular responses to tissue distortion. In: Bader DL, editor. Pressures sores: Clinical practice and scientific approach. London: Macmillan, pp 141–152
32. Conner LM, Clack KW (1993) In vivo (CT scan) comparison of vertical shear in human tissue caused by various support surfaces. Decubitus 6:20–28
33. Bosboom EMH, Nicolay K, Bouten CVC, Oomens CWJ, Baaijens FPT (2000) Assessment of skeletal muscle damage after controlled compressive loading using high-resolution MRI. In: Prendergast PJ, Lee TC, Carr AJ (eds) Proceedings of the 12th Conference of the European Society of Biomechanics, August 28–30, 2000, Dublin, Ireland. Royal Academy of Medicine in Ireland, Dublin p 179
34. Vandeberg JS, Rudolph R (1995) Pressure (decubitus) ulcer: Variation in histopathology – a light and electron microscope study. Hum Pathol 26:195–200

35. Landsman AS, Meaney DF, Cargill RS, Macarak EJ, Thibault LE (1995) High strain rate tissue deformation. A theory on the mechanical etiology of diabetic foot ulcerations. Am Pod Med Assoc 85:519–527
36. Bouten CVC, Knight MM, Lee DA, Bader DL (2001) Compressive deformation and damage of muscle cell sub-populations in a model system. Ann Biomed Eng 29:153–163
37. Bliss MR (1993) Aetiology of pressure sores. Rev Clinical Gerontol 3:379–397
38. Breuls RGM, Bouten CVC, Oomens CWJ, Bader DL, Baaijens FPT (2003) Compression induced cell damage in engineered muscle tissue: an in-vitro model to study pressure ulcer aetiology. Ann Biomed Eng 31:1357–1365
39. Bouten CVC, Oomens CWJ, Baaijens FPT, Bader DL (2003) The aetiology of pressure sores: skin deep or muscle bound? Arch Phys Med Rehab 84:616–619

Medical Perspectives in the 21st Century 2

Jeen Haalboom

Epidemiological Studies on Pressure Ulcers in The Netherlands

Pressure ulcers occur regularly in clinical practice. In a recent Dutch prevalence study [1], in which more than 38,000 patients were examined, it was reported that approximately 13% of patients in university hospitals had pressure ulcers, 23% exhibited them in general hospitals, 30% in nursing homes and 17% in home care. This is unacceptably high, but similar figures have been found in studies from other countries. For example, in a smaller prevalence study in the UK, commissioned by the European Pressure Ulcer Advisory Panel (EPUAP) in 2001, 21.8% of all patients had established pressure ulcers. Comparable data were also obtained from studies in Canada [2] and in Europe (ongoing EPUAP study). It may be concluded that pressure ulcers occur much more regularly than would normally be presumed. Indeed, the figures are so alarming that more specific data are still needed and it is therefore necessary to work with frequency data.

There are several sets of frequency data in use that illustrate the extent of 'the problem' of pressure ulcers. In the Netherlands in the period 1998–2001, annual prevalence recordings were performed, conducted by the Steering Committee on Pressure Ulcers. In particular, details were obtained related to prevalence. By contrast, there is a relative paucity of data regarding the incidence of pressure ulcers.

Prevalence is defined as the number of patients with pressure ulcers at a certain moment, i.e. point recording, usually expressed as a percentage of the total number of patients admitted to an institution. The main goal of prevalence data is to obtain an insight into the magnitude of the problem of pressure ulcers and, to a lesser extent, the factors contributing to their development. Prevalence provides a reflection of the availability and/or efficiency of the labour of nursing personnel and the use of prevention and treatment protocols. There are large differences in prevalence data among institutions and countries. In large studies in hospitals, prevalence figures ranging from 5.2 to 18.6% have been reported [3–5], with equivalent ranges in nursing homes of between 7.9 and 33.2% [6–9], and in home-care situations of between 4.9 and 29.1% [10, 11].

However, prevalence figures as found in the literature are difficult to compare mainly due to diversity in methodology. Typical methods employed have been:

1. Use of a questionnaire [5, 7, 10].
2. Retrospective analysis of patient files [6, 12].
3. Investigation of patients obviously at high risk of developing pressure ulcers [3, 4].

In addition, the use of different classification systems for pressure ulcers makes the comparison of prevalence figures very problematic. In some studies, pressure ulcers were recognized as a discolouration of the skin [13–15], in others when this discolouration was non-blancheable [16, 17] and in others when a skin defect was evident [17]. Prevalence recordings should be compared only when a distinctive internationally recognized classification system is established and regularly used [18].

The inclusion of stage 1 pressure ulcers, defined as non-blancheable discolouration of the skin, in the overall classification of pressure ulcers is an important explanation for the differences found in the literature for both prevalence and incidence between institutions and countries. In the Dutch prevalence studies 60–75% of the patients with pressure ulcers were considered to exhibit grade 1 ulcers. Thorough examination and documentation of patients is of critical importance, since somewhere within the domain of the so-called grade 1 pressure ulcer there is a turning point, the watershed between full recovery and the progressive development of more severe pressure ulcers.

As far as the method of prevalence studies is concerned it is important that, without exception, all patients in an institution are examined. The three methods detailed above all underestimate the true prevalence. They suppose that all patients with pressure ulcers are known to the nursing staff or that every patient with pressure ulcers is registered in the nursing file. If the only patients examined are those with a perceived increase in risk of developing pressure ulcers, it is wrongly assumed that patients without such an increased risk all do not have pressure ulcers. Further analysis of the 1999 prevalence study in the Netherlands showed that out of all patients examined, 3112 had one or more pressure ulcers [1]. However, using the Braden risk assessment tool, 37% of these patients did not have an increased risk. It could be assumed that all patients with stage 3 and 4 ulcers should be known to the nursing staff. For patients with ulcers stages 1 and 2 this was not the case. Of the 37% of patients without an increased risk, no less than 61% demonstrated stage 1 lesions, 25% stage 2 and, more remarkably, 14% stages 3 and 4. Thus if only patients with an increased risk had been examined, these patients would have been missed and, accordingly, the prevalence figures would have been much lower.

Until 1998 there was no insight into the scale of the problem of pressure ulcers in terms of intra- and extra-mural healthcare in the Netherlands. It was assumed that prevalence was 8–10% in hospitals and 15–20% in nursing homes [19]. In Table 2.1 the results of a Dutch prevalence study in the period 1998–2001 are presented, with respect to the type of institution and grade of pressure ulcer. The sample was considered to be representative for the whole population of healthcare institutions in the Netherlands. The first study

Table 2.1. The results of a Dutch prevalence study in the period 1998–2001

	Stage 1	Stage 2	Stage 3	Stage 4	Total
University hospitals					
1998	5.6	4.9	2.1	0.6	13.2
1999	6.0	4.1	3.2	1.0	14.4
2000	8.5	7.6	2.1	0.9	15.8
2001	5.2	6.1	2.6	1.2	18.4
General hospitals					
1998	11.5	7.4	3.4	1.0	23.3
1999	10.1	5.9	3.2	1.1	20.3
2000	10.8	6.2	3.0	1.0	20.9
2001	11.3	7.2	3.0	0.9	22.3
Nursing homes					
1998	17.5	8.5	3.7	2.7	32.4
1999	14.8	7.6	4.2	2.4	28.3
2000	19.1	7.7	3.5	1.8	32.1
2001	20.8	7.3	3.7	1.6	33.4
Home care					
1998	10.1	5.9	4.4	0.9	21.3
1999	8.0	5.3	3.8	0.5	17.7
2000	8.5	5.0	3.1	1.1	17.7
2001	9.6	6.2	3.4	1.3	20.5
Elderly care					
1998	10.1	3.0	1.8	0.5	15.5
1999	6.4	2.6	2.3	0.3	11.6
2000	7.2	2.5	2.8	1.1	13.6
2001	10.3	3.0	1.2	0.2	14.6

showed that prevalence was much higher than was assumed, while studies in subsequent years did not reveal large changes, despite the introduction of a number of preventive measures. There is no obvious explanation for this finding, although it is possible that the increasing age of the patients with an associated increase in the severity of their illness might negate the possible positive effect of improved preventive measures. There are no large-scale prevalence studies known for intensive care situations. One study, however, revealed a prevalence of between 40 and 50% [20].

Incidence is defined as the number of new patients developing pressure ulcers in a defined period of time in relation to the total number of patients. As a rule, it is expressed as the number of patients presenting with pressure ulcers in a month or a year since admission. As with prevalence, there is no agreement about the criteria for incidence in the literature. The description of different patient populations and the use of different classifications and methods limit direct comparisons. Studies are most likely to represent so-called cumulative incidences, namely the number of new cases during the study divided by the total number of patients in the whole study. Here it is assumed that all patients participated in the study for the same period of time. In most studies, however, the admission times were not equal. Some patients died, some were discharged earlier, while other patients were admitted for prolonged periods. The use of the "incidence rate" is the preferable solution in this respect, representing as it does the number of new cases during the study per number of days, months or years that the patients participated in the study.

Incidence of pressure ulcers among hospital patients varies between 2.7% and 29.5% [21–25]. In several sub-populations even higher figures are reported. For example, in surgical patients incidence varies between 2.7% and 66% [26–33] and in intensive care patients between 5 and 50% [34–38]. In homes for the elderly incidence values of between 2.4 and 77.3% have been estimated [21–23, 37, 39–41]. No incidence data have been reported for nursing homes.

Recently in both the EPUAP and the Dutch Steering Committee on Pressure Ulcers there has been extensive debate about the comparative values of prevalence and incidence data. It was concluded that prevalence is of limited value, pointing towards the extent of the problem, without clarifying details of the factors that contribute to the development of pressure ulcers. In addition, the effects of preventive interventions are not measured using prevalence data and it is impossible to make comparisons between institutions (see Chap. 3). The tendency exists to use prevalence data to judge individual institutions, but the limitations of assessments such as the Braden risk assessment tool impart limited value to the data. A Canadian

Table 2.2. Incidence study at the University Medical Centre Utrecht ($n=400$)

Gender	Number	Mean age
Men	186 (46.5%)	57.8±17.6
Women	214 (53.5%)	
Pressure ulcers	47 (11.8%)	66.9±70
Surgical patients		
Number	234	
Pressure ulcers	32 (13.6%)	
Non-surgical patients		
Number	166	
Pressure ulcers	15 (9%)	

study showed that in one institution prevalence can change considerably with time, for the most part at a constant incidence. In a prospective study in Utrecht University Hospital, part of the prePURSE study [39, 40], the value of incidence was again illustrated.

In total 400 patients were analysed, 234 of whom were on surgical wards, and the remainder on wards for internal medicine and neurology. They were investigated three times weekly for a period coincident with their individual hospitalization or until the occurrence of a pressure ulcer. Results indicated that there were significantly more patients with pressure ulcers on the surgical wards (13.6 versus 9%). It was also shown that longer operations are associated with a higher incidence of pressure ulcers, with median values of 4.4 h and 2.9 h for pressure ulcer and non-pressure ulcer patients, respectively. In addition, the mean age of 66.9 years was significantly higher than the mean age of 57.8 years for the population as a whole.

Figures 2.1 and 2.2 illustrate the age pattern of the patients on the surgical and non-surgical wards and the time of development of the pressure ulcers, respectively. It is striking that in surgical patients pressure ulcers do not occur exclusively in the elderly, but also in the younger age group, particularly the latter undergoing extensive head and neck surgery. Figure 2.2 also shows that pressure ulcers routinely can be observed in the second week of admission [39, 40]. This contradicts the long-held supposition that pressure ulcers were caused by inadequate nursing care; rather, it strongly suggests that many pressure ulcers develop during operation and/or periods of treatment in the emergency rooms or during investigations in, for example, X-ray departments where mattresses have not been routinely adapted to these severely ill patients. This explains the high incidence in head and neck patients, operated upon in a half-sitting position, who develop ulcers in the sacral region. It is noteworthy that adaptation to the operation table diminished the incidence sharply. This finding was reported in incidence, as opposed to prevalence, surveys. Pressure ulcer care should

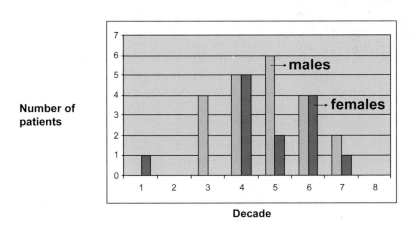

Fig. 2.1. Incidence study. Surgical patients: age distribution in decades

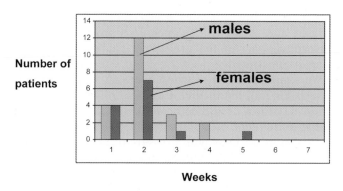

Weeks

Fig. 2.2. Incidence study. University Medical Centre Utrecht: week of development of pressure ulcers

therefore also be focused on the situations in both hospital and community settings, during which patients are vulnerable to soft tissue breakdown.

Costs of Pressure Ulcer Care

With a population of 16 million, the combined cost of the prevention and treatment of pressure ulcers in the Netherlands is approximately € 600 million per year [42, 43]. The total amounts to more than 1% of the total national costs of healthcare. Thus pressure ulcers constitute an important financial burden on the Dutch health budget, behind only the management of cancer, AIDS and cardiovascular diseases. With equivalent levels of healthcare it is only logical that in other technically advanced countries comparable amounts of money are spent per capita.

These enormous costs have attracted the increased attention of organizations managing healthcare, such as the Ministry of Health, as well as health insurance companies. When dealing with increasing costs more detailed studies involving the analysis of the generation of these costs is an important first step. It was concluded that there are distinct patterns distinguishable in pressure ulcer care, namely:

1. Prevention is cheaper than appropriate forms of treatment.
2. Costs are mainly generated by longer hospital admissions once an ulcer has become established in a patient.
3. Special devices are expensive.

Therefore in the Netherlands, at least, attention is now more focused on prevention. Prevention implies that patients at risk should be routinely monitored and managed with appropriate prophylactic measures, whereas patients not at risk should not receive special attention. Thus identification of patients at risk is critical, although it remains questionable which methods should be used in this process. Current risk assessment tools are of only limited value. These tools can be examined with respect to their specificity and sensitivity, using receiver operating characteristic (ROC) curves. Prospective studies revealed ROC curves indicating values of approximately 50%, comparable to the probability of correctly selecting the outcome when tossing a coin. Figure 2.3 shows the results of the prePURSE study involving 1,200 patients [39, 40], in which prospectively all factors of the established risk assessment instruments were recorded. The main conclusions were that surgery implied a certain risk, but that the predictive utility of the tools is, at best, limited. This finding is important, since in most institutions preventive interventions are taken, and in fact considered as good nursing practice, when a risk tool indicates increased risk. Using these instruments means that preventive measures may be adopted in patients who are not at risk but not employed in patients who really are at risk. Changing the threshold limits that define risk/no risk only provides a cosmetic solution. A complete revision of the factors associated with risk assessment is urgently needed.

Since the Waterlow tool was primarily designed to assess surgical patients, its predictive performance was slightly better than the others tested (Fig. 2.3). Risk assessment tools were developed in nursing to improve clinical skills and to analyse what could be considered to be a clinical view. This personal expertise of well-trained nurses still has an impact. In the recent Dutch Guideline on Pressure Ulcers (2002) the use of risk assessment tools is still encouraged, but in combination with "clinical view", since the combination of the two tends to identify patients better than not using either of them. It is likely that, in the near future, some more scientifically based tools will become available. However, such tools will need to accommodate the complex recent challenges associated with an ever-older population. These include more severely ill patients, many of whom are treated

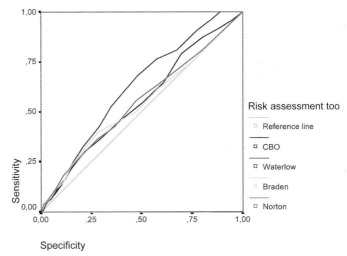

Fig. 2.3. ROC curve, defining sensitivity and specificity of risk score lists (adapted from [39])

as outpatients and who enjoy less home-care facilities. It is still uncertain whether these factors will lead to an increased risk and need to be treated as such.

In additional to the marginal scientific evidence associated with risk assessment, there are few quality studies investigating the effects of nursing and medical interventions. Indeed, studies examining the effects of beds are so rare, that medical and nursing journals tend to publish studies without the normal scientific rigour. As an example, a so-called controlled study was published in the *Lancet* in 1994 [41], investigating the effects of removing some foam blocks from a mattress. At first glance the statistics appeared to suggest that the modified mattress performed better than the control standardized hospital mattress. On closer examination, however, neither had the characteristics of both devices been specified nor was there any questioning as to why on the standard mattress the incidence of pressure ulcers was 60% (with hip fractures), although in a normal setting the value would have been predicted to be 20%. With the new tested mattress the incidence was 23%. Better? Yes, better than the previously used standard mattress, but was it any improvement on other mattresses considered to be "anti-pressure ulcer devices"? In a recent study by the College for Health Insurances in the Netherlands, no less than 200 such mattresses were listed (CVZ, 2002). The Cochrane study group concluded in 2000 that there is no evidence that any special device is better in preventing and treating pressure ulcers than any other. They did, however, stipulate that foam mattresses must be at least 80 mm thick and stated that air-fluidized beds had a tendency to perform better in high- or intensive care patients. It is obvious that the manufacturer of the block mattress advertised very aggressively and made a lot of money from the publication of the study [41]. The first step in reducing overall costs to the providers should be limitation of the number of devices after an extensive objective evaluation of all the commercially available systems. Limitation of the number of devices should decrease the price of the individual item. Indeed, experimentation in some institutions with the replacement of all old hospital mattresses by mattresses known as anti-pressure ulcer mattresses has already demonstrated that the costs of pressure ulcer care can be decreased by more than 30% in one year.

To conclude, pressure ulcers occur often and are even likely to increase in frequency in an ever-older population. Costs are largely generated by increased admission periods in institutions, and attention should be focused on the use of accurate and reliable prediction tools and well-tested preventive measures. Both the risk assessment instruments and the preventive materials need urgent testing, since their successful implementation could make a considerable impact on reducing the incidence of pressure ulcers.

References

1. Meehan M (1990) Multi-site pressure ulcer prevalence survey. Decubitus 3:14–17
2. Davis CM, Caseby NG (2001) Prevalence and incidence studies of pressure ulcers in two long-term care facilities in Canada. Ostomy Wound Management 47:28–34
3. O'Dea K (1993) Prevalence of pressure damage in hospital patients in the UK J Wound Care 2:221–211
4. Barrois B, Allaert FA (1995) A survey of pressure sore prevalence in hospitals in the greater Paris region. J Wound Care 4:234–236
5. Zulkowski K (1999) MDS + Items not contained in the pressure ulcer RAP associated with pressure ulcer prevalence in newly institutionalized elderly. Ostomy/Wound Management 45:24–33
6. Shiels C, Roe B (1998) Pressure sore care. Elder Care 10:30–34
7. Weiler PG, Kecskes D (1990) Pressure sores in nursing home patients. Aging 2:267–275
8. Young L (1989) Pressure ulcer prevalence and associated patient characteristics in one long-term care facility. Decubitus 2:52–55
9. Inman C,Firth JR (1998) Pressure sore prevalence in the community. Professional Nurse 13:515–520
10. Oot-Giromini BA (1993) Pressure ulcer prevalence, incidence and associated risk factors in the community. Decubitus 6:24–32
11. Schue RMRM, Langemo DKRP (1998) Pressure ulcer prevalence and incidence and a modification of the Braden scale for a rehabilitation unit. JWOCN 25:36–43
12. Gruen RLS, et al (1997) Point prevalence of wounds in a teaching hospital. Aust N Z J Surg 67:686–688
13. Vandenbroecke H, et al. (1994). Decubitus in de thuis-verpleging. Het risico en de screening. Nationale Federatie van de Wit-Gele-Kruisvereniging, Brussels
14. Eckman KL (1989) The prevalence of dermal ulcers among persons in the U.S. who have died. Decubitus 2:36–40
15. Barczak CA, et al. (1997) Fourth national pressure ulcer prevalence survey. Advances in Wound Care 10:18–26
16. Berlowitz DR, et al. (1996) Rating long-term care facilities on pressure ulcer development: importance of case-mix adjustment. Ann Intern Med 124:557–563
17. Haalboom JRE, et al. (1997) Pressure sores: incidence, prevalence and classification. In Parish LC, Witkowski JA, Crissey JT (eds) The decubitus ulcer in clinical practice. Springer, Berlin Heidelberg New York, pp 12–23
18. Gunning-Schepers LJ, et al. (1993) Decubitus in Nederland. Een onderzoek naar de mogelijkheden om het voorkomen van Decubitus in Nederland te meten. Instituut voor Sociale Geneeskunde, Universiteit van Amsterdam, Amsterdam
19. Bours G, Halfens R (1999) Decubitus komt nog veel te veel voor. TVZ 20:608–611
20. Xakellis GC, Frantz RA, Lewis A, Harvey P (1998) Cost-effectiveness of an intensive pressure ulcer prevention protocol in long term care. Adv Wound Care 11:22–29
21. Severens J (1999) Kosten van decubitus in Nederland. Afdeling MTA, Universitair Medisch Centrum St. Radboud, Nijmegen

22. Panel for the Prediction and Prevention of Pressure Ulcers in Adults (1992) Pressure ulcers in adults: prediction and prevention. Clinical practice guideline. Agency for Health Care Policy and Research, Public Health Service, U.S. Department of Health and Human Services, Rockville. AHCPR Publication No. 92-0047

23. Goodridge DM, Sloan JA, LeDoyen YM, McKenzie JA, Knight WE, Gayari M (1998) Risk-assessment scores, prevention strategies, and the incidence of pressure ulcers among the elderly in four Canadian health-care facilities. Can J Nurs Res 98:23–44

24. Bergstrom N, Braden B, Kemp M, Champagne M, Ruby E. (1996) Multi-site study of incidence of pressure ulcers and the relationship between risk level, demographic characteristics, diagnoses, and prescription of preventive interventions. J Am Geriatr Soc 44:22–30

25. Allman RM, Goode PS, Patrick MM, Burst N, Bartolucci AA (1995) Pressure ulcer risk factors among hospitalised patients with activity limitation. JAMA 273:865–870

26. Clark M, Watts S (1994) The incidence of pressure sores within a National Health Service Trust hospital during 1991. J Adv Nurs 20:33–36

27. Grous CA, Reilly NJ, Gift AG (1997) Skin integrity in patients undergoing prolonged operations. J Wound Ostomy Continence Nurs 24:86–91

28. Hoyman K, Gruber N (1992) A case study of interdepartmental cooperation: operating room-acquired pressure ulcers. J Nurs Care Qual [Suppl]:12–17

29. Kemp MG, Keithley JK, Smith DW, Morreale B (1990) Factors that contribute to pressure sores in surgical patients. Res Nurs Health 13:293–301

30. Schoonhoven L (1998) Incidentie van decubitus op de operatietafel. 1-66. Internal report, Utrecht University

31. Baudoin C, Fardellone P, Bean K, Ostertag EA, Hervy F (1996) Clinical outcomes and mortality after hip fracture: a 2-year follow-up study. Bone 18:149S–157S

32. Bertelink BP, Stapert JW, Vierhout PA (1993) The dynamic hip screw in medial fractures of the femoral neck: results in 51 patients. Ned Tijdschr Geneesk 137:81–85

33. Stordeur S, Laurent S, D'Hoore W (1998) The importance of repeated risk assessment for pressure sores in cardiovascular surgery. J Cardiovasc Surg Torino 39:343–349

34. Thomas TA, et al. (1999) An analysis of limb-threatening lower extremity wound complications after 1090 consecutive coronary artery bypass procedures. Vasc Med 4:83–88

35. Keller P, Wille J, Ramshorst B van, Werken C van der (2002) Pressure ulcers in intensive care patients: a review of risks and prevention. Intensive Care Med 28(10):1379–1388

36. O'Sullivan KL, Engrav LH, Maier RV, Pilcher SL, Isik FF, Copass MK (1997) Pressure sores in the acute trauma patient: incidence and causes. J Trauma 42:276–278

37. Olson B, Langemo D, Burd C, Hanson D, Hunter S, Cathcart ST (1996) Pressure ulcer incidence in an acute care setting. J Wound Ostomy Continence Nurs 23:15–22

38. Langemo DK, Olson B, Hunter S, Hanson D, Burd C, Cathcart ST (1991) Incidence and prediction of pressure ulcers in five patient care settings. Decubitus 4:25–30

39. Schoonhoven L, Haalboom JRE, Bousema MT (2002) Prospective cohort study of routine use of risk assessment scales for prediction of pressure ulcers. BMJ 325:797–799
40. Schoonhoven L (2003) Prediction of pressure ulcers: problems and prospects. PhD thesis, University of Utrecht, ISBN 90-393-3264-9
41. Hofman A, Geelkerken RH, Wille J, Hamming JJ, Hermans J, Breslau PJ (1994) Pressure sores and pressure decreasing mattresses: a controlled clinical trial. Lancet 343:568–571

Medico-Legal Implications

Courtney Lyder

3

Introduction

The medico-legal implications of pressure ulcer development are burgeoning throughout the world. Increasingly, pressure ulcers are being used as a quality indicator of care. Hence, the development of pressure ulcers can constitute a failure in the healthcare system. In the United States, the federal government believes that pressure ulcers are an excellent surrogate for how well the healthcare team is functioning. Thus, a high incidence of pressure ulcers usually can be correlated with high incidence of other care issues (e.g. falls, restraint usage, urinary incontinence). One aspect of the increasing view of pressure ulcer development as a marker for quality care has been the increasing level of pressure ulcer litigation against clinicians and their employers (hospitals, nursing homes, etc.).

This chapter will review various aspects of the medico-legal implications of pressure ulcer development. More specifically, it will review pressure ulcers as a political agenda; the legality of pressure ulcers; regulatory and reimbursement aspects of pressure ulcers; necessity of chart audits related to pressure ulcers; and pressure ulcers as a quality measure.

The Politics of Pressure Ulcers

In the past 10 years, there has been a fundamental paradigm shift in how governments and consumers of healthcare have thought about pressure ulcer development. In part, this has occurred because of a greater need of governments to control burgeoning healthcare costs associated with an ever-increasing older adult population. Although the true cost associated with pressure ulcer prevention and development remains unknown, these ulcers can significantly increase healthcare expenditures. For example, in the Netherlands pressure ulcer treatment is conservatively estimated from a low of $ 362 million to a high of $ 2.8 billion, 1% of the total Dutch healthcare budget [1]. In the UK, the costs of pressure ulcers have ranged annually from £ 180 million to £ 321 million, or 0.4–0.8% of healthcare spending [2] (see Chap. 2). The financial costs to the National Health Service (NHS) are also substantial. Preventing and treating pressure ulcers in a 600-bed general hospital costs between £ 600,000 and £ 3 million a year, excluding litigation costs [3]. In the United States, it has been conservatively estimated that the treatment cost alone ranges anywhere between $ 1.68 billion to $ 6.8 billion or more than 1% of the total U.S. healthcare budget [4]. These estimates do not account for pain, suffering, or potential days of lost income. Thus, pressure ulcers are an expensive health problem.

The increasing accountability of healthcare clinicians to prevent and manage these wounds more effectively has led to an explosion of national guidelines on pressure ulcer. These national guidelines on prevention and treatment were developed by various healthcare providers and organizations as a method of streamlining and providing consistent pressure ulcer care. The earliest national guidelines were derived from the Netherlands and the United States [5]. Moreover, several governments have established national centres which have addressed quality pressure ulcer care. In the UK, the National Institute for Clinical Excellence released national guidelines on pressure ulcer risk management and prevention [6]. These guidelines were in part derived from the Royal College of Nursing. The NICE guidelines provide both a clinician and patient versions. The NICE guidelines are quite similar to the guidelines of the U.S. Agency for Health Care Policy and Research (now the U.S. Agency for Health Care and Quality) for pressure ulcer prevention in that both clinician and patient versions exist [4, 7].

Coupled with the growing needs for governments to manage their health expenditures more effectively, healthcare consumers have become increasingly aware through the media (internet, television) that pressure ulcers can be prevented and effectively treated. Thus, a more informed general public has led to the increasing need for healthcare providers to be educated on proper pressure ulcer care. One potentially negative consequence of an informed general public has been the increased scrutiny by the legal and/or government body to litigate or sanction penalties when care is not optimized.

Litigation

There remains a steady increase in litigation related to either the development of pressure ulcers or failure to effectively manage them. This is fuelled by ever-increasing media attention to patients suffering from these ulcers. Moreover, in recent years there has been an effort by professional health organizations and ministries of health to educate the consumer on pressure ulcers. Although most cases may be settled through an inquiry by a health trust, there appears to be an increase of consumers seeking financial remedies.

A growing number of health professionals view the development of pressure ulcers as evidence of negligent care by a healthcare provider or health system. In one study by Tsokos et al. [8], 11.2% of 10,222 corpses in Germany were found to have a pressure ulcer. This study found that the majority of physicians did not associate the potential fatal outcome of pressure ulcers and fatalities (e.g. sepsis) related to the development of these ulcers. Moreover, the investigators stated that the prevalence of pressure ulcers is a good parameter of quality nursing and medical care, thus the field of legal medicine can contribute significantly to general quality control of standards of nursing and medical care.

The assumption that pressure ulcers result from poor care by the medical and/or nursing staff has led to a flood of litigation. These lawsuits often lead to significant financial outlays by healthcare providers and/or healthcare institutions. In a retrospective study investigating the lawsuit judgment in cases of patients developing pressure ulcers on admission to hospitals, it was found that a significant number of medico-legal cases of pressure ulcer development could easily have been avoided at little expense to the healthcare institution. Thus, if the healthcare institution had provided systematic and comprehensive preventative measures it could have potentially avoided many lawsuits. The investigators found that the damages awarded varied from £ 3,500 to £ 12,500, although there have been cases with damages in excess of £ 100,000 [9].

In the U.S. pressure ulcer litigation has become rampant. In fact, it has become common for plaintiff attorneys to advertise on televisions and newspapers; they have even begun to advertise on roadside billboards. In a study investigating typical pressure ulcer awards in the U.S., sums ranging from $ 5,000 to $ 82,000,000, with a median award of approximately $ 250,000, have been reported [10]. Most revealing in this study was that the average age of the plaintiff was 72 years. This indicates that an increasing number of older adults are bringing legal cases against healthcare providers and health institutions. The following case study highlights elements of how healthcare providers and healthcare institutions can be easily exposed to litigation.

"83 y.o. male was admitted to hospital with history of congestive heart failure, right cerebral vascular accident, early stage dementia, urinary and faecal incontinence. A pressure ulcer risk assessment scale was completed indicating that the patient was at mild risk for pressure ulcers. The patient was placed on a standard mattress with a 4 inch solid foam overlay, turned every two hours while in bed and chair. On Day 2 of hospital admission, a nurse indicated an "erythematic" area on left hip and heel. She intervened by gently massaging the two erythematic areas with lotion and turned the patient on the right side. By Day 5, a Stage 2 pressure ulcer was noted on the left hip and a Stage 1 pressure ulcer was noted on the left heel. A hydrocolloid dressing was placed on the Stage II pressure ulcer, and nothing was ordered for the Stage I pressure ulcer. The charts noted that a tissue viability nurse would be consulted. By Day 8, a Stage III pressure ulcer was noted on left hip and heels. The Tissue Viability Nurse changed all of the wound care orders".

This case highlights some common errors made by the hospital staff. To identify a couple of areas of concern, the patient was at extreme high risk for pressure ulcers since he had multiple health conditions that rendered him immobile (congestive heart failure, right cerebral vascular accident, early stage dementia, urinary and faecal incontinence). Moreover, the risk assessment tool showed only mild risk. This is an important factor, indicating that the tool may have been completed incorrectly. Further, no pressure ulcer risk assessment tool has 100% sensitivity and specificity [11] (see Chap. 2). The patient was only placed on a standard mattress with a foam overlay. Given the patient's risk level, a dynamic surface (alternating air mattress, etc.) might have been more appropriate. Further complicating this patient's condition was the massaging of the erythematic area on the patient's left hip and heel. Research indicates that massaging a red spot may actually deepen the devitalized area [12]. Further, although a hydrocolloid dressing was ordered for the stage 2 pressure ulcer, nothing was ordered for the stage 1 ulcer (e.g. removing load from the heel). In this case study, it was obvious that additional preventive measures were not instituted; thus these pressure ulcers could perhaps have been avoided.

The above case scenario could occur anywhere in the world. Thus, any healthcare provider could be exposed to litigation when caring for a patient with a pressure ulcer. It appears that several key factors must be met to bring a pressure ulcer case to court. Most cases involve negligence; in other words, the healthcare professional and/or healthcare institution failed in providing care. There are three major factors that must be fulfilled to prove negligence. These three factors are accountability, causation and breach of standard of care [13]. When all three are met, the verdict will be for the plaintiff.

The first key factor is accountability. Hence, the plaintiff was owed a duty of care, and this duty of care was breached. Moreover, the breach of care resulted in permanent damage or injury, and the plaintiff is owed compensation due to the injury. This factor is easily acknowledged since any patient that enters a hospital, nursing home or home care setting is owed a certain level of care by healthcare providers. Since pressure ulcers can develop when preventive measures are not implemented, it is very easy to meet this standard.

The second factor is causation. Thus, the harm suffered by the patient was a foreseeable consequence of the breach of the duty of care. Although the majority of patients that develop pressure ulcers do not die due to the pressure ulcer, pressure ulcers (especially stage 3 and 4 ulcers) can increase the potential for infections (sepsis, cellulites). Pressure ulcers may also be quite painful. Proving causation can be quite easy, especially when the medical record is void of good documentation of the type and quality of care provided. The absence of good documentation on the preventative services provided or treatments carried out can make it easy for a plaintiff attorney to show that lack of care caused the formation of the pressure ulcer.

The final factor is the standard of care by staff. It is important to note that the standard of care is not at the level of an expert, but rather that of an average healthcare professional. Most often, expert practitioners are used to determine the expected skill mix of the average healthcare provider related to wound care. A physician expert would be used to determine the physician skill mix and a nurse expert would be used to determine a nurse skill mix. When the expert resides in a country that has developed national guidelines on the prevention and treatment of pressure ulcers, quite often these will be used to determine the appropriateness of pressure ulcer care. One study investigating the impact of implementation and subsequent compliance with practice guidelines in mitigating exposure to litigation found that of 49 plaintiff cases with compensations worth $ 14,418,770, use of guidelines could have saved the defendant $ 11,389,989 [14].

It appears that national guideline recommendations can be costly to implement for many healthcare institutions. One study found that the cost of implementing support surface equipment varies widely, from over £ 30,000 for some bed replacements to less than £ 100 for some foam overlays [15]. According to the UK National Health Service many clinical areas will already have access to equipment, but this is not always the case – especially for the pressure-redistributing overlays/mattresses on operating tables, which are supported by relatively recent and convincing evidence for use in high-risk individuals. Local decisions need to be made about the access and purchase of equipment in the light of available resources [15]. Consideration also needs to be given to the ongoing costs of equipment maintenance and replacement, given that the average daily cost of managing a pressure ulcer ranges from £ 38 to £ 196 with little variation by stage of ulcer [16].

Documentation

One major factor in decreasing the exposure to litigation appears to be the adequacy of documentation. Comprehensive documentation is also requisite for reimbursement of services and products in some countries. Moreover, good documentation justifies the medical necessity of services and products. Regulatory agencies, independent of healthcare setting, provide requisite documentation to justify continuation of pressure ulcer care. Good documentation should reflect the care required in the prevention and/or treatment of pressure ulcers [17]. Essential documentation should include the following, independent of healthcare setting:

Prevention of Pressure Ulcers

1. Risk assessment tool (e.g., Waterlow, Norton, Braden tools)
2. Daily skin assessment
3. Repositioning (off loading) and turning schedules
4. Use of support surfaces to address pressure redistribution (both bed and chair)
5. Control of moisture from perspiration and urinary and faecal incontinence
6. Nutritional assessment and supplementation when appropriate
7. Education of patient and/or family

Treatment of Pressure Ulcers

1. Regular assessment/reassessment of the wound (daily, weekly, etc.)
2. Characteristics of the ulcer
   a) length
   b) width
   c) depth
   d) exudate amount
   e) tissue type
   f) pain
3. Local wound care
4. Wound-bed preparation
5. Repositioning (off loading) and turning schedules
6. Use of support surfaces to address pressure redistribution (both bed and chair)
7. Control of moisture control from perspiration and urinary and faecal incontinence
8. Nutritional assessment and supplementation when appropriate
9. Use of adjunctive therapies (negative-pressure wound therapy, electrical stimulation, etc.)
10. Education of patient and/or family

Regulation and Reimbursement

It is universally accepted that patients receiving care in hospitals, nursing homes or the community should be free of pressure ulcers or, if ulcers exist, care should be provided to treat them effectively. The majority of healthcare settings are under the auspices of the national ministry of health, which has broad parameters for operating the various trusts (usually determined by geographical locations) within a specified country. With the socialized healthcare still prevalent in European and South American countries, quality pressure ulcer care is most dependent on the resource allocation by the specific healthcare trust. To this end, the quality of pressure ulcer care (as measured by support surfaces, types of dressings, adjunctive therapies used) may vary greatly dependent on the trust. The Canadian and Mexican models for pressure ulcer care are quite similar to the European model. Thus, pressure ulcer regulation and resource allocation for the acquisition of dressings, support surfaces, and adjunctive therapies (e.g. negative-pressure wound therapy) are dependent on the provincial trusts. In these systems, one trust may provide superior wound care based on the amount of resources that are allocated to pressure ulcer care. It should be noted that complaints by a health consumer or family are usually addressed by the individual trusts.

Probably the most regulated country with regard to pressure ulcer care is the United States. With the federal government being the largest health insurer (through Medicare), regulations exist for all settings related to re-imbursement and survey process for ensuring quality pressure ulcer care. Although a given state may have additional regulations, all states must follow the federal regulations. For example, in nursing homes, the quality for pressure ulcers is ensured by the federal survey process guidelines [18].

These guidelines state that:

1. A resident who enters the facility without a pressure ulcer does not develop pressure ulcers unless the individual's clinical condition is such that they were demonstrably unavoidable.

2. A resident having pressure ulcers receives necessary treatment and services to promote healing, prevent infection and prevent new ulcers from developing.

Federal and/or state surveyors visit all 19,000 nursing homes in the U.S. to ensure compliance with the federal mandate. The inspections are unannounced and may occur at any time of the day (10% of visits must occur in the evening or night time). To assist the surveyors in evaluating whether a nursing home is compliant with the federal mandate, an investigative protocol is followed that covers all areas of pressure ulcer care (assessments, prevention, documentation, treatment, etc.). If the nursing home has been found to be non-compliant, then monetary penalties are calculated based on the seriousness of the violation. The maximum penalty for non-compliance is $ 10,000 per day [18]. If the violation is serious enough, the nursing home can be closed immediately. For example, if a survey team finds more than one resident with Stage 3 or 4 ulcers that they believe were avoidable, then the nursing home can lose all financial support from the federal and/or state governments.

Some have argued that the survey team only has to prove that the pressure ulcer developed after admission to the nursing home, whereas the nursing home must prove that the pressure ulcer was unavoidable [19]. Given that all aspects of care are usually not documented, proving unavoidability is difficult. It should be noted that all nursing home survey results are in the public domain and can be accessed on the government website. This places more pressure on nursing homes to reduce their pressure ulcer rates, since it may affect the decision by families to place their loved ones in a particular home.

In an attempt to understand the magnitude of adverse events in U.S. hospitals, the federal government has developed a monitoring program to track multiple patient safety issues. One of the first clinical indicators under study is pressure ulcers. In this program, the development of pressure ulcers in a hospital could be classified as a medical error. Presently, the data are being collected; however, this initiative will have potentially significant regulatory and legal implications for U.S. hospitals.

Until December 2002, Japan used the universal health coverage paradigm, similar to Europe and Canada. However, in January 2003 Japan introduced a modified prospective payment system on a select group of health conditions for hospitalized patients [20]. The new system is considered a hybrid between the European universal coverage and the American prospective payment system. Pressure ulcers were selected as one of the health conditions to be pilot tested. Hospitals will need to begin to track pressure ulcer incidence and outcomes of interventions. Moreover, hospitals are now required to have an interdisciplinary wound team (comprising at least physicians and nurses). All patients with pressure ulcers must be evaluated and a plan of care instituted. Although the defined acceptable rate of pressure ulcers has not been released, hospitals exceeding this incidence rate will incur monetary penalties [20].

Benchmarking

The ability to benchmark incidence or prevalence rates for any disease condition is critical to assess the health status from a national, regional, local or institutional level. Without obtaining incidence or prevalence data, it is difficult to ascertain the effectiveness of preventative or treatment interventions (also see chapter 2). Thus, chart audits have become extremely popular throughout the world. In the past 10 years, numerous studies have published incidence and prevalence data on pressure ulcers. Both measure disease frequency. Incidence measures the proportion of people at risk for the disease (pressure ulcer) who eventually acquire the disease (pressure ulcer) over a specific period of time [21]; it conveys the likelihood that an individual in that population will be affected by the condition. Prevalence is the proportion of people who have the disease (pressure ulcer) in a specified population at risk [22, 23]. Studies usually report point prevalence, which is the prevalence rate for a specific point in time (what is the prevalence of pressure ulcers for today?). Period prevalence refers to a prevalence rate over a given time (what is the prevalence of pressure ulcers over a 3-month period?) [24]. The National Pressure Ulcer Advisory Panel has published a comprehensive monograph on the prevalence and incidence of pressure ulcers in the U.S. This document also presents step-by-step guidance on how to conduct studies on both incidence and prevalence of pressure ulcers [25].

The prevalence and incidence rates appear to differ greatly depending on the healthcare setting studied and within countries. In Canada, researchers noted a point prevalence rate of 25.7% for pressure ulcers in hospital, nursing home and community care settings [26], while in Japan a point prevalence rate of 6% is common in hospital and nursing homes [27]. In the United Kingdom, point prevalence rates have ranged from 8.5 to 32.1% for hospitals and 2.5 to 6.1% in the community [28–30]. A study investigating period prevalence of pressure ulcers in 11 German hospitals found a range of 12–53.5%, with an average of 28.3% [31].

In the United States more studies exist that report the incidence of pressure ulcers. In attempting to understand whether or not there has been an overall decrease in the incidence of pressure ulcers in the United States, the

National Pressure Ulcer Advisory Panel collected data from the published research literature over a 10-year period (1990 to 2000). They found incidence rates of 0.4–38% for hospitals, 2.2–23.9% for nursing homes and 0–17% for home care [25].

When benchmarking published data on either incidence or prevalence of pressure ulcer it is imperative to ensure that you are comparing similar data points as well as patient or unit populations. For example, an incidence rate of 20% for a hospital may be significant or not, depending on what particular medical units were involved. If this information is not available, comparisons among hospitals, nursing homes, etc. will be very difficult to make and should be avoided.

Pressure Ulcers as a Quality Measure

There has been little discourse on whether or not pressure ulcers should be used as an indicator of quality care. In fact, some have noted that the development of pressure ulcers results from a breakdown in the institutional system of care delivery because the prevention of pressure ulcers requires the cooperation and skill of the entire medical team. There is abundant literature that suggests that a large proportion of pressure ulcers can be prevented through systematic risk factor identification, skin assessments, use of effective support surfaces, and education of patients and staff. Implementation of a pressure ulcer prevention program is effective in decreasing the incidence of pressure ulcers in hospitals. However, few studies have been published that demonstrate the implementation prevention guidelines in their entirety, which is most likely due to the complex and interdisciplinary nature of pressure ulcer prevention. Several studies have reported the implementation of components of recommendations from the AHCPR guidelines. Gunningberg et al. [32], investigating the incidence of pressure ulcers in 1997 and 1999 among patients with hip fractures, attributed the significant reduction in incidence (from 55% in 1997 to 29% in 1999) to performance of systematic risk assessment on admission, accurate staging of pressure ulcers, use of pressure-reducing mattresses, and continuing education of staff. Another study, involving implementation of a comprehensive prevention program consisting of a risk assessment tool, uniform skin care, pressure-reducing support surfaces, repositioning schedules, standardized nutritional assessment and support, and staff education, found significant reductions in pressure ulcer incidence during a 5-month period [33]. Similar results have been noted elsewhere [34, 35]. Although these studies support the benefit of a comprehensive approach, no study could be found that has implemented all recommendations of the AHCPR prevention guidelines or any other national guidelines. Moreover, the sustainability of pressure ulcer reductions has not been studied for long periods.

Pressure ulcers may indicate a potential problem within the healthcare organization, but some ulcers may be unavoidable. There is a paucity of literature that suggests an acceptable rate for pressure ulcer development. Lyder suggested that a rate of 5% should be allowed, since not all risk factors have been identified nor has any study been published that consistently implemented a respective country's pressure ulcer prevention guidelines [11]. The discourse on avoidability versus unavoidability remains heated; however, little guidance can be found in the world literature beyond the assumption that the pressure ulcer may be deemed unavoidable if all preventative guidelines have been implemented and the ulcers develops.

Conclusion

There remain numerous medico-legal issues related to pressure ulcers. Given the burgeoning world of electronic information technology, cutting-edge information on pressure ulcer care can readily be transmitted throughout the world. The ever-increasing knowledge level of the general public, primarily conveyed by the mass media, will most likely lead to increasing legal claims against healthcare providers and healthcare institutions. Healthcare providers will need to educate themselves on currently acceptable practices related to pressure ulcer prevention and treatment. This will also lead to more accountability within the healthcare community and in turn to increased documentation of care provided. The key to providing optimum pressure ulcer care will be good documentation that clearly articulates the needs for services and products implemented. Moreover, good documentation will clearly identify assessment of the patient, interventions instituted and outcomes achieved.

As governments continue to quantify health expenditures related to pressure ulcers, there will be increased pressure on healthcare systems to address this costly problem. Many experts believe that the healthcare team has some capacity to thwart the development of pressure ulcers. Therefore, many countries may experience increased regulations related to pressure ulcer care, as already seen in Japan and the United States.

References

1. Severens JL, Habraken JM, Duivenvoorden S, Frederiks CM (2002) The cost of illness of pressure ulcers in the Netherlands. Adv Skin Wound Care 15:72–77
2. Touche R (1993) The cost of pressure sores. Reports to the Department of Health. Department of Health, London, UK
3. http://www.nice.org.uk/pdf/clinicalguidelinepressuresoreguidancercn.pdf
4. Panel for the Prediction and Prevention of Pressure Ulcers in Adults (1992) Pressure ulcers in adults, prediction and prevention: Clinical practice guideline. Public Health Services Agency for Health Care Policy and Research, Rockville, MD, publication 92-0047. United States Census Bureau Statistics, Washington DC

5. http://www.epuap.org
6. http://www.nice.org.uk/page.aspx?o=94726
7. U.S. Department of Health and Human Services (1994) Healthy People 2010 (conference edition in two volumes). Washington, DC: January 2000
8. Tsokos M, Heinemann A, Puschel K (2000) Pressure sores: epidemiology, medico-legal implications and forensic argumentation concerning causality. Int J Legal Med 113:283–287
9. Franks PJ (2001) Health economics: The cost to nations. In: Morrison MJ (ed) The prevention and treatment of pressure ulcers. Mosby, St Louis, pp 52–53
10. Bennett RG, O'Sullivan J, DeVito EM, Remsberg R (2000) The increasing medical malpractice risk related to pressure ulcers in the United States. J Am Geriatr Soc 48:73–81
11. Lyder C (2003) Exploring pressure ulcer prevention and management. JAMA 289:223–226
12. Lyder C (2002) Pressure ulcer prevention and management. Annu Rev Nurs Res 20:35–61
13. Dimond B (1999) Pressure ulcers and litigation. Nursing Times 99:61–63
14. Goebel RH, Goebel MR (1999) Clinical practice guidelines for pressure ulcer prevention can prevent malpractice lawsuits in older patients. JWOCN 26:175–184
15. www.guideline.gov/summary.aspx?ss=15&doc_id=2953&nbr=2179
16. Bennett G, Dealey C, Posnett J (2004) The cost of pressure ulcers in the UK. Age Aging 33:230–235
17. Lyder C (2003) Regulation and wound care. In Baranoski S, Ayello E (eds). Wound care essentials: practice principles. Springhouse, Springhouse, pp 35–46
18. Health Care Financing Administration: Investigative Protocol (2000) Guidance to surveyors – long term care facilities. Rev 274. U.S. Department of Health and Human Services
19. http://www.nurses.info/law_for_nurses_journals.htm
20. http://www.mhlw.go.jp/english/
21. Hulley S, Cummings S (1988) Designing clinical research: an epidemiologic approach. Williams and Wilkins, Baltimore, MD
22. Baumgarten M (1998) Designing prevalence and incidence studies. Adv Wound Care 11:28
23. Berquist S, Frantz R (1999) Pressure ulcers in community-based older adults receiving home health care. Prevalence, incidence, and associated risk factors. Adv Wound Care 112:339–351
24. Hennekens CH, Burling JE (1987) Epidemiology in medicine. Little Brown, Boston, MA
25. Cuddigan J, Ayello EA, Sussman C, Baranoski S (Eds) (2001) Pressure ulcers in America: prevalence, incidence, and implications for the future. National Pressure Ulcer Advisory Panel, Reston, VA
26. Foster C, Frisch S, Denis N, Forler Y, Jago M (1992) Prevalence of pressure ulcers in Canadian institutions. CAET J 11(2):23–31
27. Mino Y (2001) Pressure ulcers in bedridden elderly subjects. Jpn J Geriatrics 39:253–256
28. Torrance C, Maylor M (1999) Pressure sore survey: part one. J Wound Care 8:27–30
29. Allcock N, Wharrad H, Nicolson A (1994) Interpretation of pressure-sore prevalence. J Adv Nurs 20:37–45

30. Hallett A (1996) Managing pressure sores in the community. J Wound Care 5:105–107
31. Gunningberg L, Lindholm C, Carlsson M, Sjoden P (2001) Risk, prevention and treatment of pressure ulcers – nursing staff knowledge and documentation. Scand J Caring Sciences 15:257–263
32. Lyder C, Shannon R, Empleo-Frazier O, McGee D, White C (2002) A comprehensive program to prevent pressure ulcers: exploring cost and outcomes. Ostomy/Wound Management 48:52–62
33. Xakellis GC, Frantz RA (1996) The cost-effectiveness of interventions for preventing pressure ulcers. J Am Board Fam Pract 9:79–85
34. Regan MB, Byers PH, Mayrovitz HN (1995) Efficacy of a comprehensive pressure ulcer prevention program in an extended care facility. Adv Wound Care 8:51–52

Patients at Risk for Pressure Ulcers and Evidence-Based Care for Pressure Ulcer Prevention

NANCY BERGSTROM

4

Populations at Risk

Pressure ulcers are a common problem in most healthcare settings. The elderly, those with spinal cord injury or other neurological deficits or degenerative processes, trauma patients, and those with any condition that limits the ability to move freely in response to the perception of discomfort are at risk for pressure ulcers. Newly recognized is the development of pressure ulcers as an end-of-life issue. The incidence of pressure ulcers is somewhat difficult to determine since there is no national registry of ulcers and many ulcers may remain unreported [1]. The incidence, projected from compiling reports of the incidence of pressure ulcers reported in research studies, is believed to be from 0.4 to 38% for hospitalized patients; 2.2 to 23.9% for long-term care; and as high as 17% in home care [2, 3]. The cost of pressure ulcers must be tabulated with consideration for costs of treatment, costs to the patient and the family, and the costs to society that are influenced by loss of time from work, costs of litigation and medical malpractice and more. Cost calculations to date are imprecise and tend to focus only on the cost of care, but several quality reports demonstrate that it costs less to prevent pressure ulcers than to treat them.

Specific Risk Factors

Prolonged pressure caused by the weight of the body on muscle and skin over the bony prominences results in occlusion of blood vessels providing nutrients to the tissue, resulting in tissue death and necrosis. The amount and duration of pressure that can be tolerated without pressure ulcers has been studied in laboratory animals and humans, with a parabolic relationship demonstrated between the amount of pressure and the duration of exposure to pressure, with low pressure tolerated over longer intervals and high pressure tolerated over much shorter times [4–6]. Another early study demonstrated that there are different tissue injury thresholds for muscle and for skin, with muscle being more sensitive to the effects of pressure [7]. The precise amount of pressure necessary for pressure ulcer formation is variable and is likely to be influenced by the integrity of the tissue to which pressure is being applied.

The list of factors associated with pressure ulcer risk is long, numbering more than 100, and includes medical diagnoses, co-morbidities and previous medical events (e.g. fractured hip, spinal cord injury, cerebrovascular accident, diabetes, previous pressure ulcer, cardiovascular disease, cancer, amputation) [8–10]; patient demographic characteristics (e.g. age, sex, race, marital status, socioeconomic status); anthropometric characteristics (e.g. height and weight, body mass index, triceps skin fold thickness, percent weight loss); physiological status (e.g. blood pressure, body temperature, glucose levels and control, tissue perfusion); nutritional status (e.g. serum albumin or pre-albumin, poor dietary intake); functional status (e.g. inability to control bladder and bowel function [11], number of deficits in activities of daily living, ability to feed self, activity and mobility levels); cognition (e.g. mental status, levels of consciousness) [12]; psychological status (e.g. stress, depression); social behaviour (e.g. substance abuse including drugs, smoking and alcohol); knowledge and adherence (e.g. educational level, knowledge of care requirements); and nursing care or facility characteristics (available RN and nursing assistant time, size or location of facility) [13], and more.

Braden and Bergstrom [14] developed a conceptual scheme, based on a review of the literature, to create a framework for organizing risk factors (see Fig. 4.1). The conceptualization suggests that there are two major factors associated with pressure ulcer risk: the amount and duration of exposure to pressure and the ability of the tissue to tolerate the pressure. In the

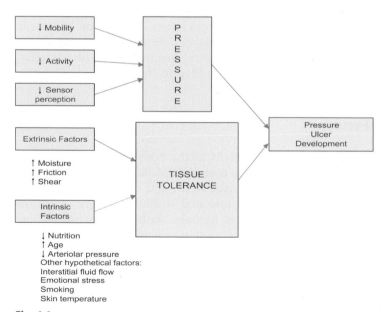

Fig. 4.1. A conceptual scheme for the study of the aetiology of pressure sores which demonstrates linkages between key pressure ulcer risk factors (duration and intensity of pressure) and other risk factors [adapted from 14]

clinical situation, pressure is influenced by mobility, activity and sensory perception. Mobility refers to the ability to turn and move about in bed. Persons who have a spinal cord injury, a fractured hip or are unconscious will not be able to move about and relieve pressure; thus, without assistance the time of exposure to pressure is increased. Activity refers to the ability to get out of bed, removing all pressure from non-weight-bearing surfaces (e.g. during ambulation) or shifting weight bearing to different pressure points (ischial tuberosities) during sitting. Sensory perception is the sum of the ability to perceive and the ability to act upon sensory information based on exposure to pressure. Individuals with a spinal cord injury, nerve damage, or a stroke may be insensate in specific body areas and be unable to detect discomfort associated with hypoxemia of local tissues exposed to pressure. Other individuals may be unable to appreciate or communicate discomfort associated with pressure due to dementia or other factors.

Tissue tolerance for pressure is defined as the ability to withstand the effects of pressure without developing a pressure ulcer. Tissue tolerance may be influenced by intrinsic and extrinsic factors. Intrinsic factors occur within the individual, while extrinsic factors impinge on or cause deterioration of the external layers of the skin. Extrinsic factors most frequently include exposure to moisture from urinary or faecal incontinence, perspiration or other drainage resulting in maceration of the skin. One of the most frequently reported risk factors across many epidemiological studies of risk factors is urinary and/or faecal incontinence. Exposure to friction and shear also disrupts the skin. Studies have shown that persons subjected to friction develop pressure ulcers at lower pressures than those not exposed to friction [15]. Friction can occur from skin rubbing against rough surfaces, for instance, when being pulled up in bed, sliding across sheets or moving repetitively as may occur with spasticity. Shearing forces occur when the skin adheres to bed linens while the underlying tissues slide down, causing vessels vertical to the skin to torque or tear, resulting in deep tissue injury. Nutritional status is an intrinsic risk factor causing the skin and underlying tissue to be more or less vulnerable to the effects of pressure. One prospective study identified dietary intake of protein and calories to be more indicative of pressure ulcer development than serum albumin and other biochemical or anthropometric markers [16], and most studies identify one or more nutritional markers as being pivotal to pressure ulcer development.

Evidence-Based Care

The United States Public Health Service, Agency for Health Care Policy and Research (AHCPR) mandated the development of clinical practice guidelines for selected areas of patient care during the early 1990s. Guidelines were developed in areas where the problem was frequently occurring or had a severe impact on patients or healthcare, where the cost of care was high and where there was a great deal of variability in practice. Multidisciplinary guideline development panels were convened to synthesize the scientific literature and make recommendations for practice based on the evidence. Two guidelines that emerged were: Pressure Ulcers in Adults: Prediction and Prevention [2] and Treating Pressure Ulcers [17]. The hallmark of these guidelines was a comprehensive review of the literature, creation of evidence tables, grading of evidence, and guideline recommendations based on evidence and clinical expertise. The guidelines had broad evaluation both in public forums and through clinical testing and organizational review prior to release.

The AHCPR guidelines for pressure ulcers were developed a decade ago and there have been any number of attempts to re-evaluate or rewrite the guidelines or to make influential statements regarding patient care. Notably, the American Medical Directors Association, re-evaluated the guidelines and rewrote them with a greater focus on the nursing home population (1994), but did not conduct a substantial review of the literature. The National Pressure Ulcer Advisory Panel, in the United States, wrote influential statements on the assessment of pressure ulcers in dark-skinned individuals and wrote a position statement on staging healing ulcers that took a stance against reverse staging. One group, the Cochrane collaboration, developed a synthesis statement on support surfaces, reviewing only randomized controlled trials and ignoring other research methods. This review, likewise, did not consider covariates of outcome success. The European Pressure Ulcer Panel [18] and an Australian panel wrote more comprehensive guidelines grading evidence in a manner very similar to the US guidelines and concluding with nearly identical guideline recommendations. Small differences appear between the guidelines. The Australian guidelines were developed based on the principles of comprehensive review supported by the Joanna Briggs Institute for Evidence Based Practice. The guidelines, Pressure Ulcer Prevention and Treatment following Spinal Cord Injury, sponsored by the Paralyzed Veterans of America (2000) are the closest in methodology to the AHCPR guidelines. Interestingly, all of these efforts follow the same or a very similar template of recommendations and most support the same or similar recommendations as are summarized below.

Additionally, a number of articles have also been written for the stated purpose of updating the guidelines [19, 20]. Yet, few substantive changes have been detected. An article in the *Journal of the American Medical Association* [21] recently stated that of all the guidelines developed in the early 1990s, the pressure ulcer guidelines remain most relevant. Sadly, there have not been major advances in the area of pressure ulcer prediction and prevention, but there have been some advances in treatment. Most of the new body of knowledge clusters around confirmation of risk factors, development and testing of dressings and support surfaces, and development and testing of vacuum-assisted therapy, electrical stimulation or topical substances. There have been few randomized controlled trials, even fewer studies that looked at the efficacy of preventive interventions or specific treatments and even fewer investigations of the effectiveness of guideline recommendations across settings. Several quality assurance-type studies demonstrated that guideline-based care reduced the incidence of pressure ulcers and saved money [22, 23], but more recent evidence shows that US hospitals, physicians and nurses have many opportunities to improve care related to pressure ulcer prediction and prevention [24]. The area of pressure ulcer prevention and treatment is in need of scientific advancement, as outlined in statements by Bergstrom and colleagues at the conclusion of the AHCPR guideline development process (1994) and more recently by the National Pressure Ulcer Advisory Panel [25].

Evidence-Based Care for Prevention

Recommendations for the prediction and prevention of pressure ulcers that appear in most guidelines, representing the best evidence combined with the best clinical judgment of international experts, are detailed below. Figure 4.2 shows a visual display of the conceptual organization, procedural flow, decision points and preferred management as described in the AHCPR guideline [2].

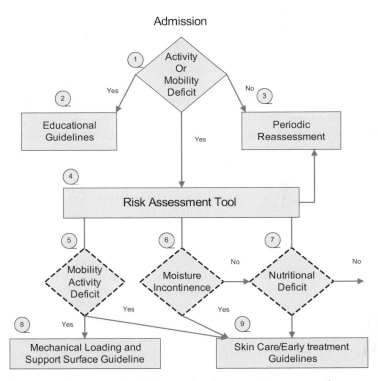

Fig. 4.2. An algorithm presenting an overview of approaches for preventing pressure ulcers

Risk Assessment

Most guidelines recommend that bed- or chair-bound individuals should be assessed for risk of developing pressure ulcers on admission to a care setting and at periodic intervals that make sense based on the rapidity with which the patient's condition is expected to change within the setting. Most guidelines detail the list of risk factors associated with pressure ulcers. Mor demonstrated that as the number of risk factors increase, the incidence of ulcers increases [1]. In order to use a list of risk factors to guide assessments, a check list of risk factors should be generated and clinicians should denote the presence or absence of the risk factor, coupled with clinical intuition as to the point at which risk is present and must be treated. The list of risk factors does not offer guidance to the specific cut-off point for risk or to specific treatments that should be instituted, and while favoured by several of the guidelines over formal risk assessment, this method has never been tested for reliability, validity or clinical utility.

Risk assessment tools based on conceptual risk factors that cut across many diagnoses, patient characteristics, physiological states and other risk factors are easier to use with consistency. One commonly used one-page risk predictor tool, the Braden Scale for Predicting Pressure Sore Risk (copyright Braden and Bergstrom, 1988) [26–28] assesses an individual for the presence and severity of risk factors and derives a score for overall risk. This total risk score identifies those requiring preventive interventions, but training and clinical judgment is pivotal to the successful use of this or any other clinical tool. The subscale scores direct attention to specific risk factors needing attention and the level of intervention needed. The Braden Scale has been tested more and with better results than the Norton, and Waterlow scales, the next most frequently used tools [29, 30]. The use of a formal risk assessment tool may level the playing field, providing experienced and less experienced clinicians with an opportunity to consider risk factors consistently. Regardless of the method used for risk assessment, clinical judgment is essential. Formal risk assessment tools are designed to detect those most commonly occurring risk factors, but specific patient-centred factors may increase or decrease that risk. The only purpose of risk assessment is to identify persons at risk and to facilitate the development of a plan of care.

Bergstrom and colleagues [31] demonstrated that in the absence of formal, documented risk assessment, conscientious physicians and nurses were likely to underestimate who was at risk and were likely to under prescribe basic preventive strategies such as turning or the use of support surfaces. Bates-Jensen and colleagues [32] likewise demonstrated that subjects with an admission risk assessment were more likely to have documented preventive interventions (76%) than those without risk assessment (14%). It is critical that the plan of care be developed and instituted promptly based on patient risk factors. Gifford and colleagues demonstrated that earlier development of a plan of care resulted in fewer ulcers (unpublished data). Risk assessment helps to identify mobility and activity and sensory deficits which require attention to mechanical loading and support surfaces, as well as good skin care. Identification of excessive moisture or nutritional deficits focuses attention on preventing and managing these deficits and directs the caregiver to provide good skin care.

Skin Assessment

Skin assessment should be done on admission and daily thereafter, with the results being documented. It is important, when assessing dark-skinned individuals, to employ careful visual inspection with good lighting and tactile inspection of vulnerable areas (AHCPR, 1992; http://www.npuap.org). Tactile inspection is done to detect changes in temperature, and to detect induration. While there are no published data to support the efficacy of this practice, early identification of abnormal findings provides an opportunity to redouble preventive efforts.

Skin Care. It is important to maintain personal hygiene, keeping the skin clean and dry, minimizing factors that cause dryness, such as low ambient humidity, bath water that is too warm, harsh soaps and too frequent bathing. Moisturizing lotions should be used to prevent dryness and cracking of the skin. Preferences of the patient for frequency and method of bathing should be considered.

Moisture. Minimize exposure of the skin to moisture from incontinence, perspiration or wound drainage. Assess and treat causes of urinary and faecal incontinence and provide opportunities for bowel and bladder training when appropriate. When exposure to moisture continues, use underpads or briefs that wick moisture away from the skin, or use moisture barriers to protect the skin. While there is evidence to show that the new disposable briefs do wick away moisture, clinical observation and judgment dictate that the skin be exposed to air at intervals to prevent the accumulation of moisture and heat.

Managing Pressure

The goal of managing pressure is to reduce pressure and the length of time tissue over bony prominences is exposed to pressure with the potential for ischaemia or decreased blood flow. Exposure to the effects of pressure should be minimized through the use of appropriate support surfaces, frequent repositioning, the use of pillows and wedges and through avoiding lying directly on the trochanter and sitting with the head of the bed elevated for extended periods of time. While there are many studies in the literature that test support surfaces, studies comparing surfaces with like properties are rare. Studies have shown that high-density foam replacement mattresses tested against a variety of static surfaces such as overlays, in studies of variable rigor, demonstrate that the replacement mattresses are generally superior to standard, plastic-covered mattresses and standard foam or circulating air overlays [33]. The properties of the support surface, including life expectancy of the surface, pressure redistribution, effectiveness of skin moisture and temperature control, product service requirements, fail-safety, infection control, flammability, and contribution to friction, should be studied uniformly in tests of such surfaces [19]. An algorithm for clinical decision making that appeared in the AHCPR (1992) guideline is presented in Fig. 4.3.

In addition to selecting the appropriate surface upon which to care for the patient, it is important to focus on other interventions, since pressure ulcers have been reported to develop even when the patient is cared for on a pressure reducing support surface.

Patients should be turned at least every 2 h according to a written schedule according to the plan of care and goals for the patient even when a special mattress or bed is used. The every 2 h rule emerged from the work of Norton and associates [34] with elderly persons in the early 1960s. An observational study demonstrated that those who were turned every 2–3 h developed fewer ulcers than those turned every 8 h or less often. The evidence supporting this guideline recommendation is weak, but it has become the standard of care world wide and should be continued until new evidence emerges that different intervals are appropriate. One study by Defloor [35] suggests that when foam replacement mattresses are used, turning every 3–4 h may be as effective as turning every 2 h on a standard hospital mattress. The study did not evaluate these findings in relation to level of patient risk. All at- risk patients were considered to be at high risk, and since the data have not been replicated, caution should be used when considering these data for practice implications. This is clearly an area requiring additional investigation. Pillows, wedges and other materials that aid in maintaining position and providing support should be used as needed.

When the patient can be turned from side to side without lying on a pressure ulcer, static surfaces may be sufficient to prevent pressure ulcers. When the patient has multiple ulcers or when the patient cannot be turned due to physiological instability, a low-air-loss or air-fluidized bed should be considered. An algorithm to support decisions for support surface selection appears in Fig. 4.3. It should be noted that, pressure ulcers may develop when the patient is on an air-fluidized bed.

Heels should be elevated on a pillow sufficient to raise the heels off the support surface, providing complete pressure relief [36]. Relief of heel pressure is important even on support surfaces purporting to reduce pressure. Abu-Own and colleagues [37] demonstrated that even on a low-air-loss surface, heel blood flow decreases in healthy subjects and patients when resting on the support surface.

Furthermore, patients should be positioned according to the 30° rule to avoid lying directly on the trochanter. The head of the bed should not be elevated above 30° for longer than necessary since the trochanter and ischial tuberosities place a great deal of pressure on the overlying tissues in these positions. Studies by Colin and associates [38, 39] confirm that pressure on the trochanter decreases $tcPO_2$ and increases $tcPCO_2$ to the underlying tissues, as does sitting with the head of the bed elevated.

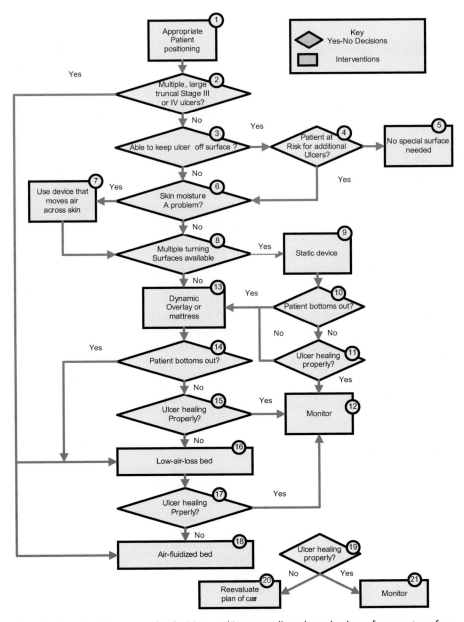

Fig. 4.3. An algorithm to guide decision making regarding the selection of support surfaces [adapted from 51]

Lifting devices that facilitate moving patients up in bed or turning them from side to side should be used to reduce exposure to friction and to prevent injury to carers. Donuts or rubber rings, because they create areas of reduced pressure, should not be used. Cushions that reduce pressure during seating and increase sitting stability should be used, but time in the sitting position should be minimized.

Nutrition for Prevention

Maintaining and improving the nutritional status of patients is thought to increase the tissue tolerance for pressure by maintaining tissue integrity and providing substrates for repair of damaged tissues. Retrospective studies have demonstrated an association between low serum albumin and low haemoglobin, decreases in body weight over short periods of time, and very low or very high body mass index. One prospective study of dietary intake found that the current dietary intake of protein and calories was a more important predictor of pressure ulcer development than either serum albumin or anthropometric indices [16]. There are no studies reported in the literature that show that a specific level of nutritional support can prevent ulcers. Attempts to study the role of dietary intake in the prevention of pressure ulcers must be carried out in conjunction with other preventive measures though to appreciate changes in pressure ulcer development or healing. Until such studies are available, every effort should be made to assess dietary intake and nutritional requirements on admission and at intervals consistent with changes in patient condition, to provide adequate food to meet nutritional needs and to engage in creative approaches to stimulating dietary intake. When intake is inadequate, dietary supplementation should be considered to improve dietary intake, as long as this supplementation is not contraindicated by other care requirements or advanced directives that preclude the use of feeding tubes. Surprisingly, little research has been done to inform practice in the area of nutritional support related to pressure ulcers.

Evidence-Based Care for Managing Pressure Ulcers

There are several components to the management of pressure ulcers included in most guidelines. These components include accurate and ongoing wound and patient assessment, wound care including cleansing, debridement, selection of dressings and adjuvant therapies.

Pressure ulcers should be assessed on admission and at every dressing change, considering and documenting the dimensions (length, width, depth, shape), location, presence of eschar or necrotic tissue, amount and odour of exudates and presence or absence of granulation tissue. Pressure ulcers should be staged according to the recommendations of the National

Pressure Ulcer Advisory Panel (http://www.npuap.org.) or a similar standard statement, and a formal documentation tool such as the Pressure Sore Status Tool (PSST) [40] or the Pressure Ulcer Scale for Healing (PUSH) [41] should be used to ensure consistency in documentation. Once the wound is assessed, a plan of care should be devised and written. Ongoing assessment, at every dressing change or once a week, whichever is the shorter interval, should guide the clinician's decisions to continue or change the plan of care. Continuity of care is important, but assessment of progress determines when to continue or when to alter the plan of care.

Cleansing. The wound should be cleansed initially and at every dressing change to reduce bacterial burden and to remove devitalized tissue and other wound exudates. Normal saline without a preservative should be used to irrigate wounds since it is reported to be non-cytotoxic. Cleansing agents with preservatives or inert carriers may be cytotoxic, and should be avoided, along with, antiseptics (e.g. Betadine) that may be toxic to regenerating cells. Hellewell and colleagues [42] reported the toxicity of several wound cleansers, finding that antiseptics were the most cytotoxic. Irrigation of the wound with the cleansing agent may be achieved with squeeze bottles, syringes, battery-powered devices or the like. Since the goal of cleansing is to remove exudate and sloughing tissue from the wound, it is recommended that some gentle mechanical force or pressure be used to cleanse the wound, rather than simply spraying the wound and patting it dry. Rodeheaver [20] recommended pulsatile lavage to loosen wound debris combined with gentle suction to remove cleansing agents and debris. When wounds are populated with significant eschar, whirlpool therapy can be considered for cleansing. One small study of 23 patients by Burke and colleagues [43] demonstrated improved wound healing of stage 3 and 4 ulcers with daily whirlpool treatments. It is important that appropriate infection control protocols are in place to maintain the cleanliness of whirlpools. Throughout the wound cleansing and dressing stages, strict attention must be paid to implementing precautions to protect against blood-borne pathogens.

Debridement. Debridement, or the removal of necrotic tissue and wound debris, should be done when cleansing alone is not sufficient to remove devitalized tissue from the wound bed. Debridement is appropriate when wound cleansing is inadequate to remove sloughing and devitalized tissue from the ulcer and should be carried out with consideration of the status of the ulcer and the condition of the patient. An exception to the debridement recommendation is when large heel ulcers covered by eschar present without erythema of surrounding tissues, fluctuance or drainage. These heel ulcers should not be debrided, but rather be evaluated frequently.

When debridement is necessary, the method most appropriate for the given patient's condition should be selected. Autolytic, mechanical, chemical or sharp debridement may all be appropriate. Autolytic debridement is achieved using an occlusive or semi-occlusive dressing that retains moisture and liquefies necrotic tissue by phagocytosis, and tissue enzymes. Mechanical debridement is achieved non-selectively using physical force such as wet-to-dry dressings, lavage, whirlpool and other methods to loosen foreign materials and contaminated tissues and healthy tissue as well. Chemical debridement employs topical proteolytic or collagenolytic enzymes to loosen and liquefy eschar, slough and wound debris. It is important that clinicians reassess the wound periodically to determine when debridement is complete and to discontinue treatments that may destroy granulating tissue. Sharp debridement selectively removes necrotic tissue, using sterile instruments, but without anaesthesia and with little or no bleeding. This is closely related to surgical debridement, in which much more aggressive excision may be done. Sharp and surgical debridement are the most appropriate when the bacterial load of the wound may evolve into spreading cellulites and sepsis. In all cases, it is important to consider the pain and discomfort to which the patient is exposed and to manage the pain effectively.

Dressings. The basic principle in the selection of a dressing is to remember that wounds heal better in a moist environment. The goal of care is to select a dressing that keeps the wound bed moist, the surrounding tissue dry and controls exudate without desiccating the ulcer bed. Deep wounds and wounds with sinus tracts and undermining should be packed loosely to eliminate dead space. There is no research supporting the use of one specific brand of dressing over another, despite the number of new dressings brought to the marketplace. It has, however, been demonstrated that dressings maintaining a moist wound environment are associated with better healing than dry dressings [44, 45]. Moisture-retaining dressings have been associated with a reduction in needed caregiver time and overall cost effectiveness [46]. It is important to remember that wet-to-dry dressings are not a variant of a moist wound environment; as the dressings dry, they provide indiscriminate mechanical debridement. In the future, smart dressings that notify of prolonged exposure to pressure, exposure to moisture, or specific substrates or bacteria in the wound may emerge; if so, they will be a welcome addition to care.

Adjuvant Therapies. A number of adjuvant therapies to promote wound healing have good evidence to support clinical implementation, and others are currently emerging. Electrical stimulation has demonstrated efficacy for promoting closure of stage III and IV ulcers when combined with other care [48–50]. Vacuum-assisted therapy is showing promise for promoting healing of stage III and IV ulcers, but no data have emerged to clearly demonstrate the efficacy and to direct clinicians regarding the end point of therapy. The lack of controlled studies prevents the recommendation of most adjuvant therapies. Manufactures and clinicians can contribute to pressure ulcer care by focusing on controlled studies.

Future Research

It is clear from the recommendations of guideline panels and most authors writing about pressure ulcers that there is a need for multi-site efficacy studies of specific products and treatment modalities. These studies must have adequate statistical power to draw conclusions and make recommendations for practice. Studies testing the efficacy of like products (similar mattresses, dressings, adjuvant therapies) from different manufacturers would be particularly helpful in clinical selection of the best, most cost-effective products.

Standard care plans should be developed based upon specific risk factors. These care plans should be tested for efficacy and to characterize the patient's response to the care plan. Characterization would provide additional information about circumstances for using the plan of care, the efficacy for specific individual characteristics and the time to healing. Testing a protocol or a comprehensive care plan would provide data that would permit conclusions about the effectiveness of the treatments, the degree of compliance with recommendations, and outcomes of clinicians. Most efficacy data only support the selection of one product over another, but effectiveness research also needs to evaluate a composite of treatments performed for prevention or treatment to permit evaluation of outcomes when protocols are used.

Recent data suggest that increased time for nurses to provide care results in improved patient outcomes. This relationship between staffing and patient outcomes needs to be tested in prospective studies where interventions can be documented. It is important to evaluate the role of other therapists and providers as well, in order to determine judicious use of consultants and consultant recommendations.

A long list of important studies that would contribute to knowledge development and clinical practice in the area of pressure ulcers could be generated. This is a fruitful area for new and seasoned investigators alike. The challenge is in identifying those studies that will most rapidly advance the science and provide an opportunity for more enlightened practice. Guideline summaries that synthesize the literature to date and point to gaps in the current knowledge base would provide an excellent starting point.

References

1. Mor V et al. (1998) Benchmarking quality in nursing homes: the Q-Metrics system. Can J Qual Health Care 14:12–17
2. Bergstrom N, Allman RM, Carlson CE, et al. (1992) Pressure ulcers in adults: predication and prevention. Clinical practice guideline, Number 3. AHCPR Publication No. 92-0047. Agency for Health Care Polich and Research, Public Health Service, U.S. Department of Health and Human Services, Rockville, MD
3. Cuddigan J, Ayello EA, Sussman C, Baranoski S (eds) (2001) Pressure ulcers in America: prevalence, incidence, and implications for the future. National Pressure Ulcer Advisory Panel, Reston, VA

4. Brooks EL, Duncan GW (1940) Effects of pressure on tissues. Arch Surg 40:696–709
5. Husain T (1953) An experimental study of some pressure effects on tissues with reference to the bed-sore problem. J Pathol Bacteriol 66:347–358
6. Kosiak M (1959) Etiology and pathology of ischemic ulcers. Arch Phys Med Rehab 40:62–68
7. Daniel RK, Priest DL, Wheatley DC (1981) Etiologic factors in pressure sores: an experimental model. Arch Phys Med Rehab 62:492–498
8. Allman RM, Goode PS, Patrick MM, Burst N, Bartolucci AA (1995) Pressure ulcer risk factors among hospitalized patients with activity limitation. JAMA, 273 (11), 865–870
9. Bader DL, White SH (1998) The viability of soft tissues in elderly subjects undergoing hip surgery. Age Ageing, 27:217–222
10. Nicholson PW, Leeman AL, O'Neill CJA, Dobbs SM, Deshmukh AA, Denham MJ (1988) Pressure sores: Effect of Parkinson's disease and cognitive function on spontaneous movement in bed. Age and Ageing 17:111–115
11. Schnelle JF, Adamson GM, Cruise PA, Al-Samarrai N, Sarbaugh FC, Uman G, Ouslander JG (1997) Skin disorders and moisture in incontinent nursing home residents: Intervention implications. J Am Geriatr Soc 45:1182–1188
12. Horn SD, Bender SA, Bergstrom N, Cook AS, Ferguson ML, Rimmasch HL, Sharkey SS, Smout RJ, Taler GA, Voss AC (2002) Description of the National Pressure Ulcer Long-Term Care Study. J Am Geriatr Soc 50:1816–1825
13. Needleman J, Buerhaus P, Mattke S, Stewart M, Zelevinsky K (2002) Nurse staffing and quality of care in hospitals in the United States. N Engl J Med 346:171–175
14. Braden BJ, Bergstrom N (2000) A conceptual schema for the study of the etiology of pressure sores. Rehab Nurs 25:105–110
15. Dinsdale SM (1974) Decubitus ulcers: role of pressure and friction in causation. Arch Phys Med Rehab 55:147–152
16. Bergstrom N, Braden B (1992) A prospective study of pressure sore risk among institutionalized elderly. J Am Geriatr Soc 40:747–758
17. Bergstrom N, Bennett MA, Carlson CE, et al. (1994) Treatment of pressure ulcers. Clinical practice guideline, number 15. U.S. Department of Health and Human Services. Public Health Service, Agency for Health Care Policy and Research, Rockville, MD. AHCPR Publication No. 95-0652
18. European Pressure Ulcer Advisory Panel (EPUAP) (1999) Guideline on treatment of pressure ulcers EPUAP, Oxford (available from: http://www.epuap.org, accessibility verified on 27 February 2003)
19. Maklebust J (1999) An update on horizontal patient support surfaces. Ostomy/Wound Management 45[Suppl 1A]:70S–77S
20. Rodeheaver GT (1999) Pressure ulcer debridement and cleansing: a review of current literature. Ostomy/Wound Management 45[Suppl 1A]:80S–85S
21. Shekelle PG, Ortiz E, Rhodes S, Morton SC, Eccles MP, Frimshaw JM, Woolf SH (2001) Validity of the Agency for Healthcare Research and Quality Clinical Practice Guidelines: How quickly do guidelines become outdated? JAMA 286:1461–1467
22. Horn S, Ashton C, Tracy D (1994) Prevention and treatment of pressure ulcers by protocol. In Horn S, Hopkins D (eds) Clinical practice improvement: a new technology for developing cost-effective quality health care. Faulkner & Gray, New York

23. Bergstrom N, Braden B, Boynton P, Bruch S (1995) Using a research-based assessment scale in clinical practice. Nurs Clin North Am 30:539–551
24. Lyder CH, Preston J, Grady JN, Scinto J, Allman R, Bergstrom N, Rodeheaver G (2001) Quality of care for hospitalized medicare patients at risk for pressure ulcers. Arch Intern Med 161:1549–1554
25. Cuddigan J, Frantz RA (1998) Pressure ulcer research: pressure ulcer treatment: a monograph. National Pressure Ulcer Advisory Panel. Adv Wound Care 8:46–48
26. Bergstrom N, Braden B, Kemp M, Champagne M, Ruby E (1998) Predicting pressure ulcer risk: a multi-site study of the predictive validity of the Braden Scale. Nurs Res 47:261–269
27. Bergstrom N, Braden B, Laguzza A, Holman V (1987) The Braden Scale for predicting pressure sore risk. Nurs Res 36:205–210
28. Braden BJ, Bergstrom N (1994) Predictive validity of the Braden Scale for pressure sore risk in a nursing home population. Res Nurs Health 17:459–470
29. Pang SM, Wong TK (1998) Predicting pressure sore risk with the Norton, Braden and Waterlow scales in a Hong Kong rehabilitation hospital. Nurs Res 47:147–153
30. Van Marum RJ, Ooms ME, Ribbe MW, Van Eijk J (2000) The Dutch pressure sore assessment score or the Norton scale for identifying at-risk nursing home patients? Age Ageing 29:63–68
31. Bergstrom N, Braden B, Kemp M, Ruby E (1996) Multi-site study of incidence of pressure ulcers and the relationship between risk level, demographic characteristics, diagnoses, and prescription of preventive interventions. J Am Geriatr Soc 44:22–30
32. Bates-Jensen BM, Cadogan M, Jorge J, Schnelle JF (2003) Standardized quality assessment system to evaluate pressure ulcer care in nursing homes. J Am Geriatr Soc 51:1194–1202
33. Whittemore R (1998) Pressure reduction support surfaces: a review of the literature. J Wound Ostomy Continence Nurs 25:6–25
34. Norton D, McLaren R, Exton-Smith AN (1962) An investigation of geriatric nursing problems in hospital. Churchill Livingstone, New York
35. Defloor T (2001) Wisselhouding, minder frequent en toch minder decubitus. Tijdschr Gerontol Geriatr 31:174–177
36. Sideranko S, Quinn A, Burns K, Froman RD (1992) Effects of position and mattress overlay on sacral and heel pressures in a clinical population. Res Nurs Health 15:245–251
37. Abu-Own A, Sommerville K, Schurr JH (1995) Effects of compression and type of bed surface on the microcirculation of the heel. Eur J Vasc Endovasc Surgy 9:1995
38. Colin D, Abraham P, Preault L (1996) Comparison of 90° and 30° laterally inclined positions in the prevention of pressure ulcers using transcutaneous oxygen and carbon dioxide pressures. Adv Wound Care 9:35–38
39. Colin D, Loyant R, Abraham P (1996) Changes in sacral transcutaneous oxygen tension in the evaluation of different mattresses in the prevention of pressure ulcers. Adv Wound Care 9:25–28
40. Bates-Jensen BM, Cadogan M, Osterweil D, Levy-Storms L, Jorge J, A-Samarrai N, Grbic V, Schnelle JF (2003) The minimum data set pressure ulcer indicator: does it reflect differences in care processes related to pressure ulcer prevention and treatment in nursing homes. J Am Geriatr Soc 51:1203–1212

41. Stotts NA, Rodeheaver GT, Thomas DR et al. (2001) An instrument to measure healing in pressure ulcers: development and validation of the Pressure Ulcer Scale for Healing (PUSH). J Gerontol 56:M795–799
42. Hellewell TB, Major PA, Foresman PA (1997) A cytotoxicity evaluation of antimicrobial and nonantimicrobial wound cleansers. Wounds 9:15–20
43. Burke DT, Ho CH, Saucier MA (1998) Effects of hydrotherapy on pressure ulcer healing. Arch Phys Med Rehab 77:394–398
44. Xakellis GC, Chriscilles EA (1992) Hydrocolloids versus saline gauze dressings in treating pressure ulcers: a cost effective analysis. Arch Phys Med Rehab. 73:463–469
45. Colwell JC, Foreman MD, Trotter JP (1993) A comparison of the efficacy and cost effectiveness of two methods of managing pressure ulcers. Decubitus 6:28–36
46. Bolton LL, van Rijswijk L, Shaffer FA (1997) Quality wound care equals cost-effective wound care: A clinical model. Adv Wound Care 10:33–38
47. Baker LR, Chambers R, DeMuth S (1997) Effects of electrical stimulation on wound healing in patients with diabetic ulcers. Diabetes Care 20:405–412
48. Wood J, Evans P, Schallreuter K (1993) A multicenter study on the use of pulsed low-intensity direct current for healing chronic state II and III decubitus ulcers. Arch Dermatol 129:999–1009
49. Stefanovska A, Vodovnik L, Benko H (1993) Treatment of chronic wounds by means of electric and electromagnetic fields. 2. Value of FES parameters for pressure sore treatment. Med Biol Eng Comput 31:213–220
50. Griffin J, Tooms R, Mendius R (1991) Efficacy of high-voltage pulsed current for healing of pressure ulcers in patients with spinal cord injury. Phys Ther 71:433–442
51. Kemp MG, Krouskop TA, Garber BS, Carlson CE (1992) Guideline: mechanical loading and support surfaces. Agency for Health Care Policy and Research, pp 137–148

The Measurement of Interface Pressure   5

Ian Swain

Introduction

There are a number of factors that can predispose an individual to a high
risk of developing pressure ulcers. These can be divided into external factors, including pressure, shear, time, temperature, humidity and their interactions, and internal factors, which determine the level of loading tolerated
by tissues before damage occurs [1]. The internal factors can be affected
by the underlying disease such as diabetes or certain neurological conditions in which the tissues are more liable to be damaged by a given level
of pressure and are dealt with elsewhere in this book. This chapter is primarily concerned with the external factors, in particular pressure, which
can be affected by a loss of muscle bulk and tone as in flaccid paraplegia,
or by the weight loss associated with the latter stages of cancer. Although
the majority of this chapter will deal with the interface pressures measured
on mattresses and cushions it should be remembered that pressure ulcers
can occur in other situations. They may be found on the feet due to poorly
fitting footwear, especially if the patient is diabetic, on limb stumps due to
prostheses, or under orthoses, especially if the orthosis is exerting significant force to try to prevent spinal or bony deformity.

There are, basically, only two ways associated with pressure in which a
support surface can operate in order to reduce the probability of a pressure
ulcer developing. Firstly, there are static systems which seek to minimise
the interface pressure by increasing the contact area, and secondly dynamic
systems which produce an alternating action that subjects the tissues to periods of high pressure followed by periods of low pressure during which it is
anticipated that the pressure is sufficiently low to enable blood flow to return.

The development of accurate pressure-measuring systems is important in
assessing such support systems. However their exclusive use in determining
risk of breakdown is critically dependent on a reliable indicator of safe pressure, or band of pressures, in association with time [2], that would be appropriate for all patients at risk. This remains a "holy grail" for medical engineers
involved in the prevention of pressure ulcers. Many attempts have been made
to determine the minimal degree and duration of compression that will consistently produce tissue damage [3–5]. Often quoted as a cut-off figure is
32 mmHg, which is the capillary pressure as measured by Landis [6]. However, this value, measured in 1930, was determined in a nail fold capillary at

heart level and it is therefore difficult to see how this relates to the external pressure needed to stop blood flow in capillaries when a person is sitting on a cushion or lying on a mattress. In such cases the picture is much more complicated, as there are supporting structures such as collagen and muscle fibres around the capillaries which will serve to distribute the applied load. In addition, the blood pressure in the capillary will vary due to both systemic blood pressure and the hydrostatic head of blood, which will depend upon the person's posture. What is undeniable, however, is that high pressures are sustainable for short times only and, if maintained, will lead to tissue breakdown.

Interface Pressure Measurement

History

Despite the fact that a 'safe' interface pressure cannot be easily determined, the vast majority of researchers accept that high interface pressures are a major contributory factor in the development of pressure ulcers. One of the first to do so, in 1961, was Kosiak [7], who subjected rats to a variety of different pressure/time loading regimes and looked at the rate of pressure ulcer formation. His earlier work had shown that pressure measured under the ischia on a foam cushion was of the order of 150 mmHg [8] and therefore he concluded that complete ischaemia of tissues over the bone was only a matter of time, with an unrelieved pressure of only 40 mmHg being sufficient to cause ischaemia [7]. The importance of the pressure/time relationship was further explored by Reswick and Rogers [2], who produced the famous graph shown in Fig. 5.1, which was based on 980 observations. They strongly stated, however, that this curve is a guideline, based on much experience but relatively few controlled measurements.

An early review of methods of measuring interface pressure was undertaken by Ferguson-Pell et al. in 1976 [9]. At that time pressure-measuring devices fell into three broad categories. Firstly, some devices consisted of thin sheets of various materials treated with inks or chemicals. These have the advantage of giving a map of the pressure distribution but are difficult to quantify, subject to in-plane forces and also sensitive to rate of loading and temperature. Secondly there are devices that consist of air cells which have electrical contacts on the inside. Inflation pressure is measured and increased until the surfaces of the cell part, which can be demonstrated by an indicator bulb. The inflation pressure in the cell at this point is taken to be equal to the interface pressure. The final type in use at that time were strain-gauge diaphragm transducers, some of which were commercially available for fluid measurements. In addition, research was being undertaken in a number of centres to develop thin capacitive, resistive or inductive sensors.

The conclusions from this review almost 30 years ago are still true today, namely that the sensor must give a useful output over the range 10–

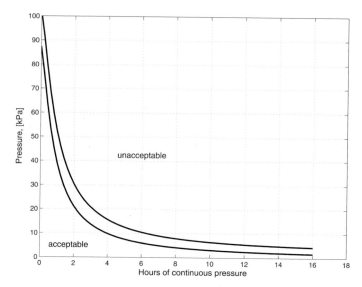

Fig. 5.1. Allowable pressures vs time of application for tissues under bony prominences. Curve gives general guidelines and should not be taken as absolute. Adapted from [2]

250 mmHg. Time dependence must be minimal or at least well defined and repeatable, and the sensor must be smaller than the radius of curvature of the body area under investigation. Finally, calibration is problematic and consideration must be given to the thickness and flexibility of the transducer, compliance of the loading interfaces and the possibility of the sensitivity of the transducer to forces other than those in the normal direction.

Any system designed to measure interface pressure will inherently have an effect on the very parameter that it is attempting to measure. There are a number of different systems that have been developed over the years ranging from single sensors, such as the original 28-mm Scimedics system (Talley Medical, Romsey, Hants, UK) which needed to be manually inflated to record pressures, to a number of systems with multi-element arrays which are capable of capturing data in real time and producing an image on a computer screen. Various researchers have advocated different systems, although to date there is no 'gold standard'.

Practical Considerations

Two main factors must be considered when measuring interface pressure. In particular the sensor must be correctly located under the relevant bony prominence, and also its presence must not introduce errors which would mask any difference between the support systems being evaluated. As will be described, interface pressure has been shown to be significantly affected both by the positioning of the subject and by any object between the subject's skin and the support surface, particularly if that object is inflexible and cannot adapt to the shape of the patient/surface interface. In practice these two factors are largely mutually exclusive, as the large-array systems have the advantage of many sensors, so that the point of maximum pressure can be determined easily, but have the disadvantage that if they are inflexible they will affect the surface, especially if the surface deforms in more than one dimension, as in the case of a low-air-loss or fluidised-bead bed. If individual sensors are used then errors will be reduced if they are smaller than the area of interest; however, they will need to be accurately positioned to record the pressure exerted on the area of interest. If the sensor is larger than the area of interest it will act as an additional support, particularly if the sensor is inflated, and will therefore significantly change the patient/surface interface. Even if the sensor is of the correct size and type and is accurately placed, it should be realised that any readings taken are only a 'snapshot' of that particular situation and will vary with time and with any change in posture of the patient.

Comparison and Analysis of Different Systems

There have been few reported comparisons of different pressure measuring systems. Allen et al. [10, 11] looked at the repeatability and accuracy of the Talley SA500 Pressure Evaluator with both the 28-mm and 100-mm sensor pads (Talley Medical, Romsey, Hants, UK). This is an electropneumatic device in which the pressure needed to inflate an air sac is increased until two contacts on the internal faces of the air sac are broken. This pressure is then recorded as the interface pressure. They also evaluated the DIPE (Next Generation, CA, USA) and found the Talley 28-mm sensor was the most accurate. Ferguson-Pell and Cardi [12] compared two arrays, the Force Sensing Array (FSA), with 225 sensors (Vista Medical, Winnipeg, Canada) and the Tekscan, with 2064 sensors, and the Talley Pressure Monitor (TPM), with 96 sensors (Talley Medical). The TPM differs from the other two, consisting of small arrays of sensors as well as individual sensors which can be directly located on the skin surface. By contrast the FSA and Tekscan are large arrays, typically 500 mm×500 mm, which cover the whole area of interest. The authors found that the TPM was the most accurate, stable and reproducible of the systems tested but was limited in its ease of use, speed and data presentation [12]. The FSA was well rated in clinical applications but demonstrated pronounced hysteresis (+19%) and creep (4%). The Tekscan system also showed substantial hysteresis (+20%) and creep (19%) but was preferred by clinicians for its real-time display capabilities, resolution and display options.

Gyi et al. [13] undertook a detailed critique of the TPM, a more recent derivative of the Oxford Pressure Monitor [14] which examines the pressure/flow characteristics of the air needed to inflate a small air sac. This has been shown to give good correlation with the Talley SA 500 [15]. These authors identified a major disadvantage of this system in that it did not give readings in real time as it samples one sensor element approximately every second and therefore each sensor is sampled only every 90 s if all 96 sensors are connected. Other findings were that the system was improved if the sensor elements were more tightly packed and that errors could occur if the sensors were placed on a curved surface, although the errors were small if the radius of curvature was less than 20 mm. In addition, if only 75% of the sensor face was covered then the reading obtained was 82% of the correct value. The authors are unaware of any other evaluations of this type and it is clear that similar studies are required to quantify errors associated with the measurement of interface pressure.

Since the studies quoted above there has been little work on the comparison of different pressure measuring systems despite the fact that a number of new systems have appeared on the market. In addition, at the time of writing this chapter, the TPM is no longer available for purchase but is still available for hire, directly from Talley. Table 5.1 shows the range of pressure-measuring equipment currently available in the UK. More information can be obtained from any of the companies' websites.

The only recent evaluation of pressure-measuring systems was by Diesing et al. [16], who compared the FSA, Novel and X sensor. Their conclusions were that all systems underestimated the force applied on a small contact area. The minimum contact area for an accurate reading was in the range between 4.5 cm^2 and 19.6 cm^2, depending upon the system. However all showed good linearity and the authors felt that all were excellent tools for clinical use but all were inclined to underestimate the pressure under small bony prominences. They also felt that it was not possible to compare pressures taken on two different systems.

Factors to Consider When Measuring Interface Pressure

As well as the inherent sources of error present in any specific measurement system, measurement of interface pressure is made more difficult by the variability that is introduced by the experimental procedures adopted. This variability is due to subject positioning, the choice of measuring system used, curvature and compliance of the subject/support surface interface, clothing etc. and is considerably greater than any inaccuracy in the measuring device itself, which is normally quoted to be of the order of 10% or 10 mmHg. Each of these will now be considered, although a more detailed account of these potential problems can be found in a recent paper by Swain and Bader [17].

Intersubject Variability

As pressure is force per unit area it is obvious that the shape of a subject will have an effect on the interface pressure. The shape of the subject will depend on the skeleton, the quantity, tone and shape of the musculature

Table 5.1. Comparison of commercially available interface pressure measuring systems

	X Sensor	FSA	Tekscan	Talley	Pressure	Novel
Principle of operation	Capacitive	Piezo-resistive	Resistive	Electro-pneumatic	Pneumatic	Capacitive
System	Seat Mattress	Seat Back Bed In shoe Orthotist	Seat In shoe Dental	Individual sensor	Individual sensor	Seat Foot Specialist e.g. bike seat hand
Sensor size (mm)	Seat 12.5×12.5 Hi-res 2.7×2.7	Bed 19×50 Foot 9×16	Foot 5×5	100 mm round 28 mm round	25 or 62.5	2.7×2.7 min 31×47 max
Sample rate	Up to 70,000 sensors s^{-1}	3,072 sensors s^{-1}	316,800 sensors s^{-1}	N/A	N/A	Up to 20,000 sensors s^{-1}
Range (mmHg)	0–220	Bed 0–200 Foot 0–1500	Seat 0–200/1,000 Foot 0–7500	20–300	0–125	Bed 0–200 Foot 0–1,800
No. of sensors	Seat 2304 Bed 10,240 Hi-res 65k	up to 32×32	over 2,000	1	1	Up to 2,304
Quoted accuracy	10% or 10 mmHg	10%	Clinically ±3% Laboratory ±1%	±2%	±3 mmHg	Typically ±5%
Output device	Computer	Computer	Computer	Handheld digital gauge	Handheld digital gauge	Computer
Web address	www.xsensor.com	www.vista-medical.nl	www.tekscan.com	www.talley-medical.co.uk	www.clevemed.com	www.novel.de

and the amount of subcutaneous fat. There have not been many studies to compare different groups although in general people with a low body mass index (BMI) are inclined to have higher interface pressures [18]. However, the effect that an individual's anatomy has on interface pressure is much more subtle, and even individuals with very similar body types can exhibit quite different interface pressures [17]. This can be demonstrated well from the baseline data on the standard King's Fund mattress obtained by the author in both Department of Health-funded and commercial trials [15, 19–22].

Therefore the range of interface pressures on various anatomical sites vary widely with the subjects' underlying anatomy, and, in my experience, it is not possible to predict the interface pressures from the person's body type.

Interface pressures were measured on the King's Fund mattress at the most common locations for pressure ulcers by the author. These readings were made using elderly ambulant volunteers and were obtained from readings made during the production of the Department of Health Evaluation Reports PS1, PS2, PS3, PS4 and PS5 [19–24] and from 20 years' consultancy work for a great number of companies.

Sacrum when semi-recumbent, backrest at 45°	62–107 mmHg (8.3–14.3 kPa)
Trochanter, side lying, hips and knees at 60°	6–156 mmHg (8.1–20.8 kPa)
Heels	107–213 mmHg (14.3–28.4 kPa)
Ischial tuberosities when sitting on 3-in. standard cushion	60–146 mmHg (8–19.5 kPa)

Variability Due to Anatomical Location and Patient Position

The human body is not a homogeneous structure and therefore the interface pressure will vary depending on the shape of the underlying bony structure at the point of interest, the amount of subcutaneous tissue covering that bone and the weight being supported. High-pressure points will therefore either be areas such as the heels when lying supine, where there is a small contact area, or the buttocks when sitting, where there is a large load combined with underlying bony prominences, the ischial tuberosities. If this contact area is further reduced by extensive loss of subcutaneous tissue, then the pressures will increase. However, when lying supine a person with normal pathology will have much lower interface pressures under the buttocks since the load is distributed over a larger area, and as the pelvis is rotated, compared to sitting, there are no obvious bony prominences in contact with the support surface. In this position more pressure will be ex-

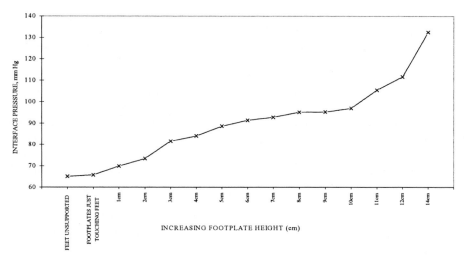

Fig. 5.2. The effect of footrest height on interface pressure

erted on the sacrum, particularly if the person is semi-recumbent. Therefore the person's posture will have a marked effect on the areas subjected to the highest pressures. For example a person sitting in a slumped position in a chair will often have the highest pressures recorded under the sacrum rather than under the ischial tuberosities.

When comparing different products, it is essential to ensure repeatable positioning of the subjects, as failure to do so can lead to errors that are greater than the underlying differences between the products. This is best demonstrated by the results obtained during the Department of Health trial on wheelchair cushions [22, 23] (Fig. 5.2).

This variability is also reported by other researchers. Koo et al. [25] found that in seated patients, interface pressure could increase from 88 to 146 mmHg (from 11.7 to 19.5 kPa) on a Roho cushion and from 106 to 221 mmHg (from 14.1 to 29.5 kPa) on a PU foam cushion as the patient varied their position in the chair from leaning forward to leaning to the right. This indicates that the more conforming the cushion, the less effect posture has on interface pressure. Hobson [26] also found that posture and body orientation had a profound effect on body-seat interface variables and that posture is a factor that deserves increased research and clinical attention.

Variability Due to Underlying Pathology

Expediency often requires that interface pressure readings are undertaken on healthy, young adult volunteers, often students, despite the fact that the vast majority of people at risk of pressure ulcers are elderly or those with chronic diseases, illness or disabilities. In those at risk there will not only be a change in shape at the patient-support interface due to loss in muscle tone, but the skin will often have inferior mechanical properties and the body will be less able to adapt to the effects of pressure due to the underlying pathology. This is particularly the case if the underlying disease affects the normal circulatory control system, such as in multiple sclerosis and spina bifida.

Of the few studies to compare the interface pressure of different groups, Brienza and Karg [27] showed that the type of cushion had a greater effect on subjects with SCI than it did with the elderly, but suggested that more research was still needed. Hobson [26] also noted that people with spinal cord injuries exhibited interface pressures between 6 and 46% higher than a control group of normal subjects. The Department of Health Evaluation Report, PS4 also measured interface pressure on a variety of users, including flaccid and spastic paraplegics, people following a cerebrovascular accident (CVA) and elderly ambulant volunteers, and showed that the ranking of products was significantly different for each of the groups. This will be considered in more detail in the section on mannequins versus normal volunteers.

Variability Due to Other Factors

A static support surface is required to conform to the shape of the body so that the load can be distributed over a larger area, hence reducing the interface pressure. In a dynamic support surface, such as an alternating pressure mattress, it is essential that nothing affects the alternating action, so that when a given cell is deflated, the interface pressure is sufficiently low to enable blood flow to return to normal levels before the next period of high pressure when the cell is reinflated. In both types of systems the properties of any covering materials between the foam, air or gel of the cushion and the subject's skin will affect the interface pressure. If the covering material is too tight and inflexible then it will be inclined to hammock across the support surface, preventing deformation of the underlying core in static systems [19] and negating the alternating action in dynamic systems.

The effect of the covering material is also of importance when advising the wheelchair- or chair-bound patient on the choice of clothing. Thus stretchy sports clothing will be far better for the patient than heavy materials like denim, which are non conforming and usually have thick seams and rivets in support areas. It is therefore essential that, as clothing will make a difference to the interface pressure, it is kept to a minimum and standardised in any product evaluations.

Correlation Between Interface and Interstitial Pressures

As briefly discussed in the Introduction, the important parameter is not actually the interface pressure but the resultant pressure that is transmitted to the tissue. If this pressure is of sufficient magnitude, it can stop blood flow and lead to tissue necrosis. It is the fact that measurement of the internal or interstitial pressure is difficult and inherently invasive that has lead to the widespread use of interface pressure as a parameter that can easily be measured in the clinical environment. Added to the difficulty in measuring interstitial pressure per se is the inherent complication that introducing a measuring device into the tissue is bound to have an effect. The exact position of the probe is critical and any location, whether just below the skin, adjacent to a bony prominence or in the middle of a muscle, will affect the results obtained.

Few studies have attempted to compare interface and interstitial pressure, and it is difficult to compare the results that different groups have obtained. In 1984 Le et al. [28], using silicon pressure transducers in pigs, stated that they measured pressures that were between three to five times greater next to the bone than the applied interface pressure on the surface of the skin. Reddy [29], however, applying pressure with a cuff in a pig model and measuring interstitial pressure with a wick catheter 2–5 mm below the skin, showed that the interstitial pressure was only 65–75% of the applied pressure but increased to 100% when the tissue was oedematous. Dodd [30] also used a pig model and showed that 28–43% of pressure was transferred to the interstitium depending upon anatomical location, with the highest readings being over the sacrum.

One of the few studies to undertake measurements on people was that by Sangeorzan et al. [31], who found that the displacement necessary to reduce TcPO$_2$ to zero was significantly less over bone than it was over muscle. Their explanation was that skin over muscle tolerates greater locally applied loads and deformations because the pressure is lower within the tissue than when similar loads and deformations are applied to skin over bone.

Uses of Interface Pressure Measurement

Pressure measurement systems can be used in two separate environments. Firstly in a clinical setting, typically associated with a seating clinic, in which interface pressure is used as an adjunct to risk assessment as well as providing an aid to clinical prescription. In this setting it can also be used to give biofeedback to the patient, providing evidence of postural factors associated with pelvic obliquity, tilt and rotation and the efficacy of pressure-relief regimens. Alternatively, it can be used in the laboratory to evaluate the relative performance of different pressure-reduction systems under controlled conditions.

Clinical

There are two roles that interface pressure measurement has in the clinical environment: firstly in patient education, and secondly to determine that a cushion is suitable for a given individual. Patient education is of vital importance when dealing with groups of people at high risk, as unless the person is themself aware of the possible consequences of poor seating, poor posture and lack of attention to skin care, they stand a greater chance of developing pressure ulcers. It is perhaps interesting to draw an analogy with patients with hypertension who regularly visit their GP and hospital clinics to have their blood pressure measured, where the information obtained is used for clinical audit and to determine the effect of any change in medication. The very act of measuring blood pressure indicates to the patient that the professionals involved are concerned and are addressing the situation. Imagine the patients' concern if their blood pressure was never measured but their medication was still changed. It is all a question of relative risk, as although it is not known that a person with a given level of hypertension will have a myocardial infarction or a CVA within a given period of time, it is known that the probability of such an event is greater. It is the same with a person who is wheelchair dependent. We do not know that a given level of interface pressure will lead to skin breakdown in a given period of time. However, we do know that the greater the period of unrelieved pressure [2, 32], the greater the risk of developing pressure ulcers. In addition, with the increase in litigation and the implementation of clinical governance in the UK, measurement and recording of interface pressure could be regarded as being as essential activity for anyone involved in wheelchair or seating clinics.

Pressure ulcer prevention clinics in which interface pressure is measured on a regular basis have been shown to be effective [33]. In such clinics interface pressure can be used to show the patients the effect of changing posture, such as leaning forward or to one side, to vary the distribution of pressure. The information can also be used by staff to determine the correct cushion for the individual and to determine the effects of changing the set-up of the wheelchair and cushion, such as changing the footrest height or the inflation pressure in a Roho cushion (Fig. 5.3 a, b) The illustrations in Fig. 5.3 c, d showing the effect of varying the footrest height in more detail. In fact, by changing the footrest height in 12 subjects the mean interface pressure increased twofold from 65 mmHg to 130 mmHg (from 8.7 to 17.3 kPa), whereas changing the type of cushion from the best to the worst saw an increase in interface pressure from 71 mmHg to 128 mmHg (from 9.5 to 17.1 kPa) [22].

The new pressure-measuring arrays are especially suitable for such applications. The ability to give a real-time representation of the pattern of pressure distribution on a monitor and the simplicity of using such systems in the clinical environment outweigh the disadvantages of the sensor mat affecting absolute pressure readings. What such systems do give is the ability to show the whole area of interest in a format that can be readily understood by the patients, greatly reinforcing any patient education programmes. Printouts of the pressure distribution can then be kept in the clinical records.

It is not just in seating that interface pressure can be used clinically. Orthotics, in particular foot orthotics, is one area where interface pressure

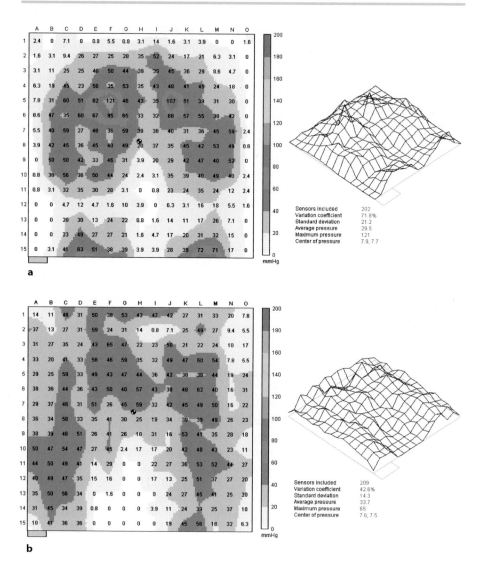

Fig. 5.3 a–b. Practical use of an interface pressure-measuring array in clinical practice

can be easily used to improve fit. Orthotic foot mats do exist for a number of the systems described above and enable the pressure-sensing surface to be placed between the customised foot orthoses and the foot to ensure that there is sufficient pressure relief over areas at greatest risk.

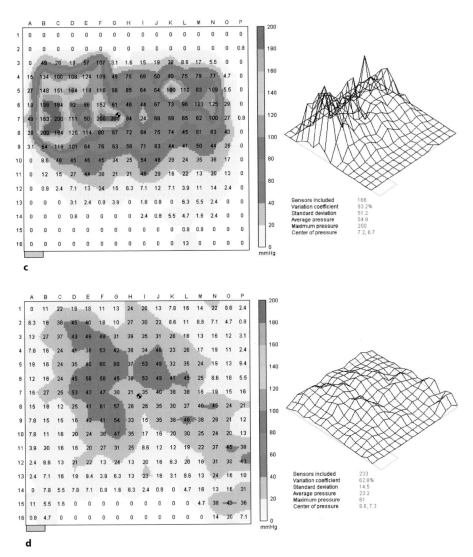

Fig. 5.3 c–d. Practical use of an interface pressure-measuring array in clinical practice

Research and Product Evaluation

The requirements on pressure-measuring systems in research and product evaluation are rather different than in the clinical setting. In research the absolute measurements are of greatest interest and therefore the accuracy and repeatability of the measurement is more important than the display of data, which will usually be determined by the researcher. For comparison between two or more commercial products, much greater care is needed to ensure that the measurement system and the way the results are presented do not distort any differences between the products. The simplest case is that of comparing two static systems. Firstly the experimental procedure has to be designed and standardised to minimise errors by controlling position and by taking multiple readings to ensure that the sensors are directly positioned under the points of interest [19–21, 23, 24, 26, 34]. In addition, falsely high readings due to creases in the sensors etc. must be avoided. Once the data have been collected the majority of researchers have used the maximum interface pressure under the area of interest as the parameter to be compared in any statistical analysis [5, 19–24, 35–39], although others have calculated an average pressure over a selected area [40]. It is noticeable that those authors who have used an average pressure find less difference between rival products. Nevertheless, even when maximum values are used, few trials report differences between product performance that are statistically significant at the 5% level.

Two studies have chosen to define other parameters calculated from the data generated by multi-sensor arrays in an attempt to give an overall impression of the relative performance of different support surfaces. Patel calculated a pressure index [41] which was based on threshold levels, whereas Shelton et al. [42] calculated a pressure index based on statistical analysis.

The possibility of presenting the data in different forms is far greater when dynamic systems such as alternating pressure mattresses are being considered, as by their very nature they will exert periods of high pressure followed by periods of low pressure. The most commonly quoted parameters are maximum, minimum and average pressures but these provide little indication as to the length of time that the pressure is at a lower value. This has led a number of researchers [33, 43] to report the amount of time the interface pressure is above or below a certain threshold, most conveniently displayed in histogram form. Although there is still considerable debate over what constitutes a safe interface pressure, there is, to date, no consensus.

Even assuming that a suitable method can be found to analyse and present the data, all the discussion above has considered a subject in a defined posture, which is not representative of real life. In particular, individuals in a wheelchair are constantly changing their position both in the short term, as they propel themselves, and in the longer term in the course of their activities of daily living. Of the few studies to have considered this, Bar [33] produced a pressure/time histogram over a prolonged sitting period and both Dabnichki and Taktak [44] and Kernozek and Lewin [37] considered the variation of interface pressure during the wheelchair push cycle. The former study indicated that the interface pressures were speed dependent and could be increased by as much as 125% compared to the situation at rest [44].

Mannequins

Design of Mannequins

Measurement of interface pressure is subject to great variability. As has been shown above, there are differences among individuals and among anatomical sites, and even when the sensor is kept on a single anatomical site on a given individual, there are differences due to small changes in posture. There are also differences due to clothing, the type of measurement system used and the interpretation of the data, i.e. is the maximum or average pressure quoted or is some form of pressure index calculated? Therefore, in order to reduce this variability when comparing products designed to reduce the incidence of pressure ulcers a number of researchers have proposed using a phantom. Initially simple domed indenters were used [36], but more recently these have evolved into anthropomorphic mannequins with an internal skeleton covered by simulated soft tissues [45, 46] (Fig. 5.4). Such mannequins are the result of extensive research and their development has involved undertaking measurements on many human volunteers in order to determine the characteristics of the materials covering the skeleton.

The European Pressure Ulcer Advisory Panel (EPUAP) [47] recommends the use of mannequins over human volunteers when undertaking comparative testing of products. The pros and cons of humans vs mannequins will be considered in the next section. However, the EPUAP recommendations for mannequins are that they should mimic the important degrees of freedom found in humans but also minimise the potential errors deriving from unplanned movements such as sagging or creep. Essential elements should include:

1. Full-body rather than partial mannequin.
2. Representative of typical height and weight of patients [various conditions: elderly, with spinal cord injuries (SCI) etc.] using such surfaces with weight distributed in correct anthropomorphic proportions, including a spectrum of heights/weights and male/female models.
3. Freely jointed at knees, hips, shoulders and neck, especially to allow use on a profiling bed.
4. Surface of mannequin to represent 3D shape of bony prominences and soft tissue coverage found in the patient group.
5. If different mannequins are developed in different centres then cross-correlation data are essential.
6. It is debatable whether the mannequin needs to be heated to determine the effects on viscoelastic products in particular.
7. The mannequin needs to produce the same ranking of products as that which would be established if a large pool of human subjects were used with a given clinical condition.

The use of mannequins is also recommended in the ISO draft document: "Test methods for determining the pressure relief characteristics of devices

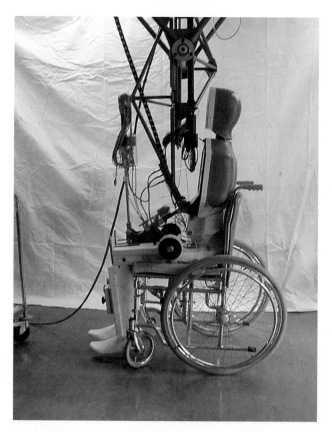

Fig. 5.4. The UCL phantom designed by Bain and Scales (photograph courtesy of Centre for Disability Research and Innovation, University College London, Stanmore)

intended to manage tissue integrity – Seat Cushions" (ISO/CD 16840-5). In this draft document it does state that the tests described are intended to differentiate performance characteristics between cushions and are not appropriate for generalised rankings or scoring cushions or for matching these characteristics with the requirements of individual users.

Mannequins Versus Normal Volunteers

Using mannequins for pressure studies has a number of obvious advantages over using human volunteers, which has led to their recommendation in the EPUAP guidelines [47]. Positioning is much more reliable as the mannequin is attached to a fixed frame and can be lowered accurately onto the support surface and sensors can be permanently attached or even imbedded in the mannequin, removing another source of error. The mannequin can also be incrementally loaded to replicate people of different

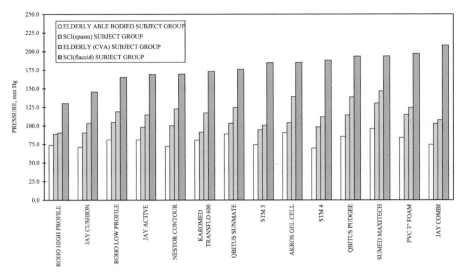

Fig. 5.5. Interface pressure readings obtained on a variety of cushions using different subject groups

weight and hence different BMI and left in position for long periods of time to determine the creep behaviour of the underlying support surface. This level of control of the experimental conditions is therefore bound to reduce errors and hence show more subtle differences between products.

However, the question that does have to be asked when using mannequins is 'Are the readings obtained relevant to the clinical situation?' In the Department of Health Evaluation Report PS4 [23] it was clearly shown that the relative performance of the cushions tested was dependent on the underlying pathology of the different groups. One of the most interesting facts that arose from this work was that irrespective of the type of cushion the interface pressures measured on the four different groups of subjects – elderly, CVA, spastic paraplegics and flaccid paraplegics – were always ranked in the same order, with the elderly volunteers exhibiting the lowest pressures and the flaccid paraplegics the highest. This is demonstrated in Fig. 5.5, in which it can be seen that for the elderly subjects the choice of cushion made comparatively little difference. By contrast, in the flaccid paraplegic group there was much greater variation and therefore the choice of the cushion made far more difference to the interface pressure. In addition, it can be seen that the ranking of the products is different among the groups. In the elderly group there is little difference between the interface pressures measured on the STM4 cushions and those on the High Profile Roho. However when considering the flaccid SCI group it can be seen that the STM4 gives significantly higher pressure readings than the Roho, and in fact is only ranked as the 10th best cushion. The same is true of other cushions. The Jay Combi is ranked as the 6th best cushion for elderly volunteers, 8th for the SCI spasm group, 14th for the SCI flaccid group and 4th for the CVA group. In contrast, the Low Profile Roho is ranked 8th for the elderly group, 11th for the SCI spasm group, 3rd for the SCI flaccid group and 4th for the CVA group. What this clearly demonstrated is that there is considerable difference among groups and that any ranking based on readings obtained in one group cannot be transferred to another. Therefore a wide variety of different mannequins will be required.

Perhaps one of the advantages of undertaking measurements on human volunteers is that there is this inherent variability. As a result a number of subjects have to be measured and statistical methods used in order to calculate mean values which, due to the large standard deviation, makes it difficult to separate different products. Conversely, the smaller standard deviation obtained with mannequin readings will make it much easier to differentiate between products, but only in terms of the readings obtained on the mannequin, which might not be true when applied to actual people. Therefore, it is the author's opinion that for the time being, until a variety of mannequins of different body types, weights, heights and disease states are available which have been shown to be representative of significant numbers of human volunteers, results obtained using mannequins should be viewed critically and not used in isolation to choose equipment for a given patient.

Conclusions

Measuring interface pressure is difficult. As a result there is bound to be considerable debate within the scientific community as to the best way to proceed. These debates will include whether to use mannequins or human volunteers, which type of sensor array is best for clinical or research applications and how the measured interface pressure relates to interstitial pressures and in turn to the formation of pressure ulcers. There are obviously no simple answers but anyone undertaking such measurements must be aware of the limitations of present techniques: only by rigorous experimental technique will they be able to make meaningful contributions to the literature.

Acknowledgements. I would like to thank all of the members of the Department of Health who have contributed to this work over the past 10 years, in particular Ellis Peters, Bill Cox Martin, Diane Norman and Wendy Wareham.

References

1. Guttmann L (1976) The prevention and treatment of pressure sores. In: Kenedi RM, Cowden JM, Scales JT (eds) Bedsore biomechanics. Macmillan, London, pp 153–159
2. Reswick JB, Rogers JE (1976) Experience at Rancho Los Amigos Hospital with devices and techniques to prevent pressure sores. In: Kenedi RM, Cowden JM, Scales JT (eds) Bedsore biomechanics. Macmillan, London, pp 301–310

3. Husain T (1953) An experimental study of some pressure effects on tissues, with reference to the bed sore problem. J Path Bact 66:347–358

4. Kosiak M (1961) Etiology of decubitus ulcers. Arch Phys Med Rehab 42:19–29

5. Meijer JH, Germs PH, Schneider H (1994) Susceptibility to decubitus ulcer formation. Arch Phys Med Rehab 75:318–323

6. Landis E (1931) Micro-injection studies of capillary blood pressure in human skin. Heart 15:209–228

7. Kosiak M (1961) Etiology of decubitus ulcers. Arch Phys Med Rehab 42:19–29

8. Kosiak M, Kubicek WG, Olsen M, Danz JN, Kottke JF (1958) Evaluation of pressure as a factor in the production of ischial ulcers. Arch Phys Med Rehab 39:623–629

9. Ferguson-Pell MW, Bell F, Evans JH (1976) Interface pressure sensors; existing devices, their suitability and limitations. In: Kenedi RM, Cowden JM, Scales JT (eds) Bedsore biomechanics. Macmillan, London, pp 189–197

10. Allen V, Ryan DW, Murray A (1993) Repeatability of subject/bed interface pressure measurements. J Biomed Eng 15:329–332

11. Allen V, Ryan DW, Lomax N, Murray A (1993) Accuracy of interface pressure measurement systems. J Biomed Eng 15:344–348

12. Ferguson-Pell M, Cardi MD (1993) Prototype development and comparative evaluation of wheelchair pressure mapping systems. Assistive Technol 5(2):78–91

13. Gyi DE, Porter JM, Robertson NKB (1998) Seat pressure measurement technologies: considerations for their evaluation. Appl Ergonomics 27:85–91

14. Bader DL, Hawken MB (1986) Pressure distribution under the ischium of the normal subject. J Biomed Eng 8:353–357

15. Norman D, Dunford C, Swain ID (1995) Assessment of support surfaces – Mistral Mattress and Bodipillo Overlay. J Tissue Viab 5:115–117

16. Diesing P, Hochman D, Boenick U (2002) Numerical accuracy of pressure mapping systems – a comparative evaluation. 6th EPUAP Meeting, Budapest, Hungary, 2002. European Pressure Ulcer Advisory Panel, Churchill Hospital, Oxford, England

17. Swain ID, Bader DL (2002) The measurement of interface pressure and its role in soft tissue breakdown. J Tissue Viab 4:132–146

18. Kernozek TW, Wilder PA, Amundson A, Hummer J (2002) The effect of body mass index on peak seat-interface pressure in institutionalized elderly. Arch Phys Med Rehab 83:868–871

19. Swain ID, Stacey PO, Dunford CE, Nichols R (1993) Evaluation, PS1 Foam mattresses. Medical Devices Directorate, Department of Health

20. Swain ID, Stacey PO, Dunford CE, Nichols R (1994) Evaluation, PS2 Static overlays. Medical Devices Agency, Department of Health

21. Swain ID, Stacey PO, Dunford CE, Nichols R (1995) Evaluation, PS3 Alternating pressure overlays. Medical Devices Agency, Department of Health

22. Swain ID, Peters E (1997) The effects of posture body mass index and wheelchair adjustment on interface pressures. Evaluation Report MDA/97/20, Medical Devices Agency, Department of Health

23. Peters E, Swain ID (1997) Evaluation of wheelchair cushions, static and dynamic. PS4, Medical Devices Agency, Department of Health

24. Peters E, Swain ID (1998) Evaluation of pressure relieving ward chairs. PS5, Medical Devices Agency, Department of Health

25. Koo TKK, Mak AFT, Lee YL (1996) Posture effects on seating interface biomechanics; comparison between two seating cushions. Arch Phys Med Rehab, 77:40–47

26. Hobson DA (1992) Comparative effects of posture on pressure and shear at the body seat interface. J Rehab Res Devel 29:21–311
27. Brienza DM, Karg PE (1998) Seat cushion optimisation: a comparison of interface pressure and tissue stiffness characteristics for spinal cord injured and elderly patients. Arch Phys Med Rehab 79:388–394
28. Le KM, Madsen BL, Barth PW, Ksander GA, Angell JB, Vistnes LM (1984) An in-depth look at pressure sores using monolithic silicon pressure sensors. Plast Reconstr Surg 74:745–756
29. Reddy NP, Palmieri V, Cochran GV (1981) Subcutaneous interstitial fluid pressure during external loading. Am J Physiol 240:R327–329
30. Dodd KT, Gross DR (1991) Three dimensional tissue deformation in subcutaneous tissue overlying bony prominences may help to explain external load transfer to the interstitium. J Biomech 24:11–19
31. Brienza DM, Karg PE, Geyer MJ, Kelsey S, Trefler E (2001) The relationship between pressure ulcer incidence and buttock cushion interface pressure in at-risk elderly wheelchair users. Arch Phys Med Rehab 82:529–533
32. Sangeorzan BJ, Harrington RM, Wyss CR, Czerniecki JM, Matsen FA (1989) Circulatory and mechanical response of skin to loading. J Ortop Res 7:425–431
33. Dover H, Pickard W, Swain I, Grundy D (1992) The effectiveness of a pressure clinic in preventing pressure sores. Paraplegia 30:267–272
34. Bar CA (1988) The response of tissue to applied pressure. PhD thesis, University of Wales
35. Swain ID, Nash RSW, Robertson JC (1992) Objective assessment of the Nimbus and Pegasus airwave mattresses. J Tissue Viab 2:43–45
36. Rondolf-Klym LM, Langamo D (1993) Relationship between body weight, body position, support surface and tissue interface pressure at the sacrum. Decubitus 6:22–30
37. Bain DS (1998) Testing the effectiveness of Patient Support Systems: the importance of indenter geometry. J Tissue Viab 8:15–17
38. Kernozek TW, Lewin JE (1998) Seat interface pressure of individuals with paraplegia: influence of dynamic wheelchair locomotion compared with static seated measurements. Arch Phys Med Rehab 79:313–316
39. Brienza DM, Karg PE, Brubaker CE (1996) Seat cushion design for elderly wheelchair users based on minimization of soft tissue deformation using stiffness and pressure measurements. IEEE Trans Biomed Eng 4:320–327
40. Kernozek TW, Breyen P, Piccanatto B (1996) Influence of hip and ankle position on the seat pressure distribution disabled elderly. Phys Ther 76:S22
41. Patel UH, Jones JT, Babbs CF, Bourland, JD, Graber GP (1993) The evaluation of five specialist support surfaces by use of a pressure sensitive mat. Decubitus 6:28–37
42. Shelton F, Barnett R, Meyer E (1998) Full-length interface pressure testing as a method for performance evaluation of clinical support surfaces. Appl Ergonomics 29:491–497
43. Rithalia SVS, Gonsalkorale M (1998) Assessment of alternating air mattresses using a time based interface pressure threshold technique. J Rehab Res 35:225–230
44. Dabnichki P, Taktak D (1998) Pressure variation under the ischial tuberosity during a push cycle. Med Eng Phys 20:242–256
45. Barnett RI, Shelton FE (1997) Measurement of support surface efficiency. Adv Wound Care 10:21–29

46. Bain DS, Scales, JT, Nicholson GP (1999) A new method of assessing the mechanical properties of patient support systems (PPS) using a phantom. A preliminary report. Med Eng Phys 21:293–301
47. Support Surfaces Working Group (2002) Draft guidelines for the laboratory evaluation of pressure distributing support surfaces. European Pressure Sore Advisory Panel Review 4(1)

Susceptibility of Spinal Cord-Injured Individuals to Pressure Ulcers

6

Kath Bogie, Dan Bader

Introduction

The development of pressure ulcers due to tissue breakdown and cell necrosis is one of the most significant secondary complications of spinal cord injury (SCI). There are many factors that lead to the occurrence of tissue breakdown. Similarly, SCI affects multiple systems of the body, primarily below the level of the lesion but also with systemic effect. The most readily obvious change in an individual with SCI is altered motor function, particularly that which affects limb movement. In addition, sensory dysfunction can alter proprioception and reaction to environmental stimuli such as pain and temperature. Over time, the body will change, as muscle bulk is lost due to disuse muscle atrophy, leading to a higher proportion of fatty tissue and poor vascularity. Other systems affected include cardiovascular, respiratory, bowel and bladder function, and digestion. The extent of systemic involvement and functional ability directly affects the individuals' susceptibility to development of pressure ulcers.

In order to clinically describe individuals with SCI, the American Spinal Injuries Association (ASIA) has developed a standardized method for determining the neurological status of a patient and for classifying SCI. The ASIA impairment score has two components: neurological level of injury and neurological impairment. The first component describes the motor and sensory level of injury. The second describes the functional ability (Table 6.1). The ASIA impairment score is widely accepted as a clinical measure and as such it can be used as a broad indicator of a sub-population's risk for pressure ulcer development. The neurological level and extent of impairment are often very different from the anatomical level of injury, and the ASIA score provides a more reliable indicator of risk status than level of injury.

Just as the ASIA impairment score contains more than one component, so the development of pressure ulcers is a multi-factorial process. These factors can be classified as extrinsic factors primarily related to the interface between the individual and external environment and intrinsic factors related to the clinical and physiological profile of the individual. Changes in clinical status following injury will alter intrinsic factors that increase the risk of tissue breakdown leading to pressure ulcer development. For example, urinary incontinence will alter the micro-environment of the skin surface and make it more susceptible to maceration and breakdown.

Table 6.1. ASIA Impairment Score

ASIA grade	Neurological function		Neurological impairment
	Motor injury	Sensory injury	
A	Complete	Complete	No motor or sensory function in the sacral segments S4–S5
B	Complete	Incomplete	No motor function below the level of injury. Sensory function may be normal or impaired but is present.
C	Incomplete	Incomplete	Some motor function is preserved below the level of injury but more than half the key muscles show significant weakness
D	Incomplete	Incomplete	Motor function is preserved below the level of injury and less than half the key muscles show significant weakness
E	None	None	Normal motor and sensory function

Changes in environmental factors, such as the seating system used, will alter external factors that affect pressure ulcer risk status, as summarized in Table 6.2.

The interactions between risk factors and clinical status provide guidelines for susceptibility to pressure ulcer development both generally, e.g. for patient sub-groups such those with complete quadriplegia (ASIA grade A), and specifically for individuals.

Intrinsic risk factors in pressure ulcer development arise as a direct consequence of the SCI. Motor paralysis below the level of a spinal cord lesion reduces muscular activity and leads to loss of muscle bulk, thus reducing soft tissue coverage over the bony prominences of the pelvic region. The proportion of avascular fatty tissue increases, leading to decreased regional vascularity. Loss of normal muscle tone leads to abnormal responses to environmental stimuli, such as applied pressure, thus increasing the risk of blood flow becoming compromised. Furthermore, individuals with higher levels of SCI are likely to experience dysfunctional central control of circulation, which can lead to autonomic dysreflexia.

Table 6.2. Factors in pressure ulcer development

Factor	Classification	Cause
Disuse muscle atrophy	Intrinsic	Motor paralysis
Reduced vascularity and blood flow	Intrinsic	Motor paralysis
Impaired/absent sensation	Intrinsic	Sensory paralysis
Reduced mobility (including loss)	Intrinsic	Motor paralysis
Poor nutritional status	Intrinsic	Poor diet
Applied pressure	Extrinsic	External loading of soft tissues
Shear at the support interface	Extrinsic	Poor posture and/or poor support materials
Adverse micro-environment at support interface	Extrinsic	Numerous, including raised temperature, sweating, incontinence, infection

Motor paralysis will also directly affect a person's ability to respond unconsciously to potential noxious stimuli, e.g. fidgeting while sitting or turning while asleep. Reduced mobility also profoundly alters the individual's ability to consciously perform postural manoeuvres necessary to relieve prolonged applied pressure, from weight-shifting while sitting to walking. The loss or reduction of mobility is further compromised by sensory paralysis, leading to the absence or alteration of normal perception of environmental stimuli such as pain or temperature. Individuals with complete sensory paralysis can no longer sense where their limbs are without visual cues, i.e. they experience a loss of proprioception. These changes affect the risk of pressure ulcer development because the individual cannot sense the warning signals that prompt action to prevent tissue damage.

Thus it can be seen that many of the primary factors that increase the susceptibility of individuals with SCI to pressure ulcer development are the inter-related intrinsic changes in body characteristics and functional abilities which occur following SCI. To a large extent, these changes have been considered to be immutable. Nutritional status can be altered by adequate diet, but a complete SCI remains an irreversible lesion that does not exhibit spontaneous recovery. There is much research currently in progress to develop clinical treatments to cure SCI. This remains exploratory, and thus the current clinically applicable techniques to prevent pressure ulcers largely address extrinsic factors that can be changed, such as applied pressure and the micro-environment of the user/support interface. These approaches to pressure ulcer prevention can be classified as education focused or device focused. Educational prevention techniques include programmes that address patient and/or carer education. Device-oriented methods focus on the provision of appropriate equipment for postural support and pressure relief, such as mattresses and wheelchair seating cushions. These approaches to pressure ulcer prevention are complementary and should be reviewed periodically throughout the lifetime of the individual with SCI.

Variation in Pressure Ulcer Risk Factors Following SCI

The clinical profile of an individual with an SCI will vary both among individuals, due to different levels of lesion, and for one person over time. The individual with an SCI will undergo the ageing process with chronic motor and/or sensory dysfunction. Moreover, it has been shown that an SCI can increase the effective rate of ageing [1, 2]. As more people live longer with SCI, research has been carried out to determine the longer-term risk status for clinical complications. With specific regard to the risk of pressure ulcer development, the individual with SCI remains at increased risk at all times post injury; however, the relative risk status and the most critical risk factors will vary over the course of time. The first stage at which pressure ulcer risk is heightened is in the acute SCI phase, immediately following injury.

Risk Factors During SCI

Following traumatic injury to the spinal cord there is an immediate decrease or loss of reflex activity below the level of the lesion. This condition is known as 'spinal shock' and although it is transient, there is considerable variation in the period required for the restoration of this activity, ranging from a few days to several months. Reflex return may be particularly delayed in patients with severe but incomplete SCI [3]. In addition, there is frequently concurrent trauma to multiple systems, which must be addressed with urgency if the patient is to survive the initial insult. Thus, the treatment received in the period immediately following a traumatic SCI is critical both to initially stabilize the patient and to ensure an optimal prognosis once the acute phase is past. It is important that skin care is rigorously monitored, for the development of pressure ulcers during the immediate post-injury phase will severely impede subsequent rehabilitation.

Patients who sustain an SCI should be admitted as soon as possible to a specialized spinal injuries unit, because secondary complications will start very rapidly following SCI. Even among specialized units, the standards of care for acute SCI vary from conservative treatment to rapid spinal stabilization and remobilization. The original protocol pioneered by Guttmann takes a very conservative approach [4]. The patient is immobilized for up to 12 weeks, to allow the traumatic fracture to stabilize, before gradually commencing a rehabilitation programme. Tissue health status should continue to be monitored to avoid development of pressure ulcers. In addition to prolonging the acute phase of the hospital admission, the early develop-

Table 6.3. Demographics of acute SCI study population

Gender	Age	Level of injury	Extent of injury
Male: 73%	16–32 years	Above T6: 33%	Complete: 40%
Female: 27%	Mean: 22 years	Below T6: 67%	Incomplete: 60%

ment of pressure ulcers can negatively affect the individual's psychological adjustment to life with an SCI. The pressure-relieving characteristics of the user support surfaces, at this stage specifically the mattress and any other support pillows, should therefore be evaluated together with the positioning of the individual in the bed.

Conservative management of acute SCI, such as employed at the National Spinal Injuries Centre, Stoke Mandeville NIH Trust, is for the patient to be immobilized until the fracture is stable, as seen on radiographic assessment of the site. The patient is positioned in a supine position with the spine in alignment and lies on a foam mattress with pillows placed under the head, buttocks and ankles to relieve pressure on the high-risk pressure points of the occiput, sacrum and heels. A turning regime is employed where the patient is turned from side to side using a turning bed at 2- to 4-h intervals, with the spine maintained in alignment at all times.

A study was carried out to evaluate the efficacy of this clinical treatment protocol for maintenance of tissue health. Interface pressures and transcutaneous oxygen levels were measured at the sacrum of subjects who had sustained a traumatic SCI [5]. Fifteen individuals were admitted to the study within 9 weeks of injury. The clinical demographics of the study population are summarized in Table 6.3.

Transcutaneous oxygen levels were measured using a Radiometer TCM3 blood gas monitor (Copenhagen, Denmark). The sensor electrode was placed over the sacrum along the midline. Concurrently, interface pressures were measured on either side of the tissue gas electrode using an Oxford Pressure Monitoring system (Talley Medical, Romsey, Hants, UK). Measurements were made for a period of 25±5 min at intervals of 1–2 weeks until the subject began to remobilize in a wheelchair.

It was found that median interface pressures at the sacral region were around 30 mmHg. This implies that the practice of "gapping" patients on pillows to relieve pressures over the bony prominences is often ineffective because an adequate gap is not achieved. The simplest approach to remedy this situation is to employ clinical guidelines that indicate the minimum gap necessary around a bony region. This would generally be around 10 cm, but this may not always be feasible if there is significant spinal instability, and in such cases it would be more effective to use an active pressure relief mattress, such as a Clinitron bed, (Hill-Rom, Ashby de la Zouch, Leicestershire).

No significant relationship between transcutaneous oxygen level and time post injury was found, indicating that the risk of tissue breakdown did not alter during the period of acute immobilization for this subject group. This implies that rapid remobilization and reduced frequency of turning when in bed may be inappropriate for many individuals with acute SCI due to the prolonged effects of spinal shock. As the proportion of cases of incomplete spinal cord trauma increases and acute bed rest continues to become briefer, this has significant implications for the clinical care of acute SCI patients.

Risk Factors During Initial Rehabilitation

The initial rehabilitation (sub-acute) phase for an individual with SCI can vary in both time post injury (from a few weeks to several months), depending on the course of the acute phase, and duration (also from a few weeks to several months). The goal of initial rehabilitation post SCI is to equip the individual with the skills and equipment necessary for them to maximize their potential abilities so that they can become reintegrated in society. This goal requires much hard work by the affected individual, his or her caregivers and the whole clinical team. It is of primary importance that during initial rehabilitation every patient and carer is thoroughly educated in the aetiology of pressure ulcers and their prophylaxis. Critical skills to be learned include the ability to carry out a pressure relief regime, both through postural changes where possible and through the provision of appropriate equipment, e.g. cushions, wheelchairs, mattresses. The need for routine skin inspection and care must also be emphasized, with particular regard to pressure areas such as the ischia, sacrum and greater trochanters.

The selection of a wheelchair seating system for the person who has recently sustained an SCI must involve consideration of many diverse criteria. In some ways it is the most important part of rehabilitation. The right combination of wheelchair and support cushion will allow the user to maximize their functional potential and interact fully with their environment. In addition, it will take full account of the user's requirements with regard to particular needs and appearance. Conversely, an inappropriate seating system can lead to poor posture, reduced functional abilities and isolate the user from their environment. All these factors can, in turn, exacerbate the risk of pressure ulcer development in the rehabilitating individual.

Thus the seating requirements of each patient must be thoroughly assessed at this time so that appropriate seating and other support surfaces can be recommended. The prescription of wheelchair seating systems must be based on a comprehensive assessment of user function (actual and potential) and seated posture. The clinical profile should be considered but of greater relevance are the actual individual characteristics at the seating/support interface for a specific user.

A study was carried out to determine changes in transcutaneous oxygen response to applied pressure during the initial rehabilitation of SCI subjects [6]. All study participants had suffered traumatic SCI less than 1 year previously and were assessed while sitting on their prescribed support cushions. The initial guidelines for cushion prescription were for all patients to receive a 4-in. foam cushion, except those with complete quadriplegia who more frequently received a Sumed gel cushion. Subjects with a history of pressure ulcer development during the acute phase were prescribed a Jay Medical or Jay Active foam/gel cushion. Subjects were classified according to their level of injury as paraplegic (below T6) or quadriplegic (above T6). Transcutaneous oxygen levels were measured over the bony prominence of the ischial tuberosity using a Radiometer TCM3 blood gas monitor. Initial assessment was made once the patient was sitting up for more than 4 h a day and was repeated at intervals of 2–4 weeks until discharge. The sensors were attached with the subject in a side-lying position with hips and knees flexed to approximate their relative posture in sitting. After a 10-min equilibration period the subject was carefully transferred to the sitting posture on their support cushion. Tissue status was then monitored for a continuous period of 25±5 min with appropriate pressure relief as required.

Tissue oxygen levels under applied load tended to improve during initial rehabilitation for quadriplegic subjects and to deteriorate for those with paraplegia. These counter-intuitive findings support the reports of others, such as Noble [7], that quadriplegics develop pressure ulcers less frequently than paraplegics, particularly than those with flaccid paraplegia. This may be because the spasticity experienced by individuals with higher level lesions means that loss of muscle bulk is slightly less than in those with no tone, i.e. with flaccid paralysis. The higher activity levels of paraplegic individuals may also be a factor since they may be more likely to neglect regular pressure relief manoeuvres due to their other activities.

Risk Factors for the Chronic SCI Population

Following initial rehabilitation, the SCI patient must maintain a high level of skin care at all times in order to prevent the occurrence of pressure ulcers. However, this economically and psychologically costly secondary complication remains one of the most common reasons for re-admission to hospital [7]. The patient with a major pressure ulcer requires an average of 180 days nursing time [8]. Allman et al. [9] found that development of a nosocomial pressure ulcer was associated with significant and substantial increases in both hospital costs and length of stay in a group of patients admitted to hospital with reduced mobility due to a primary diagnosis of hip fracture. Xakellis and Frantz [10] found that the cost of treating pressure ulcers was greatly increased when a patient required hospitalization. These studies did not focus on individuals with SCI, but it can reasonably be predicted that the outcomes would be poorer for those individuals with greater initial impairment. The most recent comprehensive figures available indicate that the cost to the health service in the UK is in excess of £ 250 million per annum in 1990 [11]. In the USA, the cost of treating pressure ulcers was estimated to be in excess of $ 1.33 billion per annum in 1994 [12]. When adjusted for inflation, this implies that current costs are around £ 416 million per annum in the UK and around $ 1.89 billion per annum in the USA.

Thus it can be seen that the prevention of pressure ulcers is a highly cost-effective goal. Pragmatically, it is also important to have clear treatment guidelines for the efficacious clinical management of pressure ulcers when they do develop. Both the European Pressure Ulcer Advisory Panel (EPUAP) and the National Pressure Ulcer Advisory Panel (NPUAP) have issued clinical guidelines for the prevention and treatment of pressure ulcers [13, 14, 15]. It is recommended that conservative treatment options, such as topical dressings, be employed whenever possible for the individual with chronic SCI who develops a pressure ulcer. In most cases early identification of a Grade I or II pressure ulcer with superficial breakdown involving only the dermal layers can be treated successfully by complete bed rest with total pressure relief over the affected area combined with appropriate dressings, as the healing period is relatively short. There are many types of topical dressings and antibiotics that can be employed to promote wound healing [12]. The common goal is to produce a moist wound environment that will promote cell proliferation.

In some cases, tissue breakdown is so extensive that conservative treatment alone is not appropriate. Grade III or IV pressure ulcers involve total breakdown of the dermal and epidermal layers, sometimes extending to the underlying muscle, that requires a prolonged period of bedrest to heal. This cannot be considered acceptable. The presence of necrotic tissue (eschar) will impede wound healing and such tissue may be removed by surgical intervention, specifically sharp debridement. Excision of sloughy tissue and cleansing of the ulcer to stop infection should permit the development of granulating tissue.

Split skin grafts may be employed to promote healing in the early stages for pressure ulcers with limited muscular involvement. However if the pressure ulcer exhibits areas of deep tissue breakdown, e.g. extending to the bone with surrounding undermining and fibrotic margins (Grade IV and some Grade III ulcers), more radical surgical treatment is required. The overall goal of surgical procedures is to excise and close the ulcer. A number of tissue-flap procedures have been developed to achieve wound coverage. Myocutaneous flaps and island fasciocutaneous flaps are most widely used [16, 17], with fasciocutaneous flaps also being found to be successful on some non-healing pressure ulcers [18].

The principal procedure employed at the National Spinal Injuries Centre is simple excision of the ulcer and bony prominence followed by direct closure. The ulcer is excised in toto with the bony prominence underneath. The wound is then closed in layers with a primary skin closure. A retrospective review of surgical patients with pressure ulcers treated at the National Spinal Injuries Centre by excision and closure was carried out. All patients admitted during a twelve year period (1980–1992) and treated by the same surgeon (IN) were studied and evaluated. A total of 400 operational procedures involving 218 patients were performed. There was a 2.25% incidence of multiple ulcers, leading to an overall total of 409 ulcers repaired surgically over the twelve year period.

The retrospective review of surgical cases showed that some patients experienced more than one surgical procedure during the period. It was important to differentiate between possible causes of repeated tissue breakdown and therefore two classes of repeated procedure were defined. Revision of a pressure ulcer was defined as a repeated surgical procedure at the same site within 1 year of the original procedure. This was considered to indicate that the original wound had failed to heal adequately. In contrast, recurrence of tissue breakdown was defined as a surgical procedure at the same site between 1 and 5 years after the original procedure.

During the 12-year review period 73 patients (33.5%) were treated on two or more occasions. In 37 of these cases this was due to bilateral and/or multiple ulcers being repaired by a series of surgical procedures. Surgical revision was found to have been required in 24 cases (6.0%). Recurrence of tissue breakdown was found to have occurred in 15 cases. One patient had two episodes of tissue breakdown at the same site 3 and 6 years after initial surgery. One other patient had recurrent breakdown over bilateral trochanteric regions after a 4.5-year interval. Thus a total of 18 ulcers (4.5%) recurred during the 12-year review period.

The relative prevalence of the 409 pressure ulcers treated by surgical excision and closure is summarized in Table 6.4, together with revision and recurrence rates. When these cases were classified according to the site of the initial pressure ulcer, revision rates appeared to be higher for the sacrum and greater trochanter than for the ischium. The reverse situation was seen with recurrence rates. Ischial ulcers were twice as likely to exhibit repeated breakdown requiring surgical repair as those occurring at the sacrum or greater trochanter.

Twenty-one (9.6%) patients had two or more episodes of tissue breakdown at different sites separated by periods greater than 1 year, e.g. initial breakdown of the ischial region with a second breakdown of the sacral region 4 years later. However, it was noted that 10 of these patients also had a history of concurrent multiple pressure ulcers at some time during the

Table 6.4. Revision and recurrence rates classified by pressure ulcer site

Pressure ulcer site	Revisions	Recurrences
Sacrum	7 (7.0%)	3 (3.0%)
Ischium	9 (5.5%)	10 (6.1%)
Greater trochanter	8 (6.6%)	4 (3.3%)

review period. Seven patients had a history of recurrent ischial ulcers where the left or right side was specified for all ulcers. In these cases, recurrent breakdown was contralateral in four patients and on the same side in two patients. One patient exhibited recurrent ischial breakdown both contralaterally and ipsilaterally. This finding implies that prophylactic ischiectomies may be effective at preventing recurrent breakdown over the same ischial tuberosity but they may increase the risk of contralateral breakdown due to postural asymmetry.

In this review we were able to assess the operational procedures by one surgeon over a 12-year period from 1980 to 1992, thus providing longer-term follow-up information. The recurrence rate of 5.3% for all ulcers represents an overall success rate of 94.7%, with 5 years' follow-up, for sacral, ischial and trochanteric ulcers closed by direct excision and closure. This compares favourably to other surgical techniques for the repair of pressure ulcers.

A prospective study was carried out to evaluate any changes in transcutaneous gas levels pre-operatively and to determine whether tissue health status is altered in unloaded and loaded soft tissues post-operatively. Transcutaneous gas levels were monitored in subjects who underwent surgical excision and closure of pressure ulcers during the period June 1989 to December 1990. Ethical approval for this study was obtained from the Aylesbury Vale Authority Research Ethical Committee. Twenty-one subjects were included in this study on meeting the selection criteria, i.e. normal haemoglobin levels pre-operatively, absence of systemic degenerative conditions and provision of informed consent. Three cases in this group had bilateral ulcers, leading to a total of 24 ulcers. The clinical demographics of this study population are shown in Table 6.5.

Tissue health was assessed pre-operatively once the area of tissue breakdown was free of slough and necrotic tissue. The sensor electrode of the Radiometer TCM3 blood gas monitor was located 20–50 mm from the margin of the wound over superficially healthy skin. Transcutaneous gas levels were monitored for a period of 25±5 min in order to determine a stable unloaded tissue response.

The pressure ulcer was then repaired by total excision of the necrotic tissue, ulcer and underlying bony prominence followed by primary closure. An elliptical incision was made around the ulcer, followed by excision of the

Table 6.5. Clinical demographics of surgical study population: summary of subject profiles

Gender	Age	Level of injury	Duration of injury	Location of ulcer(s)
Male: 76%	16–80 yrs	Above T6: 33%	Acute: 14%	Ischium = 58%
Female: 24%	Mean: 42 years	Below T6: 67%	Chronic: 86%	Sacrum = 13% Trochanters = 29%

whole ulcer, making sure that the pseudo-epithelial lining of the ulcer was excised in toto. The underlying bony prominence was exposed and excised. In ulcers with undermined cavities, the boundaries of the cavity are easily identified by packing it with ribbon gauze and thus changing it into a pseudotumour. Dissection was then carried out to remove the whole lining.

Table 6.6. Clinical demographics of surgical study population: individual subject profiles

No.	Gender	Age	Level	Duration[a]	Location of ulcers	Previous surgical repair
1	M	50	A	Chronic	R ischium	N
2	M	27	B	Chronic	L ischium	N
3	M	42	B	Chronic	Sacrum	N
4	F	80	A	Chronic	L ischium	Y
5	M	59	A	Chronic	R ischium	Y
6	M	43	A	Acute	Sacrum	N
7	M	19	A	Chronic	L posterior trochanter	N
8	F	71	B	Chronic	L ischium	N
9	M	57	B	Chronic	R ischium	N
10	M	37	A	Chronic	B. posterior trochanters	N
11	M	19	B	Chronic	L ischium	Y[b, c]
12	F	36	B	Chronic	L ischium	N
13	F	22	B	Chronic	Bilateral ischia	–[c]
14	F	22	B	Chronic	R ischium and perineum	–[c]
15	M	16	B	Acute	Bilateral trochanters	N
16	M	38	B	Chronic	L posterior trochanter	N
17	M	19	B	Acute	Sacrum	N
18	M	50	B	Chronic	R ischium	N
19	M	72	A	Chronic	L trochanter	N
20	M	43	B	Chronic	L ischium	Y[b]
21	M	58	B	Chronic	L ischium	N

[a] Acute, less than 2 years post-injury; Chronic, more than 2 years post-injury.
[b] Previously repaired by rotation flap.
[c] Full surgical history not available.

The wound was then closed in as many layers as possible. This makes closure of the ulcer achievable without undue tension. A suction drain was always left for a few days in order to drain the deep area.

The sutures were usually removed in two stages at 10 and 11 days post-operatively. Twenty-four hours following removal of all sutures, transcutaneous gas levels in unloaded tissues were again assessed. The monitoring site was 20–50 mm medial to the mid-point of the suture line.

A further assessment of tissue response under load was carried out following remobilization in the wheelchair for 19 subjects. Transcutaneous gas levels were monitored at the same site as for the post-operative assessment. Regional interface pressures at the subject support interface were monitored simultaneously using the Oxford Pressure Monitoring system. The sensors were located using the same experimental protocol followed for the study of initially rehabilitating SCI subjects (see above). Sensors were attached over the region of the surgical repair with the subject in a side-lying position with hips and knees flexed to approximate their relative posture in sitting. The tissue gas electrode was located 20–50 mm medial to the mid-point of the suture line and the pressure sensors were placed either side. After a 10-min equilibration period the subject was carefully transferred to the sitting posture on their standard support cushion. Tissue status was then monitored for a continuous period of 25 ± 5 min with the appropriate pressure relief as required.

The distribution of pressure ulcer locations found in the long-term review was reflected in the study of transcutaneous gas levels in surgical subjects, with ischial ulcers representing 58% of cases.

The unloaded transcutaneous oxygen pressure ($TcPO_2$) in normal healthy subjects is considered to be in the region of 80 mmHg [19]. The risk of tissue necrosis increases as the blood supply becomes inadequate and $TcPO_2$ falls. Unloaded $TcPCO_2$ is around 35 mmHg. If tissue health becomes compromised due to inadequate blood supply, $TcPCO_2$ will start to increase due to the accumulation of noxious by-products from tissue respiration. Pre-operatively, $TcPO_2$ was generally found to be in excess of 30 mmHg, and $TcPCO_2$ levels were abnormally high in a number of cases. Thus soft tissues surrounding regions of necrotic tissue may have slightly compromised tissue gas levels due to a reduced clearance of tissue waste, even though they may appear visually normal. Post-operatively $TcPO_2$ levels in unloaded tissues were generally observed to be in excess of 30 mmHg and $TcPCO_2$ was within the normal range for an increased number of subjects. Thus transcutaneous gas levels in unloaded tissue surrounding a repaired wound were similar to those found in other healthy soft tissues. This may be due to the operation itself stimulating blood flow, or it may simply be that regional blood flow improves as a result of the removal of necrotic tissue.

Future Developments in Pressure Ulcer Research:
Decrease in the Susceptibility of the Individual with SCI

Despite the development of many support devices and the application of many training programs the incidence of pressure ulcers remains unacceptably high, particularly in the SCI population. Furthermore, there remain a significant number of individuals with SCI who exhibit chronic recurrence of tissue breakdown despite the use of high-performance support cushions.

Device-orientated prevention techniques continue to be developed and refined. Active pressure-relief mattresses often incorporate temperature sensors to control the micro-environment, and this type of technology is now starting to be applied in wheelchair cushions. In addition, 'smart' cushions have been developed that monitor the duration of applied pressure, i.e. static sitting time, and issue an alarm when the user should perform a pressure-relief manoeuvre.

Advanced technologies and new pharmacological approaches are being explored that can affect the intrinsic clinical status of the individual with a SCI. The long-term application of implanted electrical stimulation devices offers a unique means to alter the intrinsic characteristics of paralysed muscle, leading to sustained improvements in regional tissue health. These changes can reduce the risk of pressure ulcer development by increasing regional blood flow and improving interface pressure distribution [20]. In addition, electrical stimulation can be applied to dynamically alter conditions at the seating support interface through stimulated muscular contractions, thus facilitating periodic changes in interface pressure.

The use of anabolic steroids has also been investigated for both the treatment and prevention of pressure ulcers in the SCI population. Any individuals with chronic 'non-healing' pressure ulcers exhibit concurrent malnutrition and weight loss. The anabolic steroid, oxandrolone, has been found to be effective on pilot studies of wound treatment. A significant majority of individuals exhibited healing of pressure ulcers after treatment for up to 6 months [21, 22]. Demling and De Santi found that optimizing nutrition alone was ineffective. However, when this was supplemented with oxandrolone therapy there was an increase in weight gain by around 1.8 kg/week (4 lb/week), which was significantly correlated with wound closure. Weight gain due to oxandrolone is primarily lean body mass, i.e. muscle tissue. No side effects have been noted with oxandrolone and this approach may therefore be applicable for pressure ulcer prevention in malnourished individuals at high risk for pressure ulcer development. Further study is necessary to determine the safety and efficacy of oxandrolone for long-term therapy.

In addition to altering the intrinsic susceptibility of individuals with SCI the incidence of pressure ulcers may be decreased by more effective delivery of care. Current clinical management is predominantly based on the ethos that pressure ulcers are avoidable given adequate preventative care, and the fact that they continue to occur at high rates is seen to imply that the patient is to some degree negligent. However, the validity of the underlying assumptions of this care model warrants further investigation.

Adequate preventative care implies that individuals at risk of pressure ulcer development are receiving both appropriate education and appropriate equipment. A recent survey of the prevalence of pressure ulcers in 5,000 hospitalized patients throughout Europe, carried out by the EPUAP, indicates that the first criterion is frequently not met [23]. The survey included all hospital inpatients, and it could be argued that individuals with SCI are not typical and will receive adequate prophylactic care. On the other hand, it can be seen from the studies presented in this paper that clinical expertise and standard treatment guidelines are not in themselves sufficient. They should be considered the starting point for effective prevention of pressure ulcers, rather than the end point.

The majority of specialized SCI rehabilitation units will provide educational programs for in-patients with acute SCI or when people are re-admitted for continuing care. However, the fact that an individual requires inpatient hospital care for treatment of a complication such as a pressure ulcer generally implies a failure in the educational process, since the problem has not been managed at an early stage. The incongruity is illustrated by the findings of a recent survey by Walter et al. [24], who found that 38% of participants reported having current problems with a pressure ulcer but only 21% of these individuals wanted to discuss their problem with a therapist. A satisfaction rate of around 80% among this group would appear somewhat unexpected.

Various approaches to improving educational awareness have been proposed. Some are based on refining the existing models of care through the development of more accurate scales for predicting pressure ulcers [25]. Others seek to modify the model through the incorporation of new technology and increased patient involvement with their care.

Initial studies have shown that the use of telehealth interventions may improve the tracking and management of pressure ulcers [26]. It was found that video monitoring combined with access to a telephone helpline will increase the number of reported pressure ulcers. However, the majority of this increased incidence is due to the reporting of Grade I and II pressure ulcers that are rarely reported in standard care models. Thus, the telehealth intervention produced an increased rate of health care utilization but this was generally to deal with less severe complications and could therefore be more cost effective. It was also found that people who employed telehealth were more likely to return to work. This has led to the hypothesis that telehealth may promote self-efficacy among users with SCI. Future work is required to investigate the role of telehealth on both physiological and psychological variables affecting the risk of SCI individuals for pressure ulcer development.

Changing the medical model to include the patient in his or her own care is another component in the future development of approaches to decreasing susceptibility to pressure ulcer development. Contingency management is a behavioural methodology that has been widely used in the treatment of substance abuse. The general protocol is reinforcement of positive patterns of behaviour through a reward system, such as financial compensation or vouchers, with the overall objective of the individual internalizing the behaviour patterns so that they no longer need the rewards in order to carry them out. Contingency management procedures have been designed for patients with high rates of non-compliance in skin care [27]; however, there is some controversy over the use of monetary rewards [28]. Further work is necessary to determine the long-term efficacy of this approach to behavioural modification.

Even as the incidence of and prognosis for SCI changes with improved prevention and the possibility for a cure, so the susceptibility to pressure ulcer development in the current SCI population is changing with new developments in many fields. Behavioural techniques and technological developments can alter the risk status of individuals by changing environmental factors. Implanted technologies and pharmacological agents have the potential to alter clinical risk factors, in particular by reversal of disuse muscle atrophy. The development of these multi-factorial preventative approaches expands the possibilities for reducing the future incidence of pressure ulcers in the spinal cord-injured population.

References

1. Charlifue SW, Weitzenkamp DA, Whiteneck GG (1999) Longitudinal outcomes in spinal cord injury: aging, secondary conditions, and well-being. Arch Phys Med Rehabil 80(11):1429–1434
2. Thompson L (1999) Functional changes in persons aging with spinal cord injury. Assist Technol 11(2):123–129
3. Little JW, Ditunno JF, Stiens SA, Harris RM (1999) Incomplete spinal cord injury: neuronal mechanisms of motor recovery and hyperreflexia. Arch Phys Med Rehabil 80:587–599
4. Guttmann L, Cope Z (eds) (1953) The treatment and rehabilitation of patients with injuries of the spinal cord. Her Majesty's Stationery Office, London
5. Bogie KM, Nuseibeh I, Bader DL (1992) Transcutaneous gas tensions in the sacrum during the acute phase of spinal cord injury. Proc Instn Mech Engrs 206:1–6
6. Bogie KM, Nuseibeh I., Bader DL (1995) Early progressive changes in the seated spinal cord injured subject. Paraplegia 33:141–147
7. Noble PC (1981) The prevention of pressure sores in persons with spinal cord injuries. In: Monograph 11, International Exchange of Information in Rehabilitation. Rehabilitation Fund Inc., New York
8. Hibbs P (1990) The economics of pressure sore prevention. In: Bader DL (ed) Pressure sores – clinical practice and scientific approach. Macmillan Press, London, pp 35–42
9. Allman RM, Goode PS, Burst N, Bartolucci AA, Thomas DR (1999) Pressure ulcers, hospital complications, and disease severity: impact on hospital costs and length of stay. Adv Wound Care 12(1):22–30
10. Xakellis GC, Frantz R (1996) The cost of healing pressure ulcers across multiple health care settings. Adv Wound Care 9(6):18–22
11. Cochrane G (1990) The severely disabled. In: Bader DL (ed) Pressure sores – clinical practice and scientific approach. Macmillan Press, London, pp 81–96

12. Bergstrom N, Bennett MA, Carlson CE, et al. (1994) Treatment of pressure ulcers. Clinical practice guideline No. 15. US Department of Health and Human Services, Agency for Health Care Policy and Research. Rockville MD. AHCPR publication No. 95-0652

13. European Pressure Ulcer Advisory Panel (1998) Guidelines on prevention of pressure ulcers. Br J Nurs 7:888–889

14. European Pressure Ulcer Advisory Panel (1999) Guidelines on treatment of pressure ulcers. EPUAP review 1:31–33

15. Garber SL et al. (2000) Consortium for Spinal Cord Medicine, Pressure ulcer prevention and treatment following spinal cord injury: a clinical practice guideline for health-care professionals. Paralyzed Veterans of America, NPUAP 2000 clinical guidelines

16. Lee HB, Kim S, Lew D, Shin K (1997) Unilateral multilayered musculocutaneous flap for the treatment of pressure ulcer. Plast Reconstr Surg 100(5):340–345

17. Erocan AR, Apaydin I, Emiroglu M et al. (1998) Island VY tensor fascia lata fasciocutaneous flap coverage of trochanteric pressure ulcers. Plast Reconstr Surg 102(5):1524-1531

18. Yamamoto Y, Tsutsmida A, Murazumi M, Sugihara T (1997) Long-term outcomes of pressure ulcers treated with flap coverage Plast Reconstr Surg 100(5):1212–1217

19. Bennett L, Kavner D, Lee BY, Trainor FS, Lewis JM (1984) Skin stress and blood flow in sitting paraplegic patients. Arch Phys Med Rehab 65:186–190

20. Bogie KM, Reger SI, Levine SP (2000) Therapeutic applications of electrical stimulation: wound healing and pressure sore prevention. Assistive Technol 12(1):50–66

21. Spungen AM, Koehler KM, Modeste-Duncan R, Rasul M, Cytryn AS, Bauman WA (2001) Nine clinical cases of nonhealing pressure ulcers in patients with spinal cord injury treated with an anabolic agent: a therapeutic trial. Adv Skin Wound Care 14(3):139–144

22. Demling R, De Santi L (1998) Closure of the "non-healing wound" corresponds with correction of weight loss using the anabolic agent oxandrolone. Ostomy Wound Manage 44(10):58–62, 64, 66 passim

23. European Pressure Ulcer Advisory Panel (2001) The prevalence of pressure ulcers in European hospitals [online publication]. EPUAP Review 3, 2001: available online at: http://www.epuap.org/review3_3/index.html

24. Walter JS, Sacks J, Othman R, Rankin AZ, Nemchausky B, Chintam R, Wheeler JS (2002) A database of self-reported secondary medical problems among VA spinal cord injury patients: its role in clinical care and management. J Rehabil Res Dev 39(1):53–61

25. Salzberg CA, Byrne DW, Cayten CG, Kabir R, van Niewerburgh P, Viehbeck M, Long H, Jones EC (1998) Predicting and preventing pressure ulcers in adults with paralysis. Adv Wound Care 11(5):237–246

26. Phillips VL, Temkin A, Vesmarovich S, Burns R, Idleman L (1999) Using telehealth interventions to prevent pressure ulcers in newly injured spinal cord injury patients post-discharge. Results from a pilot study. Int J Technol Assess Health Care 15(4):749–755

27. Mathewson C, Adkins VK, Jones ML (2000) Initial experiences with telerehabilitation and contingency management programs for the prevention and management of pressure ulceration in patients with spinal cord injuries. J Wound Ostomy Continence Nurs 27(5):269–277

28. Adkins VK, Mathewson C, Ayllon T, Jones M (1999) The ethics of using contingency management to reduce pressure ulcers: data from an exploratory study. Ostomy Wound Manage 45(3):56–58, 60–61

Prevention and Treatment of Pressure Ulcers Using Electrical Stimulation

7

Thomas Janssen, Christof Smit, Maria Hopman

Introduction

Skin-related secondary disabilities, especially pressure ulcers, are a common problem for wheelchair users such as individuals with spinal cord injury (SCI), resulting in great discomfort and significant medical care costs. Pressure ulcers typically arise in areas of the body where prolonged pressure and shear forces are being exerted on soft tissue over bony prominences, such as the sacrum and the ischial tuberosities, inhibiting blood and oxygen supply and ultimately causing tissue ischaemia and necrosis. Individuals with SCI are at increased risk for pressure ulcers due to factors such as reduced mobility, reduced microcirculation, impaired sympathetic function, atrophy of the paralysed muscles, and a disturbed muscle pump function (also see Chap. 6). In addition, due to impaired sensation, individuals are often not aware of the necessity to relieve pressure. Although it has been shown that special cushioning systems can provide an improved redistribution of pressure, as has been reviewed in Chaps. 5 and 6, pressure ulcers still are prevalent in the SCI population. The predisposition of SCI patients with flaccid paralysis to ulcer development has been outlined in Chap. 5. It is theoretically possible that electrical stimulation (ES) and ES-induced exercise can help to reduce the risk of pressure ulcers, since they have been shown to increase muscle mass, capillary density and skin and muscle blood flow (BF). The first purpose of this chapter, therefore, is to discuss how ES can contribute to reduction of pressure ulcer risk and pressure ulcer incidence. The second purpose is to evaluate how ES can be helpful in pressure ulcer healing once preventative measures have failed.

Electrical Stimulation

Technique

It is beyond the scope of this chapter to give a complete overview of ES techniques, application principles, precautions and contra-indications. In this chapter we will review briefly the general techniques of ES to induce muscle contractions and increase BF. For a more comprehensive review of

ES methodology, the reader is referred to, for example, Robinson and Snyder-Mackler [1].

The basic technique to induce muscle contractions for exercise via ES involves the use of an electrical stimulator providing impulses to skin surface electrodes placed over the muscle to simulate action potentials that would normally arise from the central nervous system. These impulses evoke action potentials in the motor neurons entering the muscle. The action potentials subsequently activate the neuromuscular junctions to release acetylcholine, evoking action potentials in all of the muscle fibres of the motor units (i.e. motor neurons and the skeletal muscle fibres they innervate), and thereby inducing muscle contractions. Thus, it is desirable to place electrodes directly over motor points, i.e. where the motor nerve enters the muscle, to obtain optimal muscle performance at relatively low ES current. Impulses are typically delivered at a frequency of 30–50 Hz to induce smooth, tetanic contractions. Contraction strength can be varied by adjusting the ES current intensity, since this directly relates (within limits) to the number of motor units activated. During a period of exercise, the muscle fibres undergo progressive fatigue and their force output decreases. To compensate for fatigue, ES current intensity must be progressively increased during the exercise period to recruit fresh, non-fatigued muscle fibres. This protocol is automatically accomplished in advanced ES systems via performance feedback circuitry. However, once the maximal current output intensity of the stimulator is reached, muscle performance will markedly decrease and become insufficient to maintain required levels of exercise. The rate of fatigue for ES-induced contractions is most likely higher than for voluntary contractions due to the non-physiological activation technique, histochemical changes in the weakened paralysed muscle fibres and reduced circulation of blood [2].

ES Modes

The two most commonly used ES-induced exercise modes in individuals with SCI are resistance exercise and endurance exercise. Research has demonstrated that the same resistance-training principles known to be effective for strengthening and inducing hypertrophy of the muscles of able-bodied individuals with voluntary exercise can be applied to ES-induced exercise of paralysed muscles. These principles include isometric contractions, as well as dynamic concentric and eccentric contractions through a safe range of joint motion, progressive "overload", several sets of exercise consisting of a relatively low number of repetitions at relatively high load resistance, and two to five sessions of exercise per week [3–6]. Most research on ES resistance exercise has been directed towards the paralysed quadriceps muscles due to their responsiveness to ES, proportional increase in force output with increasing ES current and relative ease of exercise implementation. However, it is probable that this ES technique can be adapted to provide resistance exercise for other paralysed/weakened muscles. For endurance exercise, a leg cycle ergometer (LCE) was developed in 1982 which is

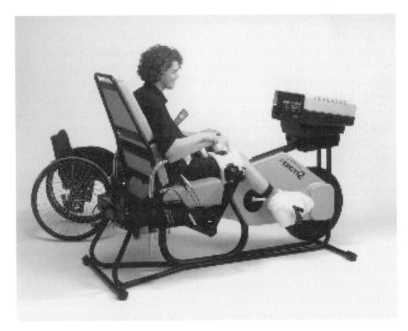

Fig. 7.1. Illustration of an individual with SCI on a commercially available leg cycle ergometer that uses electrical stimulation of paralysed muscles

pedalled via ES-induced contractions of the paralysed lower-limb muscle groups [7]. Computer-controlled ES is used to induce contractions of the paralysed quadriceps, hamstring and gluteal muscle groups during an appropriate range of pedal angles to maintain smooth cycling. When pedalling at a 50 rpm target rate, a total of 300 muscle contractions per minute are induced. To control the cyclic ES pattern and current intensity, a microprocessor that receives pedal position and velocity feedback information from sensors is incorporated. As muscle fatigue progresses during an exercise period, ES current intensity automatically increases to a maximum of about 140 mA to recruit non-fatigued muscle fibres. When maximal current is reached and additional muscle fibre recruitment is no longer possible, the pedalling rate declines and ultimately falls below 35 rpm, at which time exercise is automatically terminated. Figure 7.1 illustrates operation of a commercially available ES-LCE by an individual with SCI.

ES Characteristics for Tissue Repair

For tissue repair and enhancement of skin BF lower current levels are generally needed than for inducing muscle contractions. The total energy delivered to the affected tissue and electromagnetic changes in the wound environment depends on the current density, which is in turn determined by the electric current intensity and the electrode size, shape, and placement.

Smaller electrodes concentrate the current, while large electrodes disperse the electric charge. When electrodes are placed further apart a deeper electric current will penetrate body tissues. Monophasic pulsed current (MPC) has been shown to be superior to constant direct current (DC). In some applications of MPC the cathode is placed initially in the wound area followed by a reversal to positive polarity (anode) after several days of treatment. In some applications the reversal is done periodically throughout the healing period. Three stimulation modalities are distinguishable: low-voltage direct current (LVDC), high-voltage pulsed direct current (HVPDC) and low-voltage alternating current (LVAC) (Table 7.1).

There is considerable variability in the electrical parameters both among and within the three basic modalities. Applied currents are direct, alternating, continuous or pulsed (with different pulse frequencies), and waveforms are continuous, peaked (saw tooth), sinusoidal, square or triangular. In addition, there is at least a 1,000-fold difference in the range of magnitudes in the reported induced currents. Voltages vary; electrode placement and polarities are sometimes exchanged mid-treatment. Table 7.2 shows common stimulation characteristics for various electrical stimulation applications for tissue repair. Despite these striking differences, most of the diverse electrical adjuvant treatments are reported to be beneficial [8–10].

Table 7.1. Comparison of electric treatment modalities (from Scheffet et al. [8])

Electrical	Treatment modalities		
	LVDC	HVPDC	LVAC
Voltage magnitude available	low (< 8 V)	high (6–200 V)	low (< 10 V)
Current type	DC	DC	AC
Average current intensity	20–999 μA	0.3–2.5 mA	15–25 mA
Waveform	Monophasic rectangular	Monophasic with sharp high peaks	Unbalanced biphasic/peaks
Pulse duration	100 μs	45–100 μs	250 μs
Pulse frequency (per second)	< 60	80–130	40–85
Treatment regimen (hours/day)	2–4	0.75–1	2
Electrode proximity placement	In wound	In wound	Edge of wound
Electrode reversal	Yes	Yes	No

Table 7.2. Common stimulation characteristics for various electrical stimulation applications for tissue repair (From Cullum et al. [9])

Application	Type of stimulation	Phase dura-tion current	Amplitude	Treatment duration
Oedema control	1. Pulsed or burst mode AC	>100 contraction	Rhythmic muscle	– [a]
	2. High voltage, pulsed, negative polarity	2–50 threshold	90% of motor	30 min/4 h
Improvement of vascular status	1. Pulsed or burst mode AC	2	Sensory level	– [a]
	2. Pulsed or burst	>100	>10% MVC	10 min
Wound healing	1. DC	NA	<1 mA	1–2 h b.i.d.
	2. Pulsed	2–150	< Motor threshold	45 min

[a] Undetermined

ES-Induced Exercise and Pressure Ulcer Risk

Muscle Size

One of the factors that may contribute to the development of pressure ulcers in SCI individuals is muscular atrophy, which is particularly severe in the muscles below the lesion level. Counteracting this atrophy could be a way to reduce pressure ulcer incidence. In SCI, voluntary muscle contractions that would prevent muscle atrophy are not possible below the lesion, but contractions in the paralysed muscles can often be induced using ES, potentially counteracting muscle atrophy. Indeed, several training studies incorporating progressive ES-induced resistance exercise techniques have shown that atrophy of the paralysed muscles can be partially reversed [4, 5, 11–13]. Using computer tomography (CT), Pacy et al. [14] indicated that the mid-thigh muscle area of four men with SCI was increased by 27% after 10 weeks of ES knee extension (KE) exercise, an increase which coincided with a significantly higher quadriceps muscle protein synthesis rate. Moreover, Taylor et al. [15] showed that quadriceps muscle size returned to normal levels in individuals with SCI following ES training consisting of KE exercise.

Similarly, ES-LCE training in individuals with SCI has been shown to elicit hypertrophy of the muscles employed as indicated by increased thigh circumference [5, 7, 16–20]. Moreover, the degree of muscle hypertrophy is most likely greater than indicated by circumference measurements since it has been shown that local adipose tissue (included in girth measurements) can be substantially reduced by ES-induced KE exercise [14, 21] and ES-LCE exercise [14]. Mohr et al. [22] showed that after 1 year of ES-LCE exercise, thigh circumference had increased by 4%, while the cross sectional area of the thigh muscles, as measured by MRI, had increased by 12%. Studies using the more sophisticated CT technique have confirmed significant increases in quadriceps area [13, 14, 18, 23, 24]. For example, Sloan et al. [23] found an increase of 4.5 cm^2 (+9.4%) in quadriceps area in nine subjects with SCI following a relatively short period of 3 months of ES-LCE training.

Even though most research has focused on the thigh area, limited data are also available on a more relevant area for pressure ulcer prevention in those with SCI, i.e. the gluteal region. Rischbieth et al. [25] showed increased circumferential dimensions across the buttocks of a man with tetraplegia by up to 21% after 24 months of regular ES-induced leg cycling, indicating a marked increase in gluteal muscle mass. Similarly, Hjeltnes et al. [26], using CT, revealed that only 2 months of ES-LCE training in individuals with long-standing SCI resulted in significant increases in cross-sectional areas of the quadriceps (+38%), hamstrings (+17%), and gluteus maximus (+27%). An important study was performed by Baldi et al. [27], who used dual-energy X-ray absorptiometry (DEXA) to find that ES-LCE exercise during the first 6 months post injury could prevent the gluteal muscle atrophy that was seen in a non-exercising control group (Fig. 7.2). This control group lost an average of 27% of gluteal lean mass during this period, whereas the ES-LCE group showed an increase of 5–10%. Although a third group that underwent unloaded ES-induced contractions of the gluteal muscles showed less atrophy than the control group, atrophy still occurred (5–10%), suggesting that dynamic loaded contractions may be necessary to fully prevent muscle atrophy after an SCI.

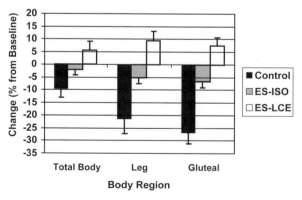

Fig. 7.2. Changes in lean body mass of the total body, legs, and gluteal area after 6 months of ES-induced isometric exercise of the gluteal muscles (*ES-ISO*) or ES-induced leg cycling (*ES-LCE*) in patients shortly after the SCI. (Results from Baldi et al. [27])

Thus, ES-induced resistance and cycling exercise appears to have a marked effect on reversing the disuse atrophy of paralysed muscles, or retard the rate of its progression. When started early after injury, ES-LCE could even be helpful in preventing muscle atrophy.

Peripheral Circulation

In inactive tissue, circulation is generally reduced. In particular in those individuals who are confined to a bed or wheelchair, muscle activity is chronically reduced, resulting in structural changes to the vascular bed supplying the muscles. BF to tissue is governed by perfusion pressure and vascular resistance. Since mean arterial pressure and venous pressure are normally maintained within narrow limits, BF control is largely accomplished by variation in vascular resistance. Vascular resistance is essentially under dual control: (1) systemic through the autonomic nervous system and humoral factors, and (2) locally by the conditions in the immediate vicinity of the blood vessels. Leg vascular resistance is dramatically enhanced in individuals with SCI. This may be caused by structural factors, such as a decrease in number of arterioles and capillaries and/or a decrease in the diameter of the resistance vessels, as well as by functional changes, involving endothelium-derived factors and/or sympathetic vascular regulation. Hopman et al. [28] showed a markedly lower femoral artery BF in SCI individuals than in an able-bodied group, which coincided with a significantly smaller femoral artery diameter. The resulting poor peripheral circulation could be a contributing factor to the development of pressure ulcers.

Acute Adaptations. A way to counteract these problems is to increase muscle activity, which would augment BF and, if performed for a longer period, reverse the vascular atrophy. Exercise bouts performed voluntarily have been shown to increase BF to the active muscles at the onset of exercise, adapting to a steady value appropriate for the metabolic demand [29, 30]. However, voluntary exercise is not always possible, such as in individuals with paralysis, patients who are unconscious, or many bedridden patients. ES could be helpful in this respect to induce the needed exercise. Several studies have indeed shown that this induced exercise, in parallel to voluntary exercise, can increase BF to the stimulated muscles [31–34]. Originally developed as an alternative prophylactic technique for deep vein thrombosis, Glaser et al. [35] demonstrated that rhythmic patterns of ES-induced isometric contractions (e.g., 1.5–2.5 s on-off duty cycle) of calf and thigh muscles could activate the skeletal muscle pump to significantly increase circulation, as indicated by stroke volume and cardiac output increases (+12–30%) in able-bodied persons and those with SCI during rest in a sitting position. Several subsequent studies indeed confirmed that this rhythmic ES technique can enhance peripheral and central circulatory responses, which may not only reduce pressure ulcer risk, but can also alleviate venous pooling and excessive oedema in the legs, as well as orthostatic hypotension [36–38]. A recent study by Janssen and Hopman [39] showed that not only ES-induced tetanic but also twitch contractions could be used to augment BF in the femoral artery of supine individuals. Also, during ES-induced knee extension exercise, marked increases in muscle BF, measured by Doppler ultrasound and positron emission tomography, of able-bodied individuals and individuals with SCI have been noted [40, 41].

Even though most research has focused on BF in the femoral artery, indicative of thigh muscle BF, limited data indicate that ES can also augment BF in the gluteal area. Using a radioactive tracer method, Levine et al. [32] measured BF under the ischial tuberosities of seated able-bodied individuals and individuals with SCI during ES of the gluteal muscles. All subjects showed an augmented BF during ES-induced contractions, which led the authors to conclude that ES can help prevent pressure ulcers.

While ES-induced activity appears necessary for augmenting muscle BF, skin BF and concomitant oxygen tension levels may also be increased by lower-intensity ES that does not induce muscle contractions. For example, a study by Kaada [42] revealed that low-intensity transcutaneous electrical nerve stimulation (TENS) induced prolonged skin vasodilation. Also, in individuals with SCI, improved perfusion as a result of high-voltage pulsed galvanic ES applied to the back at spinal level T6 coincided with a 35% higher sacral transcutaneous oxygen tension [43]. Hence, both muscle and skin BF can be augmented by using various types of ES.

Chronic Adaptations. From the above, it is clear that ES and ES-induced exercise can elicit acute increases in skin and muscle BF. What about adaptations when this induced exercise is performed chronically? Indeed, ES-induced exercise training has been shown to markedly increase resting BF in the femoral artery of individuals with SCI [15, 44, 45]. For example, Taylor et al. [15] showed that thigh BF, which was approximately 65% of normal levels before the training period, returned to normal levels in a group of patients with SCI who participated in a training programme for the Odstock functional ES standing system. In addition, a study by Hopman et al. (2002) revealed that the increased leg vascular resistance found in patients with SCI was reversible towards normal values by training the paralysed legs using ES of the muscle. Also, Kainz et al. [46] showed that after an 8-month period during which the quadriceps muscle of 16 patients with chronic SCI, including 7 patients with denervated muscles, was stimulated daily using surface electrodes, muscle BF had increased by circa 80%. This improved muscle BF, as measured with radioactive thallium-201, was probably due to concomitantly improved muscle work and muscle size, as indicated by an increased cross sectional area of the muscle (CT) and muscle fibres (biopsy), and an increase in aerobic muscle enzymes by a factor of 5–8. Also, skin BF (measured by xenon-133 clearance) at the start of the training period, increased by approximately 75% as a result of the stimulation. Moreover, all 16 patients showed a reduction in the oedema of the lower extremities, indeed suggesting an improved peripheral circulation. It is important to notice is that only activated muscles demonstrated an augmented BF, indicating that it is essential to stimulate those areas that are at risk of developing pressure ulcers.

Moreover, a case report by Twist [47] indicated that several weeks of ES-KE and ES-LCE exercise was effective for reducing acrocyanosis, discolouration, swelling, toe ulceration, and discomfort in one individual with tetraplegia. Pedal and popliteal pulses appeared strengthened, which suggested that venous, arterial, and lymphatic circulation had all improved.

Hence, skin and muscle BF appear chronically augmented after ES-induced exercise training. From animal studies it is known that a chronically increased BF stimulates cells of the endothelium to induce structural vascular changes, resulting in increased vessel diameters [48], and the same could be expected after ES-induced exercise in humans. Indeed, a recent study by Gerrits et al. [44] showed that the diameter of the femoral artery had increased by 8% after only 6 weeks of ES-LCE training in men with chronic SCI. In addition, a study by Chilibeck et al. [49] revealed that the capillary-to-fibre ratio in the vastus lateralis muscle of individuals with SCI yielded a 39% increase, from 0.75 ± 0.14 to 1.04 ± 0.20, after 8 weeks of ES-LCE training. In contrast, daily ES without loading the muscle seems to be insufficient to improve the vascular bed [50, 51].

Seating Pressure

Since prolonged mechanical loading at the skin as well as the muscle level appear to be important factors in the aetiology of pressure ulcers, reducing this loading may be critical in preventing pressure ulcers. In wheelchair users, reductions in seating pressure can be realised by regular weight-relief lifts actively performed by the user. However, not all users are capable of performing these lifts, or performing them on a regular basis, thereby increasing the risk of prolonged mechanical loading. An interesting technique that may be helpful in this respect was proposed by Ferguson et al. [52], who applied ES to the quadriceps muscles of nine seated individuals with SCI while their lower legs were restrained. Results indicated that the average ischial pressure was reduced by 44 and 27 mmHg for the right and left buttocks, respectively, which contributed to the authors' conclusion that this mode of ES could be a useful prophylactic aid in pressure ulcer management.

A different approach to induce changes in seating pressure that may be beneficial in pressure ulcer prevention was proposed by Levine et al. [53], who applied ES to induce isometric contractions of the gluteal muscles of seated wheelchair users with SCI. It was concluded that ES produced marked changes in the shapes of the buttock tissue, which may assist in preventing pressure ulcers over the seating surface. The additional advantage of the latter technique is that circulation and muscle size changes may also occur in this high-risk area.

Pressure Ulcer Incidence

From the above sections, it is clear that ES and ES-induced exercise can have positive effects on factors reducing the risk of pressure ulcer development: muscle atrophy can be (partially) reversed, skin and muscle BF can be augmented, and seating pressures can be reduced. Hence, it may be predicted that regular ES-induced exercise can reduce pressure ulcer incidence. In fact, many individuals indicate that they suffer less from pressure ulcers while participating in an ES exercise program. Although not confirmed by controlled experimental studies, Petrofsky [54] reported that the incidence of pressure ulcers was reduced by 90% in a group of over 100 individuals with SCI participating in a 2-year ES exercise program, consisting of ES-induced resistance, endurance or standing exercise. However, the lack of controlled studies, mainly due to the difficulty of including sufficient subjects in these cumbersome investigations, presents a serious problem. Thus a definite statement can still not be made on whether ES-induced exercise can actually prevent pressure ulcers.

Treatment of Pressure Ulcers by ES

Pressure Ulcer Treatment

Several scientific, clinical and economic studies have proven that the incidence and prevalence of pressure ulcers are sufficiently high to warrant concern, even when presumably adequate preventive measures have been taken [55–59]. Conventional treatment of pressure ulcers incorporates three main strategies: (1) local treatment of the wound using dressings and other topical applications; (2) pressure relief using beds, mattresses or cushions, or by repositioning the patient; and (3) treating concurrent conditions that may delay healing (e.g. poor nutrition, infection).

However, the conventional treatment of pressure ulcers is almost always problematic. These wounds heal very slowly or not at all, and thus treatment usually takes months. It is often very physically and mentally stressful for patients who are hospitalised, bedridden, or wheelchair bound to decrease pressure on the damaged and surrounding areas. In addition, this treatment is very expensive, with estimated annual treatment costs in the USA of billions of dollars [8, 60].

For these reasons, considerable research has been directed at improving the conventional treatment, the importance of which has been highlighted by government services, (para-)medical practitioners and patient groups [10, 58, 61]. Alternative and adjuvant therapies such as ES, ultrasound, magnetic fields, topical hyperbaric oxygen and laser therapies have all been studied for clinical and cost effectiveness. For most of these therapies there is only limited scientific evidence available, and conclusions about their contribution to wound healing should be drawn cautiously. None of these therapies has yet been proven to be the best option, and therefore there is currently no standard in clinical practice of wound treatment.

From previous sections it could be argued that some effects of ES, such as improved circulation, might also contribute to accelerated wound healing. However, most studies on clinical effectiveness of ES in wound healing have to deal with methodological problems and as a consequence they vary considerably in scientific quality. Nevertheless, all studies show results suggesting only positive effects of ES on wound healing, as will be described in the following sections.

Potential Wound Healing Mechanisms

In general, the rationale for using ES is based on the fact that the human body has an endogenous bioelectric system that enhances healing of bone fractures and soft-tissue wounds. When the body's endogenous bioelectric system fails and cannot contribute to wound repair processes, a chronic pressure ulcer will fail to heal. Therapeutic levels of electrical current may then be delivered into the wound tissue from an external source [60].

Neutrophils, macrophages, fibroblasts and epidermal cells involved in wound repair carry either a positive or a negative charge. When these cells are needed, ES facilitates galvano-taxic attraction of these cells into wound tissue and thereby accelerates healing (Figs. 7.3 and 7.4) [10, 60]. Several studies have shown that apart from attracting neutrophils and macrophages, ES has also a stimulatory effect on cells, resulting in more receptor sites for growth factors, stimulation of growth of fibroblasts and granulation tissue, and prevention of post-ischaemic oxygen radical-mediated damage [60, 62, 63]. Furthermore, Weiss et al. [64] and Sheffet et al. [8] found that the number of mast cells in healing human wounds decreased following exposure to ES, indicating that these cells, which are associated with conditions of abnormal fibrotic healing, are inhibited from migrating into the area.

On an organic level, ES increases BF and reduces oedema, as the major colloidal protein in blood, albumin, is negatively charged and is repelled by negative polarity, causing a shift in tissue fluids. Thereby it has been a clinical observation that negative polarity facilitates debridement of necrotic wound tissue, stimulates neurite growth, and induces epidermal cell migration [65]. ES also inhibits bacteria from growing and from migrating into the wound [66, 67]. As these effects are contributory to accelerated wound healing, it seems likely that ES has a clinical additional positive effect. Various experiments have been performed to assess the effects of ES on the clinical repair processes of skin.

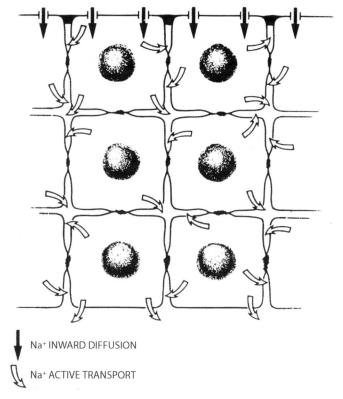

↓ Na⁺ INWARD DIFFUSION

↳ Na⁺ ACTIVE TRANSPORT

Fig. 7.3. Sodium ions enter the outer (*top*) cells of the epithelium via specific channels in the outer membrane, migrating along a steep electrochemical gradient. Once in the cell, they can diffuse to other cells of the epithelium via the gap junctions that join the cells of the epithelium, and they can be actively transported from all of these cells via electrogenic "pumps" that are present in all of the plasma membranes of the epithelium except the outer membrane that has the Na+ channels. This results in a transport of Na+ from the water bathing the epithelium to the internal body fluids of the animal, and the generation of a potential of the order of 50 mV across the epithelium. Tight junctions between cells at the outer edge of the epithelium minimise the escape of the positive charge transported inwards and therefore minimise the collapse of the potential generated by the epithelium's electrogenic Na+ transport [75]

Effects of ES Treatment on Wound Healing

Animal Studies. Many controlled studies of soft tissue healing using animal models have indicated that ES applied as either LVDC or HVPDC is effective [68–70]. An oft-cited study by Assimacopoulos et al. [69], for example, used several rabbit models, and one of the conclusions drawn was that 100 μA applied in continuous negative current shortened wound healing time by 25%. In addition, Young [71] reported that application of HVPDC following a 12-h period of tourniquet-induced ischaemia prevented the gangrene observed in the legs of untreated dogs. Animal models may not

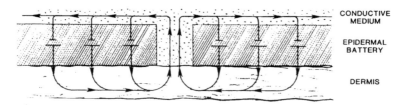

CONDUCTIVE
MEDIUM

EPIDERMAL
BATTERY

DERMIS

Fig. 7.4. When a wound is made in an epithelium, the potential across the epithelium drives a current (considered to be a flow of positive charge) through the subepidermal region and out of the wound. This current returns to the battery via some conductive path outside the epithelium. In amphibians and, possibly, mammalian cornea and oral epithelium, and skin that is kept moist by an occlusive dressing, this is simply the fluid bathing the epithelium. In mammalian skin, this conductive path normally is between the living and dead layer of the epidermis [75]

be directly applicable to wound healing problems of humans. In the majority of animal experiments, the wound was created by a sharp surgical incision and all animals were healthy. In clinical practice, skin problems often occur in patients having vascular or neurological impairment and wounds and pressure ulcers do not resemble surgical incisions.

Clinical Studies and Meta-analysis. Several clinical studies on patients, using high-quality methodology incorporating a meta-analysis, in fact confirm the findings from animal studies. In 1969, Wolcott et al. [72] treated 75 chronically ischaemic skin ulcers in a series of 67 patients suffering from neurological disease. After division of the patients into two groups, the wounds of the patients in the treatment group were subjected to direct current (LVDC, 200–1000 µA) for 6 h per day. The control group received the conventional treatment. Wound volume was determined by measuring length, width and depth. All wounds combined in both groups decreased in volume by an average of 13.4% per week. However, the wounds in the treated group healed at 27% per week, suggesting a markedly improved result following ES treatment.

Similarly, Gault and Gatens [73] treated 106 chronic ischaemic ulcers of 76 elderly patients with neurological disease using LVDC stimulation (200–1000 µA) for 6 h per day. Untreated wounds healed at a rate of 14.7% per week, whereas treated ulcers healed at a rate of 30% per week. More recently, Gentzkow et al. [67] studied 40 non-healing stage III and IV pressure ulcers in 37 patients, ranging in age from 29 to 91 years. They utilised LVDC for 30 min twice daily over a period of 4 weeks. At the end of the treatment period, the treatment group showed an average change of 49.8% in wound-healing area, versus 23.4% in the control group. A separate analysis identified factors that affected healing: individuals who had a metabolic condition (such as diabetes) and females showed improved healing, whereas individuals who had tunnels undermining the wound or a more advanced-stage wound showed less healing.

Subsequently, Wood et al. [74] conducted a larger randomised clinical trial on the efficacy of pulsed LVDC, applied 3 times per week over a few hours for a period of 8 weeks, or until the wound fully healed. Seventy-one older subjects with stage II and III pressure ulcers who had shown no significant improvement in 5 weeks were randomly assigned to the treatment group or to a control group that received conservative wound treatment. Results showed that treatment increased the healing rate significantly: 58% of ulcers in the treatment group healed in 8 weeks, compared with a 3% healing rate in the control group.

Recently, Gardner and co-workers [61] performed an extensive meta-analysis on effects of ES on chronic wound healing. Fifteen studies, including 24 ES samples and 15 control samples, were analysed. The average rate of healing per week and the 95% confidence intervals were calculated. Rate of healing per week was 22% for ES samples, and 9% for control samples. The 95% confidence intervals of ES (18–26%) and control (3.8–14%) samples did not overlap, indicating a significant improvement of ES treatment over control treatments. ES was more effective against pressure ulcers (net effect = 13%), than venous ulcers or other type of wounds. The samples were subsequently grouped by type of ES device and chronic wound and reanalysed. However, findings regarding the relative effectiveness of different types of ES device were inconclusive.

The small scale of most of the randomised clinical trials and different treatment outcome measures precludes comparisons of efficacy between the various electric current treatment modalities. Data pooling also is not feasible because of the diversity in electric current treatment parameters [8]. Several studies, however, suggest that placement of the anode in a direct-current circuit directly over the wound enhances tissue healing. Support for the use of the anode over the wound with direct-current amplitudes below 1 μA for enhancement of wound healing is strong [9, 61].

Conclusion

In conclusion, several studies have shown that ES and ES-induced exercise can have positive effects on factors reducing the risk of pressure ulcer development: muscle atrophy can be partially reversed, skin and muscle BF can be augmented, and seating pressures can be reduced. Therefore, it is plausible that regular ES-induced exercise can reduce pressure ulcer incidence. However, the lack of controlled studies is a serious problem, preventing a definite statement on whether ES-induced exercise can actually prevent the incidence of pressure ulcers.

When prevention has failed, treatment of pressure ulcers is necessary. However, physicians are often not familiar with treatment options such as the use of physical therapies, e.g. ES, ultrasound and laser therapy. ES has long been a largely unknown and poorly understood treatment modality for chronic wound healing [61]. Treatment of pressure ulcers is generally empirical, and seems often based on dogma and rhetoric, rather than on evidence-based results. In protocols of scientific and medical advisory boards, ES is not recommended for treatment in wound healing, largely due to a lack of evidence of its efficacy. The sample size of most current studies was indeed small; the number of methodologically good quality studies is limited, and absence of controls and the different ways of reporting make comparison among studies difficult. Consequently, reflecting the limitations of the evidence-rating system used in the US Agency for Health Care Policy and Research guidelines as discussed in Chap. 4, the authors' review of existing studies to support ES treatment does not result in a high rating.

We wonder what conclusions should be drawn for clinical practice. Is it justified to conclude that based on the limited scientific evidence ES should never be used in clinical practice, or only on a small scale? We believe not. When viewed collectively, the efficacy studies and the 'mechanism of action' studies, of which some are described above, provide a strong indication that ES has a direct positive effect on tissue and is effective for promoting the healing of dermal wounds such as pressure ulcers. ES is also safe and relatively simple to apply. No reported study in the international literature describes adverse effects of ES on the patient or the wound. Finally, the costs of applying ES are low.

We believe that instead of focusing on the limited scientific data available for each specific type of ES device and on unanswered questions regarding, for example, the optimal ES dosage, ES should be used more often in clinical practice for pressure ulcer prevention and for wound treatment. More high-quality studies can follow to ascertain the cost effectiveness of ES.

References

1. Robinson AJ, Snyder-Mackler L (1995) Clinical electrophysiology: electrotherapy and electrophysiologic testing. Williams & Wilkins, Baltimore
2. Glaser RM (1991) Physiology of functional electrical stimulation-induced exercise: basic science perspective. J Neurorehabil 5:49–61
3. Gruner JA, Glaser RM, Feinberg SD, Collins SR, Nussbaum NS (1983) A system for evaluation and exercise-conditioning of paralyzed leg muscles. J Rehab Res Dev 20:21–30
4. Petrofsky JS, Phillips CA (1983) Active physical therapy: a modern approach to rehabilitation therapy. J Neurol Orthop Surg 4:165–173
5. Faghri PD, Glaser RM, Figoni SF, Miles DS, Gupta SC (1989) Feasibility of using two FNS exercise modes for spinal cord injured patients. Clin Kinesiol 43:62–68
6. Ragnarsson KT (1988) Physiologic effects of functional electrical stimulation-induced exercises in spinal cord-injured individuals. Clin Orthop Rel Res 53–63
7. Petrofsky JS, Phillips CA, Heaton HHI, Glaser RM (1984) Bicycle ergometer for paralyzed muscles. J Clin Eng 9:13–19
8. Sheffet A, Cytryn AS, Louria DB (2000) Applying electric and electromagnetic energy as adjuvant treatment for pressure ulcers: a critical review. Ostomy Wound Manage 46:28–33, 36–40, 42–44

9. Cullum N, Nelson EA, Flemming K, Sheldon T (2001) Systematic reviews of wound care management: (5) beds; (6) compression; (7) laser therapy, therapeutic ultrasound, electrotherapy and electromagnetic therapy. Health Technol Assess 5:1–221

10. Lee RC, Canaday DJ, Doong H (1993) A review of the biophysical basis for the clinical application of electric fields in soft-tissue repair. J Burn Care Rehabil 14:319–335

11. Hjeltnes N, Lannem A (1990) Functional neuromuscular stimulation in 4 patients with complete paraplegia. Paraplegia 28:235–243

12. Bajd T, Kralj A, Turk R, Benko H, Sega J (1989) Use of functional electrical stimulation in the rehabilitation of patients with incomplete spinal cord injuries. J Biomed Eng 11:96–102

13. Pacy PJ, Evans RH, Halliday D (1987) Effect of anaerobic and aerobic exercise promoted by computer regulated functional electrical stimulation (FES) on muscle size, strength and histology in paraplegic males. Prost Orthot Int 11:75–79

14. Pacy PJ, Hesp R, Halliday DA, Katz D, Cameron G, Reeve J (1988) Muscle and bone in paraplegic patients, and the effect of functional electrical stimulation. Clin Sci 75:481–487

15. Taylor PN, Ewins DJ, Fox B, Grundy D, Swain ID (1993) Limb blood flow, cardiac output and quadriceps muscle bulk following spinal cord injury and the effect of training for the Odstock functional electrical stimulation standing system. Paraplegia 31:303–310

16. Ragnarsson KT, Pollack S, O'Daniel W, Jr., Edgar R, Petrofsky J, Nash MS (1988) Clinical evaluation of computerized functional electrical stimulation after spinal cord injury: a multicenter pilot study. Arch Phys Med Rehabil 69:672–677

17. Arnold PB, McVey PP, Farrell WJ, Deurloo TM, Grasso AR (1992) Functional electric stimulation: its efficacy and safety in improving pulmonary function and musculoskeletal fitness. Arch Phys Med Rehabil 73:665–668

18. Block JE, Steinbach LS, Friedlander AL, Steiger P, Ellis W, Morris JM et al (1989) Electrically-stimulated muscle hypertrophy in paraplegia: assessment by quantitative CT. J Comput Assist Tomogr 13:852–854

19. Phillips CA, Danopulos D, Kezdi P, Hendershot D (1989) Muscular, respiratory and cardiovascular responses of quadriplegic persons to an F. E. S. bicycle ergometer conditioning program. Int J Rehabil Res 12:147–157

20. Sipski ML, Alexander CJ, Harris M (1993) Long-term use of computerized bicycle ergometry for spinal cord injured subjects. Arch Phys Med Rehabil 74:238–241

21. Rodgers MM, Glaser RM, Figoni SF, Hooker SP, Ezenwa BN, Collins SR et al (1991) Musculoskeletal responses of spinal cord injured individuals to functional neuromuscular stimulation-induced knee extension exercise training. J Rehab Res Dev 28:19–26

22. Mohr T, Andersen JL, Biering-Sorensen F, Galbo H, Bangsbo J, Wagner A et al (1997) Long-term adaptation to electrically induced cycle training in severe spinal cord injured individuals. Spinal Cord 35:1–16

23. Sloan KE, Bremner LA, Byrne J, Day RE, Scull ER (1994) Musculoskeletal effects of an electrical stimulation induced cycling programme in the spinal injured. Paraplegia 32:407–415

24. Bremner LA, Sloan KE, Day RE, Scull ER, Ackland T (1992) A clinical exercise system for paraplegics using functional electrical stimulation. Paraplegia 30:647–655
25. Rischbieth H, Jelbart M, Marshall R (1998) Neuromuscular electrical stimulation keeps a tetraplegic subject in his chair: a case study. Spinal Cord 36:443–445
26. Hjeltnes N, Aksnes AK, Birkeland KI, Johansen J, Lannem A, Wallberg-Henriksson H (1997) Improved body composition after 8 wk of electrically stimulated leg cycling in tetraplegic patients. Am J Physiol 273:R1072–1079
27. Baldi JC, Jackson RD, Moraille R, Mysiw WJ (1998) Muscle atrophy is prevented in patients with acute spinal cord injury using functional electrical stimulation. Spinal Cord 36:463–469
28. Hopman MTE, van Asten WN, Oeseburg B (1996) Changes in blood flow in the common femoral artery related to inactivity and muscle atrophy in individuals with long-standing paraplegia. Adv Exp Med Biol 388:379–383
29. Joyner MJ, Proctor DN (1999) Muscle blood flow during exercise: the limits of reductionism. Med Sci Sports Exerc 31:1036-1040
30. Shoemaker JK, Hughson RL (1999) Adaptation of blood flow during the rest to work transition in humans. Med Sci Sports Exerc 31:1019–1026
31. Kim CK, Strange S, Bangsbo J, Saltin B (1995) Skeletal muscle perfusion in electrically induced dynamic exercise in humans. Acta Physiol Scand 153:279–287
32. Levine SP, Kett RL, Gross MD, Wilson BA, Cederna PS, Juni JE (1990) Blood flow in the gluteus maximus of seated individuals during electrical muscle stimulation. Arch Phys Med Rehabil 71:682–686
33. Currier DP, Petrilli CR, Threlkeld AJ (1986) Effect of graded electrical stimulation on blood flow to healthy muscle. Phys Ther 66:937–943
34. Walker DC, Currier DP, Threlkeld AJ (1988) Effects of high voltage pulsed electrical stimulation on blood flow. Phys Ther 68:481–485
35. Glaser RM (1994) Functional neuromuscular stimulation. Exercise conditioning of spinal cord injured patients. Int J Sports Med 15:142–148
36. Figoni SF, Glaser RM, Rodgers MM, Hooker SP, Ezenwa BN, Collins SR et al (1991) Acute hemodynamic responses of spinal cord injured individuals to functional neuromuscular stimulation-induced knee extension exercise. J Rehab Res Dev 28:9–18
37. Davis GM, Servedio FJ, Glaser RM, Gupta SC, Suryaprasad AG (1990) Cardiovascular responses to arm cranking and FNS-induced leg exercise in paraplegics. J Appl Physiol 69:671–677
38. van Beekvelt MC, van Asten WN, Hopman MT (2000) The effect of electrical stimulation on leg muscle pump activity in spinal cord-injured and able-bodied individuals. Eur J Appl Physiol 82:510–516
39. Janssen TWJ, Hopman MTE (2003) Blood flow response to electrically induced twitch and tetanic lower-limb muscle contractions. Arch Phys Med Rehabil 84:7:982–987
40. Olive JL, Slade JM, Dudley GA, McCully KK (2003) Blood flow and muscle fatigue in SCI individuals during electrical stimulation. J Appl Physiol 94:701–708
41. Scremin OU, Cuevas-Trisan RL, Scremin AM, Brown CV (1998) Mandelkern MA. Functional electrical stimulation effect on skeletal muscle blood flow measured with H2(15)O positron emission tomography. Arch Phys Med Rehabil 79:641–646
42. Kaada B (1982) Vasodilation induced by transcutaneous nerve stimulation in peripheral ischemia (Raynaud's phenomenon and diabetic polyneuropathy). Eur Heart J 3:303–314

43. Mawson AR, Siddiqui FH, Connolly BJ, Sharp CJ, Stewart GW, Summer WR et al (1993) Effect of high voltage pulsed galvanic stimulation on sacral trans-cutaneous oxygen tension levels in the spinal cord injured. Paraplegia 31:311–319

44. Gerrits HL, de Haan A, Sargeant AJ, van Langen H, Hopman MT (2001) Per-ipheral vascular changes after electrically stimulated cycle training in people with spinal cord injury. Arch Phys Med Rehabil 82:832–839

45. Nash MS, Montalvo BM, Applegate B (1996) Lower extremity blood flow and responses to occlusion ischemia differ in exercise-trained and sedentary tet-raplegic persons. Arch Phys Med Rehabil 77:1260–1265

46. Kainz A, Kern H, Mostbeck A (1988) Zur Objektivierung der muskeldurch-blutungsfördernden Wirkung der Elektrostimulation bei Querschnittgelähm-ten (Untersuchungen mit 201 Thallium und 133 Xenon). Vasa – Supplemen-tum 26:209–213

47. Twist DJ (1990) Acrocyanosis in a spinal cord injured patient – effects of computer-controlled neuromuscular electrical stimulation: a case report. Phys Ther 70:45–49

48. Miyachi M, Iemitsu M, Okutsu M, Onodera S (1998) Effects of endurance training on the size and blood flow of the arterial conductance vessels in hu-mans. Acta Physiol Scand 163:13–16

49. Chilibeck PD, Jeon J, Weiss C, Bell G, Burnham R (1999) Histochemical changes in muscle of individuals with spinal cord injury following functional electrical stimulated exercise training. Spinal Cord 37:264–268

50. Rochester L, Barron MJ, Chandler CS, Sutton RA, Miller S, Johnson MA (1995) Influence of electrical stimulation of the tibialis anterior muscle in paraplegic subjects. 2. Morphological and histochemical properties. Paraple-gia 33:514–522

51. Martin TP, Stein RB, Hoeppner PH, Reid DC (1992) Influence of electrical sti-mulation on the morphological and metabolic properties of paralyzed muscle. J Appl Physiol 72:1401–1406

52. Ferguson AC, Keating JF, Delargy MA, Andrews BJ (1992) Reduction of seat-ing pressure using FES in patients with spinal cord injury. A preliminary re-port. Paraplegia 30:474–478

53. Levine SP, Kett RL, Cederna PS, Brooks SV (1990) Electric muscle stimulation for pressure sore prevention: tissue shape variation. Arch Phys Med Rehabil 71:210–215

54. Petrofsky JS (1992) Functional electrical stimulation: a two-year study. J Re-habil 58:29–34

55. Davis CM, Caseby NG (2001) Prevalence and incidence studies of pressure ul-cers in two long-term care facilities in Canada. Ostomy Wound Manage 47:28–34

56. Bours GJ, Halfens RJ, Abu-Saad HH, Grol RT (2002) Prevalence, prevention, and treatment of pressure ulcers: descriptive study in 89 institutions in the Netherlands. Res Nurs Health 25:99–110

57. Hammond MC, Bozzacco VA, Stiens SA, Buhrer R, Lyman P (1994) Pressure ulcer incidence on a spinal cord injury unit. Adv Wound Care 7:57–60

58. Lyder CH, Shannon R, Empleo-Frazier O, McGeHee D, White C. A (2002) comprehensive program to prevent pressure ulcers in long-term care: explor-ing costs and outcomes. Ostomy Wound Manage 48:52–62

59. Margolis DJ, Bilker W, Knauss J, Baumgarten M, Strom BL (2002) The inci-dence and prevalence of pressure ulcers among elderly patients in general medical practice. Ann Epidemiol 12:321–325

60. Kloth LC, McCulloch JM (1996) Promotion of wound healing with electrical stimulation. Adv Wound Care 9:42–45
61. Gardner SE, Frantz RA, Schmidt FL (1999) Effect of electrical stimulation on chronic wound healing: a meta-analysis. Wound Repair Regen 7:495–503
62. Unger PG, Raimastery S (1991) A controlled study of the effect of high pulse current on wound healing. Phys Ther 71:S119
63. Griffin JW, Tooms RE, Mendius RA, Clifft JK, Vander Zwaag R, el-Zeky F (1991) Efficacy of high voltage pulsed current for healing of pressure ulcers in patients with spinal cord injury. Phys Ther 71:433-42; discussion 442–444
64. Weiss DS, Kirsner R, Eaglstein WH (1990) Electrical stimulation and wound healing. Arch Dermatol 126:222–225
65. Sawyer PN (1964) Bioelectric phenomena and intravascular thrombosis: the first 12 years. Surgery 56:1020–1106
66. Biedebach MC (1989) Accelerated healing of skin ulcers by electrical stimulation and the intracellular physiological mechanisms involved. Acupunct Electrother Res 14:43–60
67. Gentzkow GD, Miller KH (1991) Electrical stimulation for dermal wound healing. Clin Podiatr Med Surg 8:827–841
68. Akai M, Oda H, Shirasaki Y, Tateishi T (1988) Electrical stimulation of ligament healing. An experimental study of the patellar ligament of rabbits. Clin Orthop 296–301
69. Assimacopoulos D (1968) Wound healing promotion by the use of negative electric current. Am Surg 34:423–431
70. Smith J, Romansky N, Vomero J, Davis RH (1984) The effect of electrical stimulation on wound healing in diabetic mice. J Am Podiatry Assoc 74:71–75
71. Young HG (1966) Electric impulse therapy aids wound healing. Modern veterinary practice. Modern Veterinary Practice 47:60–62
72. Wolcott LE, Wheeler PC, Hardwicke HM, Rowley BA (1969) Accelerated healing of skin ulcer by electrotherapy: preliminary clinical results. Southern Med J 62:795–801
73. Gault WR, Gatens PF Jr (1976) Use of low intensity direct current in management of ischemic skin ulcers. Phys Ther 56:265–269
74. Wood JM, Evans PE 3rd, Schallreuter KU, Jacobson WE, Sufit R, Newman J et al (1993) A multicenter study on the use of pulsed low-intensity direct current for healing chronic stage II and stage III decubitus ulcers. Arch Dermatol 129:999–1009
75. Vanable J Jr (1989) Natural and applied voltages in vertebrate regeneration and healing. In: Integumentary potentials and wound healing. Liss, New York, p 186

Biochemical Status of Soft Tissues Subjected to Sustained Pressure

8

DAN BADER, YAK-NAM WANG, SARAH KNIGHT, ADRIAN POLLIACK, TIM JAMES, RICHARD TAYLOR

Introduction

The breakdown of soft tissue leading to the development of pressure ulcers has implications in terms of both the overall health of an individual and the overall resources required for health care. Although the cause of the condition is multifactorial [1], it is well established that prolonged pressure ischaemia will affect the viability of soft tissues, leading to their eventual breakdown (see Chap. 1).

There are a host of external factors, generally physical, biochemical and clinical in nature, which contribute to the development of tissue breakdown and the formation of pressure ulcers [2]. However, the presence of pressures applied normally at the interface between the soft tissues and the patient support must be considered as an initiating factor. When prolonged pressure is applied to the skin, the underlying blood vessels may be partially or totally occluded, creating an anoxic environment, and oxygen and other nutrients are not delivered at a rate sufficient to satisfy the metabolic demands of the tissue. The lymphatic and venous drainage will also be impaired and thus the breakdown products of metabolism accumulate within both the interstitial spaces and the cells [3]. As energy stores diminish there is an increasing possibility of failure of some of the cellular processes and dissipation of ionic gradients across cellular membranes, resulting in cell damage [4]. In the able-bodied subject regular movement relieves these pressures at local tissue areas and there follows a period of increased blood flow after vascular occlusion, termed reactive hyperaemia. However, many immobile and disabled subjects are less able to relieve pressures, and their tissues, particularly adjacent to bony prominences such as the sacrum, are often compromised. This makes them a prime group for the development of pressure ulcers.

Previous Studies of Tissue Status Under External Loading

Over the last two decades, there has been a series of techniques that have been proposed to indicate the viability, or status, of soft tissues subjected to periods of loading. Some of these are covered in Chaps. 5 and 6. These techniques have, to date, been largely restricted to examining the response of skin layers to mechanical loading, and include measurements of blood flow using laser Doppler flowmetry [5] and reflective spectrophotometry [6, 7], both of which are discussed in Chap. 17. Advances in the latter technique have enabled distinct absorption spectra to be identified for oxygenated and deoxygenated blood in skin [7]. The authors claim that a number of other skin biomolecules, such as melanin and collagen, can also be distinguished. The most popular technique, however, is to measure transcutaneous gas tensions ($TcPO_2$ and $TcPCO_2$) at elevated skin temperatures [8–13]. It has also been employed in a clinical setting to investigate the performance of prescribed support cushions in sub-acute spinal cord-injured subjects [14]; the detailed results of this study are provided in Chap. 6. The study employed an assessment criterion for tissue viability based on the percentage time at which the $TcPO_2$ and $TcPCO_2$ values were within acceptable levels. Clear relationships were indicated between depressed levels of $TcPO_2$ and elevated levels of $TcPCO_2$, at associated high values of interface pressure [14]. However, this and related studies yielded no clear guidelines as to the precise relationship between compromised tissue gas levels for a set time period and the onset of progressive tissue breakdown that will ultimately result in a pressure ulcer.

This chapter presents a series of studies by the authors in which concentrations of metabolites are determined in sweat collected from the surface of tissues subjected to various compressive loading regimens. The sweat metabolites may be proposed as non-invasive markers of tissue status. If metabolic changes reflecting early stages of tissue degradation could be monitored it might become possible to identify patients at risk of developing pressure ulcers and to adopt appropriate preventative measures.

Sweat Analysis

An alternative method of assessing tissue status is to examine the metabolite levels in localised soft tissue areas subjected to pressure ischaemia and subsequent reperfusion. These metabolites are transferred via the sweat glands, which are simple tubular glands, and can be collected at the skin surface. Sweat is a hypotonic solution of sodium and chloride ions in water. Together with other constituents including lactate, urea and potassium, these metabolites account for about 95% of the osmotically active substances in sweat [15]. A few such studies have been reported [16–20]. The earliest study [16] used a bulky system to chemically induce sweat production. By contrast, the latter studies by the present authors [17–20] collected thermally induced sweat by absorption on thin pads, made from filter paper, attached to the skin surface. This collection system provided minimal distortion and proved ideal for use at a loaded tissue support interface.

Sweat Metabolites as a Function of Sweat Rate

The early studies compared sweat collected during periods of loading at the ischium and sacrum compared to unloaded periods at adjacent areas. They revealed that tissues subjected to partial ischaemia, specifically produced by a uni-axial indenter system, yielded a general increase in concentrations of sweat lactate, chloride, urea and urate associated with a decreased sweat rate [17]. As an example, sweat lactate and urea levels were increased by 24 and 27%, respectively, at the loaded sacrum, which yielded a 162% decrease in sweat rate compared to unloaded controls. Following the removal of loading, the levels of both sweat metabolites tended to decrease back to basal levels.

In a separate study [20, 21], sweat was collected at two adjacent sites, one loaded and one unloaded, at the sacrum of a number of able-bodied subjects. Three distinct pressures were applied. Estimations were made of both the absolute values of sweat metabolite concentrations and the ratios of the concentration at both loaded and unloaded tissue sites, thus eliminating the wide variation between subjects. The ratio for lactate is presented as a function of the three applied pressures in Fig. 8.1.

It is evident that there is a significant increase in sweat lactate ratios at applied pressures of 40 mmHg (5.3 kPa) and above. Indeed, a linear regression model applied to the lactate data, using the Spearman correlation coefficient, revealed statistical significance at the 1% level. Similar trends were also apparent with sweat urea, urate and chloride [20]. In addition, the absolute lactate concentrations for the three pressures were pooled as loaded data in conjunction with unloaded data to yield two separate relationships with the inverse of sweat rate. As illustrated in Fig. 8.2, the resulting linear models were found to be statistically significant ($p < 0.01$ in both cases).

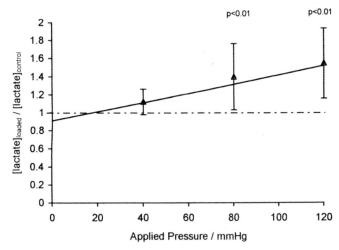

Fig. 8.1. The effect of applied pressure on the ratio of sweat lactate concentration as a result of sacral loading in a group of able-bodied subjects. Linear model: $y = 0.0046x + 0.975$; $r = 0.48$, $p < 0.01$

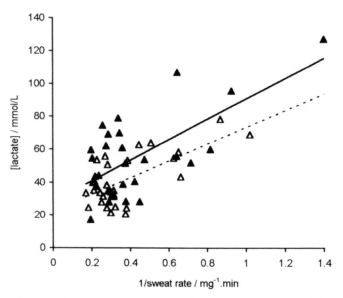

Fig. 8.2. Relationship between sweat lactate concentration and the inverse of sweat rate on the sacrum of individual subjects for both loaded sites (*continuous line*) and unloaded sites (*dashed line*). Linear model (loaded): $y=62.29x+28.53$; $r=0.67$, $p<0.01$. Linear model (unloaded): $y=51.14x+22.34$; $r=0.68$, $p<0.01$

The slopes and intercepts of the linear models were clearly higher for the loaded data than the unloaded controls, by approximately 20 and 28%, respectively. This would indicate that the increase in concentrations in sweat lactate is higher during the ischaemic loaded period than would be predicted by a decrease in sweat rate alone. Such a finding could be explained from processes such as anaerobic glycolysis. A similar response was found for sweat urea [20].

Sweat Metabolites as an Indicator of Tissue Status

The study was extended by employing two independent techniques in combination to assess the soft tissue response to applied pressure on a group of able-bodied subjects, to establish baseline data [21]. The methods involved the simultaneous measurement of the local tensions of oxygen and carbon dioxide ($TcPO_2$ and $TcPCO_2$) and the collection and subsequent analysis of metabolite concentrations of sweat samples. Adjacent loaded and unloaded sites on the sacrum were tested to allow for between-subject variation. Several parameters were selected from each of the techniques and their inter-relationships were examined. Results indicated that oxygen levels ($TcPO_2$) were lowered in soft tissues subjected to applied pressures of between 40 mmHg (5.3 kPa) and 120 mmHg (16.0 kPa) [21]. At the higher pressures this decrease was generally associated with an increase in carbon dioxide well above the normal basal levels of 45 mmHg (6 kPa). There were also considerable increases, in some cases twofold magnitude, in the concentrations of sweat lactate at the loaded site compared to the unloaded control. By comparing selected parameters, a threshold value for loaded TcPO$_2$ could be identified, representing a reduction of approximately 60% from unloaded values, as indicated in Fig. 8.3 a.

Above this threshold level there was a significant relationship between this parameter and the loaded/unloaded concentration ratios for both sweat lactate and urea [21]. Given that tissue oxygen and sweat lactate reflect different aspects of tissue ischaemia, this degree of reduction (60% in median oxygen tension) may represent a critical level for the development of tissue damage. The study also related the lactate ratio to the percentage time at which TcPCO$_2$ exceeded 50%. Figure 8.3 b indicates the presence of two distinct clusters of data. For example, when the carbon dioxide parameter exceeded 37%, the lactate ratios were well in excess of unity. The differences could be attributed to the degree of pressure-induced tissue ischaemia. Thus, under conditions of mild ischaemia elevated levels of tissue carbon dioxide may be released from loaded areas in a normal manner, resulting in TcPCO$_2$ values below 50 mmHg, whereas in severe conditions, both sweat lactate and TcPCO$_2$ will be elevated (Fig. 8.3 b).

Sweat lactate is generally thought to be derived from the sweat gland itself [15, 22]. During normal metabolism, oxidative phosphorylation is believed to be the main metabolic pathway of the eccrine sweat gland [23]. However, under conditions of ischaemia and/or in anaerobic conditions, glycolysis becomes the main metabolic pathway resulting in the formation of lactate. This explains the elevated lactate concentrations observed in the sweat collected from the experimental site and suggests that a sufficient degree of ischaemia was induced in the sacral tissue during the two loading periods.

Sweat urea is believed to be derived mainly from serum urea by the passive diffusion across the glandular wall and cell membrane, although it is still unknown whether it is also produced by the sweat gland [23]. Sweat urea levels are therefore expected to be similar to levels within the blood, and indeed this was observed in several studies, particularly at high sweat rates [24, 25]. However, it has been proposed that water reabsorption is responsible for sweat to plasma urea ratios greater than unity [26]. Low sweat rates, as observed during ischaemia, have been found to result in elevated sweat urea concentrations.

Urea is the main product of protein metabolism and can thus be an indicator of tissue damage if elevated levels are found in bodily fluids, such as urine or blood. Prolonged periods of ischaemia can lead to muscle damage, resulting in an increased serum urea level which, in turn, can result in enhanced concentrations of sweat urea [23]. These findings [21] suggest that the tissue was compromised during the loading period. It was strongly proposed by the authors that such an approach, using a series of parameters, may prove useful in identifying those subjects whose soft tissue may be compromised during periods of pressure ischaemia.

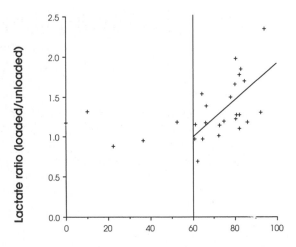

a **Percentage reduction in median TcPO2**

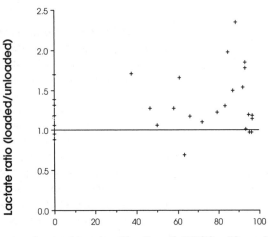

b **Percentage loading time TcPCO2 > 50 mmHg**

Fig. 8.3. Relationship between ratio of sweat lactate concentration and **a** percentage reduction in transcutaneous gas tension (TcPO$_2$) and **b** percentage of time for which transcutaneous carbon dioxide tension (TcPCO$_2$) exceeded 50 mmHg, as a result of sacral loading on individual subjects

Sweat Metabolites in Different Subject Groups

In a separate study, the potential of this technique as a clinical tool was examined in a group of 11 debilitated subjects [18]. Sweat was collected at the sacrum with the subjects either seated in a wheelchair or lying in bed. During prolonged loading for up to 10 h at relatively low levels of interface

Table 8.1. Comparative results of sweat metabolites collected from the unloaded and loaded sacrum

Test conditions/collection time/temperature/subject group		Sweat metabolite concentrations		
		Lactate (mmol.l^{-1})	Urea (mmol.l^{-1})	Urate (μmol.l^{-1})
Unloaded sacrum/ 8–14 h/ambient/ able-bodied	Median (range)	32.9 (20.6–57.2)	17.9 (9.3–38.8)	27.0 (9–42.9)
Unloaded sacrum/ 9–16 h/ambient/ debilitated	Median (range)	38.1 (20–87)	25.1 (2.4–49.9)	30.0 (6–91)
Loaded sacrum/ 8–14 h/ambient/ debilitated	Median (range)	53.0 (41.9–72.9)	32.0 (30.8–51.8)	37.0 (15.0–90.0)

pressure, ranging from 16 mmHg to 49 mmHg (2.3 kPa to 6.9 kPa), there was an elevation in the levels of some metabolites; for example, there were median increases of 39 and 28% for lactate and urea respectively. The basal levels of the sweat metabolites measured in rehabilitation subjects were compared to those reported by the authors in able-bodied subjects (Table 8.1). The median lactate and urea concentrations were 16 and 40% higher, respectively. The sweat rates were very similar (data not shown). This table also shows that the median lactate and urea concentrations increased further in the rehabilitation subjects during periods of sacral loading. The ranges of metabolite concentrations observed in the unloaded tissues of the rehabilitation subjects were similar to those in the able-bodied. The ranges represent the natural variation between individuals, with evidence for possible further changes in the rehabilitation group as a consequence of susceptibility to tissue breakdown.

Successive measurements on one individual over a period of several months showed only small variations compared to those observed in either groups of non-disabled or disabled subjects [18]. These data suggest that the technique might be applicable in a clinical setting to monitor tissue status in individual subjects subjected to external loading conditions. As such, it could be used in conjunction with monitoring other parameters such as interface pressures.

Sweat Purine Analysis in Conditions of Ischaemia and Reperfusion

It is well established that in many conditions, such as adult respiratory distress and myocardial infarction [27–29], the occurrence of ischaemia is followed by a complex biochemical response when the blood supply is re-established, and this may result in additional injury to the tissues [30]. During ischaemia–reperfusion, one aspect of biochemical changes involves the irreversible loss of high-energy phosphate (ATP). In addition, an important mechanism is triggered with the influx of molecular oxygen during reperfusion. The formation of oxygen-derived free radicals can potentially cause damage to cells, as detailed in Chap. 13. It is also evident from the literature that purine metabolism plays an important role in tissue breakdown during both ischaemia and reperfusion (see Fig. 13.1). Terminal products of purine metabolism produced during these periods, may directly produce cell injury [27]. In addition to lactate and urea, these terminal metabolites, may be useful as markers for tissue breakdown. These include the purines allantoin, hypoxanthine, inosine, uric acid and xanthine. In a previous study, increases in sweat uric acid, as determined by the uricase method, were measured in skin subjected to load-induced ischaemia and reperfusion [17]. An alternative method is required to analyse a series of purines [31].

Test Protocols

The method of sweat collection was identical to that previously used by the authors for the measurement of sweat lactate and urea [17, 18]. Briefly, this involved the use of individual circular sweat pads, 40 mm in diameter, made of pure cellulose chromatography paper (1 Chr; Whatman Paper, Maidstone, Kent, UK). The pads were covered with an impermeable, hydrophobic polypropylene sheet, cut to 50 mm diameter, to minimise the loss of sweat by evaporation. The sweat pad and the overlying plastic sheet were held in position by Micropore surgical tape (3M Healthcare, Loughborough, UK).

Sweat collection was carried out in an environmental chamber, maintained at a temperature of $38\pm1\,°C$ at a relative humidity of between 45 and 65%. These conditions were chosen in order to achieve a sufficient sweat rate. Each subject underwent an equilibrium period of 20 min in the chamber to ensure that a steady sweat rate had been attained. The subject then adopted a prone position on a bed and two pre-weighed sweat pads, approximately 100–150 mm apart, were attached to the skin above the sacrum, which had been cleaned with sterile wipes. One area was designated the control site and the other the experimental site. Loads were applied to the experimental test site via an indenter and the bed-mounted loading gantry described in a previous publication [21].

A total of eight sweat samples were collected from each subject: four from the control site and four from the experimental site. The experimental site was subjected to both ischaemia and reperfusion. During the former, the indenter applied a constant pressure (80±20 mmHg) to the skin for a period of an hour, during which two 30-min sequential sweat samples were collected. This pressure level, monitored continuously using the Oxford Pressure Monitor Mk II (Talley Group, Romsey, UK), has been demonstrated to induce significant ischaemia in soft tissues [9]. The reperfusion phase involved removing the loaded indenter and collecting two sequential samples of sweat, each over a 30-min period. Whenever the sweat pad at the experimental site was changed the pad at the control site, which remained unloaded throughout, was also changed to provide a time- and condition-related comparison.

After the prescribed period each pad was removed and sealed in a pre-weighed bottle, which was re-weighed to obtain the net sweat rate by difference. After sweat collection the sweat pad was re-weighed and frozen at –20 °C for subsequent biochemical analysis. To extract the sweat from the pads 30-ml tubes with conical bottoms were adapted by addition of a perforated separation device [17] above which the pad was placed prior to centrifugation. After centrifugation the liquid sweat was harvested from the bottom of the tube.

Biochemical Analyses

The measurements of sweat lactate and sweat urea have been described by the present authors in detail elsewhere [17–19]. Briefly, lactate was measured by a lactate dehydrogenase spectrophotometric method from NADH production at 340 nm [32] on a Cobas Fara clinical chemistry analyser (Roche Diagnostics, Lewes, UK). Sweat urea concentrations were measured via the urease–glutamate dehydrogenase method.

The determination of sweat purines involved a high-performance liquid chromatography (HPLC) system (Waters, Milford, MA, USA), consisting of two 510 pumps, a Waters 717 autosampler and a 2487 dual-wavelength absorbance detector (set at 254 and 280 nm). Both the pre-column and column were from Phenomenex, Macclesfield, Cheshire (Kingsorb 3 μm C18 column, 150×4.6 mm). Millennium Chromatography Manager Software (Waters), was used for data processing.

A 5 mmol/l phosphate, 5 mmol/l 1-heptanesulphonic acid, pH 3.3 mobile phase (sodium salt, both BDH, pH 3.3) at a flow rate of 1 ml/min was used for separation of the purine components. After 20 min a 50% methanol: water solution was introduced as the mobile phase for 1 min to rapidly remove retained components which were not of analytical interest, to reduce sample run times. A re-equilibration period of 28 min re-established the phosphate buffer prior to the next specimen injection.

Stock solutions of purines were prepared at concentrations of 0.3 mmol/l (uric acid) or 6 mmol/l (xanthine, hypoxanthine and inosine). A mixed working standard was prepared with a final concentration of 30 μmol/l (uric acid) and 100 μmol/l (xanthine, hypoxanthine and inosine). All standards and chemicals were obtained from Sigma (Sigma Chemical Co., Poole, UK).

Sweat collections greater than 100 µL were analysed neat. Smaller sweat volume specimens required dilution by a factor dependent on yield to provide the analytical volume for the HPLC method. Thus, sixfold (volumes <20 µL), fourfold (20–40 µL), twofold (40–60 µL) and 1.5-fold (60 and 80 µL) dilutions were used. All specimens from the same subject were analysed in the same batch to minimise imprecision.

Studies to validate the purine HPLC method for application to sweat were required. Identification of purine peaks within the chromatogram was based on a number of criteria listed below:

1. Each purine has a characteristic 254:280 nm peak ratio. These were observed to be almost identical in the chromatograms of standards, sweat samples and sweat supplemented with the standard. The values were also comparable to literature values [33].

2. Relative retention times for xanthine, hypoxanthine and inosine compared to uric acid were calculated and observed to be consistent in all sweat and standard specimens.

3. The peaks representing the purines of interest were observed to increase when sweat was supplemented with mixed standard.

4. Sweat and standards were treated with enzymes known to digest specific purines. Exposure of sweat and mixed standard to 1 U/ml uricase resulted in the loss of the uric acid peak. Similarly, 20.8 U/ml xanthine oxidase resulted in the loss of both the xanthine and hypoxanthine peaks.

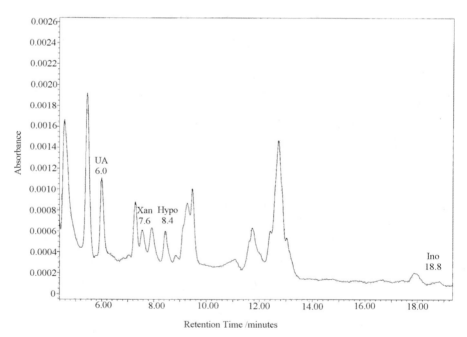

Fig. 8.4. Typical chromatogram at 254 nm of sweat sample collected at the sacrum

Cumulatively this information was used to assign the peak identification of uric acid, xanthine, and hypoxanthine in sweat to be approximately 6.0 min, 7.6 min and 8.4 min, respectively. The within-batch precision, calculated from the mean variability of four paired replicates of pooled sweat, was 9.6% for uric acid, 6.4% for xanthine and 12.6% for hypoxanthine. In the third batch of purine analysis the chromatography demonstrated a clean peak at 18.1 min, which from previous work with aqueous standards could be identified as due to inosine. A typical sweat chromatogram at 254 nm is illustrated in Fig. 8.4.

Results

Subjects producing less than 50 mg, equivalent to 50 μl, of sweat at one collection site during at least three of the four collection periods were excluded from further analysis. The quantity of sweat collected from both sites of the 13 able-bodied volunteers over the four periods is summarised in Table 8.2. It is evident that, particularly with the unloaded controls, there was a considerable variability in the sweat amounts. Close examination of these data revealed that in six volunteers there was a decline in the sweat amounts collected over the 120-min period. This decrease may be a result of fatigue of the sweat glands, as demonstrated in previous work [22]. Nonetheless, the median decrease of approximately 32% in the total

Table 8.2. Sweat amounts collected from the experimental and control sites for subjects maintained at 37 °C and high relative humidity

	Collection period							
	0–30 min ischaemia		30–60 min ischaemia		60–90 min reperfusion		90–120 min reperfusion	
	Exp. site	Control site	Exp. site	Control site	Exp. site	Control site	Exp. site	Control site
Sweat amount (mg)								
Median	182.9	218.5	199.0	215.2	188.2	164.0	174.7	127.9
Range	10.8–246.5	20.2–279.2	52.8–313.8	99.3–278.3	92.7–272.3	46.5–237.4	38.0–290.2	32.5–281.4
Sweat ratio (experimental/control)								
Median	0.78		0.92		1.26		1.27	
Range	0.12–1.21		0.39–2.30		0.44–2.52		0.49–2.96	

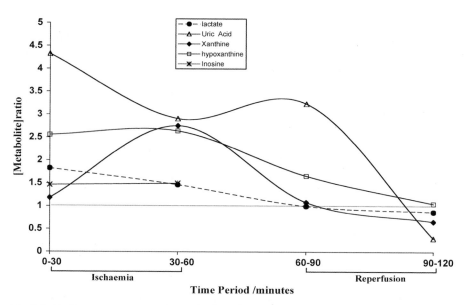

Fig. 8.5. Median sweat concentration ratios for collection at two adjacent sites on the sacrum for able-bodied subjects for lactate and four purines during four separate 30-min collection periods

group was not found to be statistically significant ($p > 0.05$). Table 8.2 also summarises the ratios of sweat rate. The results indicate that a median sweat rate ratio of experimental to control samples of below unity was exhibited during the two 30-min periods of ischaemia. However, during the periods of reperfusion, when the load was removed from the experimental site, the median ratios increased to exceed basal levels. Most of the subjects demonstrated these trends.

In many cases, the sweat purine chromatographs at 254 nm generally reflected that illustrated in Fig. 8.4. The main exception was the peak corresponding to inosine, at the highest retention time, which was not routinely easy to identify due to low signal-to-noise ratio. The absolute levels for the purines were estimated from their peak areas and these values were found to be variable both at different collection periods and between subjects. For example, uric acid concentrations ranged from 2.5 μmol/l to 75.2 μmol/l. The corresponding purine ratios were estimated and the median values and ranges are presented in Fig. 8.5, in conjunction with lactate ratios, for the separate collection periods. It can be seen that for the first ischaemic period, all metabolite concentration ratios were above unity. However, there was a wide spread in median values, which ranged from 1.18 to 4.32. All the median ratios remained at an elevated level during the second ischaemic period, although the variation was considerably less, ranging from 1.47 to 2.91. It should be noted that in the case of xanthine, ratio values were higher in the second ischaemic period.

During the first reperfusion period, the ratios for lactate and xanthine fell to approximately unity, whereas the ratios for both hypoxanthine and,

Table 8.3. Differences in uric acid, xanthine and hypoxanthine between collection periods for subjects maintained at 38 °C and a relative humidity of 45–55%

Comparison	Uric acid	Xanthine	Hypoxanthine
0–30 I vs 30–60 I	n.s.	n.s.	n.s.
0–30 I vs 60–90 R	n.s.	n.s.	n.s.
0–30 I vs 90–120 R	$p < 0.05$	$p < 0.05$	$p < 0.05$
30–60 I vs 60–90 R	n.s.	$p < 0.05$	n.s.
30–60 I vs 90–120 R	$p < 0.05$	$p < 0.05$	$p < 0.05$
60–90 R vs 90–120 R	$p < 0.05$	n.s.	$p < 0.05$

I, ischaemia; R, reperfusion; ns, $p > 0.05$.

in particular, uric acid remained significantly above unity. The ratios for all the metabolites decreased during the second reperfusion period to values approximating to or below unity. This decrease was most pronounced for uric acid, which exhibited a ratio value, 0.29, one order of magnitude lower than each of the other three periods. For both reperfusion periods, insufficient data precluded the estimation of ratio values for inosine. It should be noted that a few individual subjects did not follow these general trends for either ischaemic or reperfusion periods.

The differences between the ratios of the three purines from consecutive collection periods were examined using the Mann–Whitney U test, and the results are summarised in Table 8.3. No significant difference was found among the first three time periods (0–30, 30–60 and 60-90 min) for either uric acid or hypoxanthine, although the metabolite ratios at all these time periods were found to be statistically significantly greater than the values for the second reperfusion period (90–120 min). In contrast, for xanthine concentrations there was a statistically significant decrease between the ratio value at the second ischaemic period (30–60 min) and the first reperfusion period (60-90 min). Although further reduction was evident in the second reperfusion period, the difference was not statistically significant.

Current Perspectives on Sweat Analysis

High-performance liquid chromatography is a chromatographic technique, applicable to virtually all soluble biological molecules. However, its use in clinical chemistry laboratories is still limited due to the time required to develop reliable assays, necessary expertise of staff and the cost and speed of analysis. This technique does permit the quantitative analysis of two or more analytes simultaneously, as reported in its use for purine concentration within body fluids, such as plasma [24, 34] and urine [35]. In the present work, a protocol using HPLC was successfully established to measure the purine concentrations in sweat collected from tissues which had been subjected to periods of loading and unloading. The target purines which had been successfully identified and quantified were inosine, hypoxanthine, xanthine and uric acid, all of which are produced at various stages of ATP degradation.

High-humidity test conditions were used to produce a high sweat rate and a high yield of sweat, as evidenced by sweat amounts of greater than 100 mg for most 30-min collection periods. The concentration of biochemical constituents in sweat is influenced by sweat rate (Fig. 8.2), nutrition and both physiological and sociological factors. Each will contribute to the observed inter- and intra-subject differences observed in the present and other sweat-related studies. To identify actual differences produced as a result of the applied experimental conditions, it is essential to collect sweat simultaneously from an adjacent control site in the same individual.

The application of load to the experimental site produced a marked reduction in sweat rate at this site in comparison to the control site (Table 8.2), a finding consistent with earlier reports [15]. During the subsequent unloading periods, there was an increase in sweat rate at the experimental site with levels reaching, and occasionally exceeding, those at the control site (Table 8.2). The increased sweat lactate during the loading period is consistent with previous studies and demonstrates that, in this particular study design, tissue ischaemia has been produced.

During reperfusion two important events occur, namely reoxygenation of the ischaemic tissue and restoration of the lymph flow. The former results in aerobic metabolism and an associated dramatic decrease in lactate formation. Lymph flow is essential in the removal of the excess lactate and other waste products from the ischaemic site. Poor lymph return is believed to be associated with further breakdown [36–38]. Any further decrease in lactate levels with extended reperfusion may be due to over-compensation of the lymph flow or an increase in sweat rate observed at the reperfusion site The wash-out of lactate during reperfusion has been suggested to be a sign of adequate reperfusion [39]. In addition, the decrease of urea concentration to approximately unity [31] suggests that restoration mechanisms were successful over the 30-min period. The further decrease in urea concentration could be due to the increase in sweat rate during this period [17].

Although previous studies have made similar observations for both sweat lactate and urea, the results for sweat purines have not been previously reported [15, 19]. The only studies including uric acid involved an analytical method with a limited degree of accuracy [20]. Inosine, hypoxanthine, xanthine and uric acid are produced at progressive stages of purine metabolism (Fig. 13.1). During prolonged periods of ischaemia high-energy phosphate compounds are broken down to form these purines. Indeed, the appearance of purines in body fluids, such as blood and plasma, has been used as evidence of cellular hypoxia [35]. It is important to note that the source of purines in sweat has not been previously examined. They could arise from metabolism within the sweat gland itself or from passive diffusion into the gland. In the present study, the elevated purine levels, in particular increased uric acid concentration, indicate that significant cellular energy depletion has occurred during the ischaemic periods, with irreversible loss of high-energy phosphate compounds [27]. However, the elevated levels of xanthine and uric acid suggest the presence of molecular oxygen as it is required to form these purines (Fig. 13.1). The presence of a combination of elevated lactate, xanthine and uric acid implies that although ischaemia produced within the tissue was adequate, it was not complete. In the present study an elevated hypoxanthine concentration was also observed at the experimental site during loading (Fig. 8.5). This should be seen in the light of similar elevations in patients suffering from ischaemic diseases, such as myocardial infarction [24].

During the first recovery period, the decrease in xanthine and hypoxanthine, with slightly elevated uric acid concentrations, suggest an increased flux to the latter with a reduction in the breakdown of high-energy phosphate compounds. The increased concentration of uric acid suggests the further formation of free radicals, which have been implicated in tissue damage [40, 41]. The elevated levels of these purines suggest that the 30-min period was not sufficient for adequate recovery from the ischaemic insult (Fig. 8.5), although the lactate and urea levels suggest otherwise [31]. This implies that the sweat purines provide additional information on tissue status to that available from sweat lactate and urea alone.

During extended periods of reperfusion, the decrease in hypoxanthine ratio to unity could be an indication that the purine metabolism had effectively returned to basal levels. However, the further decrease in xanthine and uric acid concentrations suggest further degeneration of these purines, with the influx of oxygen, to produce free radicals and result in the formation of allantoin, which is the most stable oxidation product of uric acid [41]. The allantoin/uric acid ratio has been used [42] as an early indicator of oxidative stress in very young infants (see Chap. 13). Using the present protocol, however, the sweat allantoin concentrations could not be determined due to the large number of peaks in the appropriate region, corresponding to a retention time of approximately 2 min [31].

Future Potential of Sweat Analysis

A non-invasive method for measuring and monitoring tissue status is of critical importance, particularly in clinical situations. The collection and analysis of sweat is already in use for the detection of cystic fibrosis. This chapter presents the extent of the studies [15, 16, 20, 31], the most recent of which has provided a detailed profile of the effects of ischaemia on sweat biochemistry, encompassing a wider range of metabolites. Investigations have generally been focused at the sacrum, which is often loaded during supine lying and sitting and thus has a high susceptibility to pressure ulcer formation. In addition, the high sweat rate found at this site, associated with a high density of sweat glands, is of particular pertinence to the present technique.

The sweat collection system used to collect the bulk of the sweat consisted of simple chromatography paper covered with an impermeable, hydrophobic plastic sheet. This technique provides a cheap and non-invasive method of sweat collection without distorting the interface with the soft tissue covering the body. It is thus an appropriate method for clinical use. However, the collection time and sample volumes required for reliable analysis do not facilitate continuous and real-time measurements. In addition, for the successful analysis of metabolite concentrations a consistent collection in excess of 50 mg of sweat, equivalent to 50 µl, is required. Thus the technique may not prove appropriate for individuals with low sweat production, as is possible for a range of inherent factors. These can include diet, reduced physical fitness, differences in excitability of sweat glands, sleep deprivation and ethnic differences [43–45]. In addition, some individuals, including some of those with spinal cord injury, have impaired sudomotor function. Thus sweat analysis may not prove universally applicable to all subjects susceptible to the development of pressure ulcers.

Current work suggests that monitoring of sweat lactate and urea alone is not able to give a full indication of the tissue status, particularly during reperfusion. The measured purines are undoubtedly useful markers or "fingerprints", as they provide an indication of the metabolic status of the tissue during both ischaemia, when there is energy depletion, and reperfusion; as such, they may be of significant potential use to identify patients at risk of developing pressure ulcers. As highlighted in many chapters in this book, the latter can lead to a process termed reperfusion injury. It is clear that the use of a combination of markers, rather than a single marker, is required to monitor the status of soft tissues. This approach would also include sweat rate, which has been repeatedly shown to be related to specific metabolites, such as sweat lactate.

The advantages of on-line and real-time measurement should be explored. Indeed, real-time determinations of sweat lactate have been employed in previous studies to monitor physical condition [46, 47]. However, the measurement devices used were large and would not be appropriate at the orthosis–body interface. By comparison, disposable biosensors are currently in use in both clinical situations and at home to monitor blood glucose levels in diabetic patients. If the biosensor technology were available, this approach could be adopted to monitor a range of metabolites to assess the tissue status of those individuals, who may be susceptible to the development of pressure ulcers. The use of these biosensors would enable a more detailed examination of the response of the tissue to recovery. This approach could also be used in conjunction with cell and tissue model systems, as described in Chaps. 15 and 16, to identify other critical biochemical markers.

Acknowledgements. Our thanks to the many volunteers, both able-bodied and disabled, who have participated in this series of studies. Their sweat was gratefully received.

References

1. Bouten CVC, Oomens CWJ, Baaijens FPT, Bader DL (2003) The aetiology of pressure sores: skin deep or muscle bound? Arch Phys Med Rehabil 84:616–619
2. Bliss MR (1993) Aetiology of pressure sores. Rev Clin Ger 3:379–397
3. Krouskop TA, Reddy NP, Spencer W, Secor J (1978) Mechanisms of decubitus ulcer formation. Med Hypotheses 4:37–39
4. Bouten CVC, Lee DA, Knight MM, Bader DL (2001) Compressive deformation and damage of muscle cell sub-populations in a model system. J Biomech Eng 29:153–163
5. Schubert V, Fagrell B (1991) Post-occlusive reactive hyperaemia and thermal response in the skin microcirculation of subjects with spinal cord injury. Scand J Rehabil Med 23:33–45
6. Hagisawa S, Ferguson-Pell M, Cardi M, Miller SD (1994) Assessment of skin blood content and oxygenation in spinal injured subjects during reactive hyperaemia. J Rehabil Res Dev 31:1–14
7. Ferguson-Pell M, Hagisawa S (1995) An empirical technique to compensate for melanin when monitoring skin microcirculation using reflectance spectrophotometry. Med Eng Phy 7:104–110
8. Newson TP, Rolfe P (1982) Skin surface PO_2 and blood flow measurements over the ischial tuberosities. Arch Phys Med Rehabil 63:553–556
9. Bader DL, Gant CA (1988) Changes in transcutaneous oxygen tension as a result of prolonged pressures at the sacrum. Clin Phys Physiol Meas 9:33–40
10. Bader DL (1990) The recovery characteristics of soft tissue following repeated loading. J Rehabil Res Dev 27, 141–150
11. Bader DL (1990) Effects of compressive load regimens on tissue viability. In: Bader DL (ed) Pressure sores – clinical practice and scientific approach. Macmillan, Basingstoke, pp 191–201
12. Colin D, Saumet JL (1996) Influence of external pressre on transcutaneous oxygen tension and laser Doppler flowmetry on sacral skin. Clin Physiol 16:61–72
13. Colin D, Loyant R, Abraham P, Saumet JL (1996) Changes in sacral transcutaneous oxygen tension in the evaluation of different mattresses in the prevention of pressure ulcers. Adv Wound Care 9:25–28
14. Bogie KM, Nuseibeh I, Bader DL (1995) Early progressive changes in tissue viability in the seated spinal cord injured subject. Paraplegia 33:1441–1447
15. Van Heyningen R, Weiner JS (1952) The effect of arterial occlusion on sweat composition. Physiology 116:404–413
16. Hagisawa, S, Ferguson-Pell M, Cardi M, Miller SD (1988) Biochemical changes in sweat following pressure ischaemia J Rehab Res Dev 25:57–62
17. Polliack AA, Taylor RP, Bader DL (1993) The analysis of sweat during soft tissue breakdown following pressure ischaemia. J Rehab Res Dev 30(2):250–259
18. Polliack AA, Taylor RP, Bader DL (1997) Sweat analysis following pressure ischaemia in a group of debilitated subjects. J Rehab Res Dev 34(3):303–308
19. Taylor RP, Polliack AA, Bader DL (1994) The analysis of metabolites in human sweat: analytical methods and potential application to investigation of pressure ischaemia of soft tissues. Ann Clin Biochem 31:18–24
20. Knight SL (1997) Non-invasive techniques for predicting soft tissue status during pressure induced ischaemia. PhD thesis, Queen Mary, University of London

21. Knight SL, Taylor RP, Polliack AA, Bader DL (2001) Establishing predictive indicators for the status of soft tissues. J Appl Physiol 90:2231–2237
22. Sato K (1977) The physiology, pharmacology and biochemistry of the eccrine sweat gland. Rev Physiol Biochem Pharmacol 79:51–131
23. Sato K, Dobson RL (1973) Glucose metabolism of the isolated eccrine sweat gland. J Clin Investig 5:2166–2174
24. Komives GK, Robinson S, Roberts JT (1966) Urea transfer across sweat glands. J Appl Physiol 21:1681–1684
25. Whitehouse AGR (1935) Dissolved constituents of human sweat. Proc R Soc Lond B 117:139–154
26. Schwartz IL, Thaysen JH, Dole VP (1955) Urea secretion in human sweat as a tracer for movement of water within the secreting gland. J Exp Med 97:429–437
27. Fox IH, Palella TD, Kelly WN (1987) Hyperuricemia: A marker for cell energy crisis. N Engl J Med 317(2):111–112
28. Grum CM, Simon RH, Dantzker DR, Fox IH (1985) Evidence for adenosine triphosphate degradation in critically ill patients. Chest 88:763–767
29. Kock R, Delvoux B, Sigmund M, Greiling H (1994) A comparative study of the concentrations of hypoxanthine, xanthine, uric acid, and allantoin, in the peripheral blood of normal and patients with acute myocardial infarction and other ischaemic disorders. Eur J Clin Chem Clin Biochem 32:837–842
30. Granger DN, Korthuis RJ (1995) Physiological mechanisms of post-ischemic tissue injury. Annu Rev Physiol 57:311–332
31. Wang Y-N (2000) The response of soft tissues to mechanical loads at different structural levels and the implications in their breakdown. PhD thesis, Queen Mary, University of London
32. Gutman I, Wahlefeld AW (1974) L-(+)-Lactate determination with lactic dehydrogenase and NAD. In: Bergmeyer HU (ed) Methods of enzymatic analysis, 2nd English edn. Verlag Chemie/AP, Weinheim, pp 1464–1468
33. Bennett MJ, Carpenter KH (1984) Experience with a simple high-performance liquid chromatography method for the analysis of purine and pyrimidine nucleosides and bases in biological fluids. Ann Clin Biochem 21:131–136
34. Kaldor G, DiBattista WJ (1978) Isoproterenol effects on hearts of ageing rats. Aging 6:101–140
35. Woolliscroft JO, Fox IH (1986) Increased body fluid purine levels during hypotensive events: Evidence for ATP degradation. Am J Med 81:472–478
36. Hyman WA, Artigue RS (1977) Oxygen and lactic acid transport in skeletal muscles. effect of reactive hyperaemia. Ann Biomed Eng 5:260–266
37. Krouskop TA, Reddy NP, Spencer WA, Secor JW (1978) Mechanisms of decubitus ulcer formation: an hypothesis. Med Hypotheses 4:37–39
38. Miller GE, Seal JL (1985) The mechanics of terminal lymph flow. J Biomech Eng 107:376–380
39. Oredsson S, Plate G, Qvarfordt P (1991) Allopurinol- A free-radical scavenger reduces reperfusion injury in skeletal muscle. Eur J Vasc Surg 5:47–52
40. McCord JM (1985) Oxygen-derived free radicals in postischaemic tissue injury. N Engl J Med 312:159–163
41. Walubo A, Smith PJ, Folb PI (1995) Oxidative stress during anti-tuberculosis therapy in young and elderly patients. Biomed Environ Sci 8:106–113
42. Moison RMW, De Beaufort AJ, Haasnoot AA, Dubbelman TMAR, Van Zoeren-Grobbea D, Berger HM (1997) Uric acid and ascorbic acid redox ratios in plasma and tracheal aspiration of preterm babies with acute and chronic lung disease. Free Radical Biol Med 23:226–234

43. McCance RA, Puroait G (1969) Ethnic differences in the response of sweat glands to pilocarpine. Nature 221:378–379

44. Cage GW, Wolfe SM, Thompson RH, Gordon RS (1970) Effects of water intake on composition of thermal sweat in normal human volunteers. J Appl Physiol 29:687–690

45. Dewasmes G, Bothokel B, Hoeft A, Candas V (1993) Regulation of local sweating in sleep-derived exercising humans. Eur J ApplPhysiol 66:542–546

46. Laccourreye O, Bernard D, de Lacharriere O, Bazin R, Brasnn D (1993) Frey's syndrome analysis with biosensor. Arch Otolaryngol Head Neck Surg 119:940–944

47. Mitsubayashi K, Suzuki M, Tamiya E, Karube I (1994) Analysis of metabolites in sweat as a measure of physical condition. Anal Chem Acta 289:27–34

Stump–Socket Interface Conditions

Joan Sanders

9

Introduction

Each year, hundreds of thousands of people undergo a limb amputation. In the US alone, the amputation rate is approximately 84,500 to 114,000 cases per year [1, 2]. There are, in general, two reasons necessitating the surgical removal of a limb: (1) traumatic injury to the point that an extremity cannot be salvaged, for example as experienced in motor vehicle accidents or falls; (2) peripheral vascular disease, e.g. consequent to diabetes or cardiovascular dysfunction. Traumatic injury patients are typically more active and will have a greater number of years as an amputee than dysvascular patients. Thus the performance needs of a prosthesis, a mechanical device intended to replace the missing extremity, are typically more demanding for these individuals.

A prosthesis is made up of a socket that surrounds the residual limb, a terminal device (hand or foot), and an apparatus to connect and adjust the position of the socket relative to the terminal device (Fig. 9.1). Typically the socket is custom-designed for the individual patient while the terminal device and connecting apparatus are purchased commercially. It is recognized in clinical practice that proper design of the socket shape is crucial to the successful clinical performance of a prosthesis. Much of a prosthetist's effort goes into designing and fabricating the prosthetic socket.

Pressure Ulcer Problems Related to Wearing Prostheses

Though both upper-limb and lower-limb prostheses are common, it is lower-limb amputees who most often experience pressure ulcer problems from mechanical irritation with the prosthetic socket. The relatively high loads and their lengthy application times from continual weight bearing and, for the trans-tibial case, the close proximity of the bone to the socket are the reasons. The challenge to a prosthetist is to create a socket that distributes interface stresses in such a way that the prosthetic limb is stably coupled to the bony skeleton yet does not overstress soft tissues. On some patients, this is a seemingly impossible challenge. Stable residual limb–prosthesis mechanical coupling, which will induce a sense of stability to the amputee during gait, requires that high interface stresses be applied. But to avoid skin trauma, interface stresses should be kept low. The skin over the leg

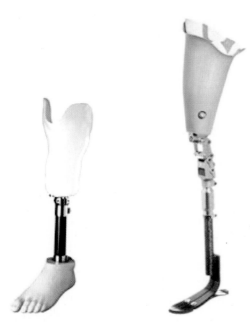

Fig. 9.1. Prosthetic limbs. A trans-tibial prosthesis (*left*) and a trans-femoral prosthesis (*right*) are shown. From Seattle Limb Systems (http://www.soginc.com/SLS) and Ossur Prosthetics (http://www.reykjavikresources.com), respectively

was not intended to tolerate the stresses of weight bearing. Skin there is very different from that on the bottom of the foot, for example.

To design an effective socket, a prosthetist must consider these conflicting design goals and achieve an effective stump–socket interface stress distribution. Using traditional socket design techniques, prosthetists concentrate stresses at load-tolerant areas, for example at the patellar tendon and popliteal fossa on trans-tibial amputees [3, 4] (Fig. 9.2). Loading at the distal third of the residual limb, often a sensitive region, however, is unavoidable. Total contact sockets [5] intended to distribute load uniformly over the stump surface have also been successful and have become increasingly popular in recent years. High distal load-bearing on the bottom of the stump is generally recognized as unfavorable since it can traumatize the soft tissues between the distal end of the bone and bottom of the residual limb. Excessive tissue trauma from distal end-bearing might necessitate surgical revision or amputation to a higher anatomical level. Stresses can be applied in two directions – pressure, which is perpendicular to the skin surface, and shear stress, which is tangential to the skin surface. Both can provide support at the stump–socket interface but above a certain level and duration can induce breakdown.

Skin responds to pressure differently than it does to shear stress. Constant pressure reduces perfusion and can lead to ischemia and tissue necrosis. Just 8 kPa (60 mmHg) pressure is sufficient to occlude skin blood flow [6]. Often, under static loading conditions underlying muscle tissue is affected sooner than skin [7, 8] due to its greater vascularity and metabolic demands. Thus soft-tissue injuries can form in deeper tissue before even being visible on the skin surface.

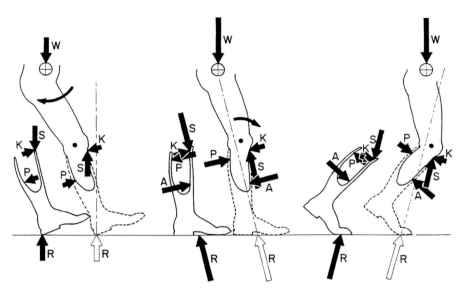

Fig. 9.2. Interface loading during gait. With a patellar-tendon-bearing prosthesis, pressures and shear stresses are concentrated at the patellar tendon bar and at the popliteal fossa. Anterior distal and posterior distal loading, however, are unavoidable. *Left panel* is during heel contact, *center panel* is during mid-stance, and *right panel* is during push-off. From: Radcliffe CW, Foort J. The patellar-tendon-bearing below-knee prosthesis. The Regents of the University of California, 1961

Skin response when shear stress is added is much dependent upon how the shear stress is applied. If shear is applied with slip between the supporting surface and the skin, then it is termed "friction". Friction can lead to blister formation, with blister fluid collecting below the granular layer and above the basal cell layer of the epidermis [9, 10]. Heat built up between the two sliding surfaces may be an important contributor to blister formation. At locations where the epidermis is very thin, an epidermal abrasion will form instead of a blister. For shear stress application without slip between the supporting surface and the skin, often termed "tangential shear," the applied force is distributed through a greater volume of tissue, thus reducing local stress concentrations and reducing the risk of injury. Heat build-up is also reduced. Skin can thus tolerate greater stresses if tangential shear is applied rather than friction [11].

Studies have been conducted attempting to quantify relationships between interface stresses and breakdown. An inverse relationship between pressure and duration in the development of a pressure ulcer was initially proposed in 1942 [7] and later studied further by a number of investigators [8, 12–18]. The results demonstrate a second-order relationship between the threshold pressure for ulcer formation and the duration of pressure application. The threshold pressure decreases quickly as duration is increased. Furthermore, soft tissue can tolerate moderately high load levels provided they are applied intermittently and not continuously. Other studies show that at a sufficiently high level of shear, shear stress will reduce the pressure necessary to cause blood flow occlusion by about one half [19]. Thus in this sense adding shear stresses is unfavorable. However, cyclic shear stresses, as occur on the stump during ambulation with a prosthetic limb, presumably allow release during each step, thus reducing the duration of occlusion and the associated detrimental effects of shear. Under frictional loading where there is slip between the support surface and skin, often unavoidable in prosthetics, quantitative evaluations demonstrate that it is more favorable to apply low frictional loads for a long time than to apply high frictional loads for a short time [20]. Therefore, concentrated frictional stresses should be avoided, and low stresses applied often are a more favorable alternative. Small amounts of fluid added to the interface, as might occur during sweating for example, will increase shear stresses. If the interface is extremely wet (flooded), however, the shear stress will decrease [21]. Thus sweat can alter the original stress distribution designed by the prosthetist. The effects of sweat at the skin–support interface are discussed in more detail in a separate chapter (Chap. 8).

While there is no doubt that interface stresses induce breakdown, it is important to recognize that soft tissues have the capability to remodel and adapt to repetitive stresses. Thus the threshold for inducing injury can be altered through practice. Clinical experience, for example, shows the effectiveness of a mobilization program for an individual with spinal cord injury who has undergone myocutaneous flap surgery to treat a pressure ulcer [22–24]. A 3-week period of pressure relief is followed by short periods of weight bearing in bed. Subsequently, range of motion is increased so as to apply tensile forces to the area, and then a sitting program is initiated, increasing weight bearing duration over time. Tissue tolerance should slowly improve. For an amputee patient with adherent scar tissue on the stump, lubricated tissue massage might be used to improve deep tissue mobilization.

Despite the relevance of soft tissue adaptation to mechanical stress, skin adaptation at the cellular and molecular level is a minimally investigated area of research [25]. A study on pigs showed that after a 1-month period of combined pressure and shear loading on the hind limb, collagen fibrils, the major load-bearing components in skin, were 20.4% larger in diameter than fibrils from unstressed control skin [26]. Similar results were obtained using an in vitro skin organ culture model [27], suggesting that the adaptation process can occur without blood flow being present. In tendon release studies, collagen fibers disaggregated and the density of nonsulfated proteoglycans increased when tension was released [28, 29]. When the tendons were repaired and tension restored, collagen fibers reappeared, the density of nonsulfated proteoglycans decreased, and the density of sulfated proteoglycans increased. Epidermal proliferation and thickening in response to repetitive mechanical loading has also been demonstrated [30, 31]. Thus distinct structural adaptations to repetitive mechanical stress have been shown.

Further investigation into the bioprocesses of adaptation is needed if the adaptive capabilities of soft tissue are to be used to maximal advantage in clinical prosthetic treatment. Molecular-based therapies might be pursued to facilitate adaptation in cases where it is impeded or lacking. A hypothesis of the detailed bioprocesses involved in skin adaptation has been suggested [32] but is currently unproven.

Given that tissue response, whether breakdown or adaptation, is so sensitive to the applied stresses, an important need in prosthetics is to quantify the magnitudes and directions of stresses applied at the stump–socket interface and to identify the prosthesis design features to which they are most sensitive. Such knowledge could enhance treatment as well as prosthetic componentry design.

Interface Stress Measurement

Interface pressures and shear stresses during ambulation with a prosthetic limb have been studied by a number of investigators using a variety of instruments (see Fig. 9.3 for an example system). Strain-gauge transducers [33–48], fluid-filled sensors [49, 50], pneumatic sensors [51–53], printed circuit sheets [54–57], and a field coil and magnet transducer [58] have been used. Only Sanders' and Williams' transducers measured both pressure and shear stress simultaneously. Results show interface pressures to approximately 415 kPa and resultant shear stresses to approximately 65 kPa [57, 59, 60]. As a reference, peak pressures on the foot during walking typically range from 700 to 870 kPa pressure [61, 62], and peak shear stresses from 24 to 70 kPa [63]. 95 kPa of suction applied for 17 min can produce a skin blister [64]. 53 kPa of frictional shear for 40 rubs on a human limb can induce a blister [20]. Thus it is of little surprise that amputees experience breakdown on their residual limbs; the stresses induced are relatively high.

Of relevance to prosthetic design is what happens to interface stresses when features of the prosthesis or amputee subject are changed. The most studied prosthesis design parameter is alignment of the prosthetic components [35, 38, 65–68]. Typically changes in peak interface stresses or interface stresses at the first peak in the axial force curve are analyzed. Results from testing trans-tibial amputee subjects, in general, show that interface stress changes at anterior sites for misaligned compared with aligned prostheses are greater than those at posterior sites [35, 66, 67]. This is a reasonable result given the much thinner layer of soft tissue over bone on anterior trans-tibial stump surfaces compared with posterior surfaces. For translational and angular misalignments that were substantial but deemed clinically safe for lab testing, pressure changes at a site up to 40 kPa [65, 68], 16 kPa [67], and 81 kPa [66] have been reported. If transducers were inserted between the limb and socket instead of flush with the interface, however, much higher pressure changes were measured: 266 kPa [35] and 147 kPa [38]. Sensor protrusion into the skin, however, may have caused erroneously high measurements in these latter studies [69, 70].

Interestingly, three studies showed that compensation for an alignment change in a positive direction was not simply the reverse of the compensa-

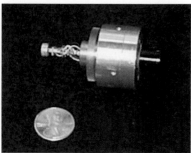

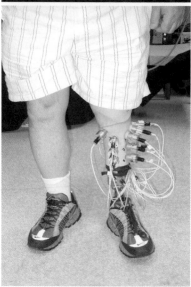

Fig. 9.3. Example of interface stress measurement system. With this system pressures and shear stresses are monitored at 13 socket sites during standing or walking. The transducers and mounts are small and lightweight (< 25 g) so as to minimize weight addition to the prosthesis

tion for the alignment change in the negative direction [35, 66, 67]. At most sites, subjects adjusted their gaits to maximize or minimize interface pressures at the clinically-deemed optimal alignment instead of at the modified alignments. This result points to the importance of an amputee's ability to compensate to prosthesis changes. Subjects adjusted their gaits to accommodate the modifications, in part by the interface conditions they sensed, and those adaptations were not predictable. Variability (standard deviation/mean) did not increase for steps at misaligned compared with aligned settings [66, 67], a result similar to that reported by Jones [71] in analysis of pylon force and moment data.

Effects of changes in socket design and componentry on interface pressures have also been studied [46, 50, 53, 54, 56]. However, most of these reports were in-depth case studies investigating the performance of one particular feature. Generalizations about socket design could not be made. Krouskop [53], however, conducted pressure studies on 18 trans-femoral subjects and noted consistent differences in the pressure distributions between quadrilateral and normal-shape, normal-alignment (NSNA) sockets.

The NSNA had distal loading around the distal femur, while the quadrilateral socket did not.

With advances in materials technology, novel interface liners have been created that can potentially help to improve interface stress distributions. Closed-cell foams are used extensively in the industry. They are typically polyethylene, urethane, or silicone-based. Liners made of polyethylene foams such as Pelite or Plastezote are easily fabricated since these are relatively moldable materials. They also are easily modified later if necessary, using grinding or heat. However, an important weakness is that they deform over time in an unpredictable way, thus altering the original interface shape. More recently, elastomeric liners have become increasingly popular. They are typically made from urethane, silicone elastomers, silicone gels, or an elastomer/gel combination. Elastomeric liners fit snugly on a residual limb, providing direct support during stance phase and, if equipped with a locking pin, suspension during swing phase. They are intended to maintain total contact with the residual limb, thus reducing localized skin tension and shear compared with a conventional closed-cell foam material. This environment should be more comfortable for the amputee. Importantly, because different products have different mechanical properties [72–74], a wide range of liners to meet a range of clinical needs are available. This variety is helpful to prosthetic fitting.

Though the stress changes induced by prosthesis or liner modifications can be relevant to fit, to date the most important feature shown to induce changes in interface stress loading is time. While for short leg-off times (minutes) interface stress changes have been measured at approximately 10%, for sessions more than 3 weeks apart differences can be higher than 50% [46, 60, 65, 66, 67]. In one study even 5-h intervals showed appreciable changes [75]. In this later study, the absolute magnitude pressure difference for 5-h intervals was comparable to that between sessions 5 weeks apart. Thus diurnal changes, not just long-term changes, can be appreciable. Limb shape changes are the most likely sources of interface stress fluctuations, and would be expected to have a strong impact given how sensitive fit is clinically to socket shape.

Problems with Changes in Stump Shape Over Time

Changes in residual limb shape occur for a number of reasons and to varying degrees, depending on the patient's activities, weight, amputation procedure, health, and other factors. Part of the challenge in prosthetic fitting is to accommodate these shape changes.

Differences in the time courses of the two types of changes, diurnal and long-term, must be recognized. Diurnal changes are cyclic, occurring over a 24-h period. In general, residual limbs shrink from the morning to the evening. The change is likely due to extracellular fluid movement, as this mechanism of transport is relatively slow compared with the blood [76,

77]. The pumping effect the socket has on residual limb soft tissues during ambulation may help drive out fluid from within the interstitial spaces over the course of a day [78]. Fluid flow entering the interstitial spaces from the vasculature is low because the prosthetic socket acts as a rigid container to prevent limb expansion, thus preventing an increase in the blood–interstitial fluid pressure difference. The result is an overall dehydration of soft tissues. At night, with no socket to constrain the tissues and the dynamic pumping effect removed, the blood–interstitial fluid pressure difference increases, interstitial fluid returns, and the limb swells back to a larger size.

Long-term shape changes are different than diurnal. They occur over weeks or months, and typically are not easily reversible. They are probably due to soft-tissue remodeling, and can be caused by a variety of factors, including limb maturation, large weight changes, muscle atrophy, and changes in the patient's vascular condition. Thus the mechanisms of diurnal and long-term shape changes are quite different, and one would expect the way they change residual limb shape to be quite different as well.

Experimental research suggests shape changes are distributed differently for diurnal variation than for long intervals [75]. In eight trans-tibial amputees, diurnal changes tended to induce a relatively uniform shrinkage over the residual limb surface. Six-month changes tended to be localized. Variance of the change in cross-sectional area down the length of the residual limb for 6-month intervals was on average 2.8 times higher than that for diurnal intervals. The differences are important because they suggest that different treatment methods might be needed to accommodate diurnal vs. long-term differences.

There are a limited number of methods to accommodate residual limb shape change. Adding/removing stump socks, filling/deflating inflatable inserts, modifying the inside socket shape, and using elastic stockinet shrinkers are examples. The former three methods add material inside the socket to replace departed tissue. Limited data collected on trans-tibial amputee subjects suggests that adding/removing stump socks of uniform thickness does not return interface stresses back to their original values before shrinkage occurred [79]. This result well illustrates one reason why prosthetic fitting is so difficult. A prosthetist must design a limb that will distribute interface stresses properly despite substantial changes in limb shape.

Most air-inflatable insert products are problematic because they tend to perform well at only a single volume level as opposed to a range of levels [80]. Thus they lack versatility. Use of liquid-filled inserts might help to overcome this problem since liquid is relatively incompressible. Whatever route is used to address this challenge, a successful approach will likely need to have some means for allowing subtle volume changes over the course of a day, preferably without the patient needing to manually make the adjustments.

Though progress is being made in interface liners and treatments for shape change, part of the challenge is that it is difficult to conduct controlled testing where just one variable, e.g. the type of liner, is changed. Other features that depend on liner performance, including the patient's stump shape, might change as well. Therefore, the quality of a design is difficult to assess quantitatively, and enhancements and improvements are slow. If an additional means to test different designs that did not have these limitations could be developed, then progress would likely proceed more quickly. Clinical testing could then be used to test only the most promising treatments. Computer modeling is one possible option.

Computer Models for the Design of Stump Sockets

Computer models have been used to try to predict interface stresses for different prosthesis designs and residual limb conditions. Several reviews exist on the topic [81–83]. An advantage of computer models over direct interface stress measurement is that they allow different sockets to be tested without subjecting an amputee's residual limb to potentially detrimental interface stress patterns. In concept, optimization strategies could be developed to interface with the computer models to design an optimal socket for each individual amputee early on in fitting.

Finite-element modeling has been the most common computer modeling method used to try to predict stresses at the stump–socket interface [44, 48, 68, 84–104]. The concept of finite-element modeling is to describe the residual limb and proposed socket design computationally as collections of small blocks or elements. Use of these small simple shapes to characterize the complex residual limb and socket makes the analysis computationally feasible. The stiffness and other material properties of the residual limb and socket, information typically derived from mechanical testing experiments, need to be specified for the analysis to be carried out. Then the mechanical interaction of each element with its neighboring elements is analyzed, based on loads applied in the computer model to the prosthesis or to the proximal residual limb reflective of standing, walking, or some other activity of interest. The computational analysis corresponds to a minimization of the potential energy in the system. The result is a complete description of the stress distribution throughout the residual limb and socket (Fig. 9.4).

The results from finite-element models are potentially very attractive and useful to prosthetists. With this tool a prosthetist can determine the interface stress loading patterns as well as stresses within different residual limb soft tissues for a number of different socket designs before ever actually putting a prosthesis on the patient. However, prosthetic computer models are still in their nascent stages, and they are not yet accurate or rapid enough for clinical use. Part of what makes these models so difficult to develop is that it is computationally very difficult to describe movement between a residual limb and prosthetic socket (pistoning). Some progress has been made using gap [68, 103] or automated contact elements [104]. Further, accurately specifying the material properties of the residual limb for each individual amputee is very challenging. Some instruments for assessment have been developed and used in clinical research [105–107]. Much progress has been made in

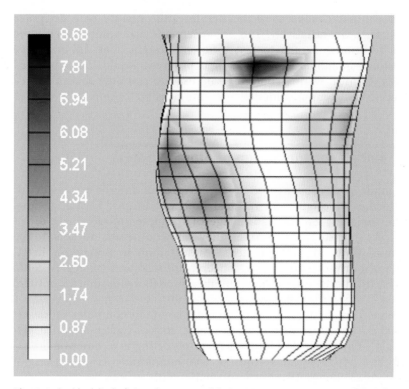

Fig. 9.4. Residual limb finite element model. Donning pressures are predicted for a trans-tibial residual limb in a patellar-tendon-bearing socket. Pressures are concentrated at the patellar tendon and tibial flares, as expected. Units are kPa

the measurement of both the socket and the residual limb shape [108]. Several imaging methods have been used, though the use of video cameras with optical or laser light sources are currently the most common [109–118]. Mesh-generation strategies to create the models quickly and easily have also been developed [119]. Thus considerable progress in finite-element modeling of residual limbs has been made since it was first attempted in 1985 [84], though quality of the models to a level acceptable for clinical practice is still in the future. Once the models are developed a range of features could be tested to establish how they affect interface stress loading, including diurnal and long-term shape change and treatments for stabilization, amputation procedure, and fluid inserts.

Future Perspectives

It is important to recognize that though interface stresses are a crucial feature of prosthetic fit and performance, ultimately it is the response of soft tissues to the stresses that determines breakdown. Several measurements related to tissue quality are possible, including transcutaneous oxygen tension [120, 121], laser Doppler flowmetry [122, 123], and thermal recovery time [124–126]. Transcutaneous oxygen tension is the partial pressure of oxygen in tissue and is typically used to determine level of amputation. Electrodes containing photoelectric sensors capable of distinguishing the wavelengths of oxygenated versus reduced hemoglobin are positioned on the skin to take the measurement. Laser Doppler flowmetry, a technique for assessing flow or perfusion in the microcirculation, is similarly used to determine amputation level. Here the Doppler effect is assessed using a low-power laser directed at the moving blood particulates. Thermal recovery time is a method under development intended to predict the risk of skin breakdown. It is the time after release of a moderate load that is required for the skin temperature difference between the stressed site and a control site to reach either a maximum or a constant value. In a population of nursing home patients, thermal recovery time was shown to correlate strongly with the risk of developing pressure ulcers, with risk defined using data on ulceration occurrence over a 1-month follow-up period [125]. The method was also used in a separate investigation to demonstrate that diabetic patients with autonomic neuropathy had an impaired thermal recovery time after pressure relief compared with normal control subjects [126]. Use of thermal recovery time or a feature from some other imaging modality may possibly quantify breakdown risk at different locations on a stump before a definitive prosthesis is designed. Such instrumentation would be very advantageous to prosthetic fitting.

The direct attachment of a prosthesis to the bony skeleton is a treatment strategy that has been pursued for over 50 years [127]. The concept is to surgically implant a strong biocompatible post within the medullary cavity of a femur or tibia that projects out through the skin. A prosthetic pylon, foot, and, in the trans-femoral case, a knee are then attached to this implant. During weight bearing, ground-reaction forces are transmitted directly to the bony skeleton. An advantage of this method of prosthesis attachment over the traditional prosthetic socket is that soft tissue loading is minimal. Thus skin breakdown problems from contact with a prosthetic socket are non-existent.

Interestingly, mechanical failure at the bone–implant interface has not proven particularly problematic in either animal [128, 129] or human [130–132] studies of direct skeletal attachment. In some patients, the bone–implant interface has proven stronger than either the bone or the prosthesis itself. There is, however, an important limitation with the treatment. The difficulty is that the skin–implant interface is a major source of bacterial penetration and migration. Achieving an effective seal between the skin and the implant is very difficult. Exit site problems are similar to those experienced by peritoneal dialysis patients, prosthetic urethra wearers, and individuals with indwelling blood access devices [133]. Epidermal cells tend to migrate on the implant rather than attach directly to it. Not only can bacteria migrate through spaces at the cell–implant interface, epidermal cells can migrate down and attempt to "grow out" the implant. The result is a site that is, to some degree, perpetually irritated. In some cases the site will be stable for a lengthy period, while in other cases it worsens and an infection develops. Once the bone–implant interface is infected, the implant typically must be removed. Thus direct skeletal attachment is an area of active research and has shown some promising results, but there are still important challenges to be overcome.

Summary

Wearing a prosthesis puts high demands on soft tissues covering the residual limb, particularly for active lower-limb amputees. A prosthetist must use clinical experience, knowledge gained from research studies on tissue response to stress, the capability of the skin to adapt, and individual tissue quality assessment to design an effective prosthesis for an amputee. If stresses at the stump–socket interface are not properly distributed, the amputee can experience blister, cyst, or ulcer formation on the residual limb, conditions that in severe cases worsen and lead to further disability.

Prosthetic interface mechanics studies have provided insight into how amputee and prosthesis characteristics alter interface stresses. Those studies highlight the importance of a person's adaptive capabilities to accommodate prosthesis modifications. An amputee uses, in part, pressure and shear sensation at the stump–socket interface to alter walking style so as to adjust to changing conditions. Results from interface stress studies suggest that while changes in prosthetic alignment, walking speed, and componentry can be accommodated for, changes in the residual limb over time, particularly stump shape and volume, are very difficult to manage. A challenge to prosthetists, amputees, bioengineers, and others in the prosthetics community is to develop effective treatments to overcome shape and volume changes and stabilize fit.

Computer models may eventually contribute towards improvement in the speed and quality of individual socket design for amputee patients. Much progress has been made in computer modeling towards limb geometry and mechanical property characterization, and towards interface specifications. However, until models are shown to accurately predict interface pressures and shear stresses, the capability to use finite element modeling in prosthetic socket design is a goal for the future.

Direct skeletal attachment of a prosthesis to the bony skeleton has been performed on a limited number of amputee patients and may represent a viable means of avoiding the stump–socket interface challenge altogether. However, another interface, the skin–implant interface, is proving problematic in direct skeletal attachment efforts. The interface, once again, will be our challenge.

References

1. Feinglass J, Brown JL, LoSasso A, Sohn M-W, Manheim LM, Shah, SJ, Pearce WH (1999) Rates of lower-extremity amputation and arterial reconstruction in the United States, 1979 to 1996. Am J Public Health 89:1222–1227
2. Dillingham TR, Pezzin LE, MacKenzie EJ (2002) Limb amputation and limb deficiency: epidemiology and recent trends in the United States. South Med J 95:875–883
3. Radcliffe CW (1962) The biomechanics of below-knee prostheses in normal, level, bipedal walking. Artif Limbs 6:16–24
4. McCollough NC, Harris AR, Hampton FL (1981) Below-knee amputation. In: Atlas of limb prosthetics: surgical and prosthetic principles Mosby, St. Louis pp 341–368
5. Hachisuka K, Dozono K, Ogata H, Ohmine S, Shitama H, Shinkoda K (1998) Total surface bearing below-knee prosthesis: advantages, disadvantages, and clinical implications. Arch Phys Med Rehabil 79:783–789
6. Holloway GA, Daly CH, Kennedy D, Chimoskey J (1976) Effects of external pressure loading on human skin blood flow measured by 133Xe clearance. J Appl Physiol 40:597–600
7. Groth KE (1942) Klinische Beobachtungen und experimentelle Studien uber die Entstehung des Dekubitus (Clinical observations and experimental studies of the pathogenesis of decubitus ulcers). Acta Chir Scand 87 [Suppl 76]:1–209
8. Husain T (1953) An experimental study of some pressure effects on tissues, with reference to the bed-sore problem. J Pathol Bacteriol 66:347–358
9. Sulzberger MB, Cortese TA, Fishman L, Wiley HS (1966) Studies on blisters produced by friction. I. Results of linear rubbing and twisting technics. J Invest Dermatol 47:456-465
10. Akers WA, Sulzberger MB (1972) The friction blister. Mil Med 137:1–7
11. Goldstein B, Sanders J (1998) Skin response to repetitive mechanical stress: a new experimental model in pig. Arch Phys Med Rehabil 79:265–272
12. Kosiak M (1959) Etiology and pathology of ischemic ulcers. Arch Phys Med Rehabil 40:62–69
13. Kosiak M (1961) Etiology of decubitus ulcers. Arch Phys Med Rehabil 42:19–29
14. Dinsdale SM (1973) Decubitus ulcers in swine: light and electron microscopy study of pathogenesis. Arch Phys Med Rehabil 54:51–56
15. Dinsdale SM (1974) Decubitus ulcers: role of pressure and friction in causation. Arch Phys Med Rehabil 55:147–152
16. Nola GT, Vistnes LM (1980) Differential response of skin and muscle in the experimental production of pressure sores. Plast Reconstr Surg 66:728–733
17. Daniel RK, Priest DL, Wheatley DC (1981) Etiological factors in pressure sores: an experimental model. Arch Phys Med Rehabil 62:492–498
18. Daniel RK, Wheatley D, Priest D (1985) Pressure sores and paraplegia: an experimental model. Ann Plast Surg 15:41–49
19. Bennett L, Kavner D, Lee BK, Trainor FA (1979) Shear vs pressure as causative factors in skin blood flow occlusion. Arch Phys Med Rehabil 60:309–314
20. Naylor PDF (1955) Experimental friction blisters. Br J Dermatol 67:327–342
21. Naylor PDF (1955) The skin surface and friction. Br J Dermatol 67:239–246
22. Griffith BH (1963) Advances in the treatment of decubitus ulcers. Surg Clin North Am 43:245–260

23. Herceg SJ, Harding RL (1978) Surgical treatment of pressure ulcers. Arch Phys Med Rehabil 59:193–200
24. Daniel RK, Faibisoff B (1982) Muscle coverage of pressure points – the role of myocutaneous flaps. Ann Plast Surg 8:446–452
25. Sanders JE, Goldstein BS, Leotta DF (1995) Skin response to mechanical stress: adaptation rather than breakdown – a review of the literature. J Rehabil Res Dev 32:214–226
26. Sanders JE, Goldstein BS (2001) Collagen fibril diameters increase and fibril densities decrease in skin subjected to repetitive compressive and shear stresses. J Biomech 34: 1581–1587
27. Sanders JE, Mitchell SB, Wang YN, Wu K (2002) An explant model for the investigation of skin adaptation to mechanical stress. IEEE Trans Biomed Eng 49:1626–1631
28. Flint M (1972) Interrelationships of mucopolysaccharide and collagen in connective tissue remodelling. J Embryol Exp Morphol 27:481–495
29. Gillard GC, Reilly HC, Bell-Booth PG, Flint MH (1979) The influence of mechanical forces on the glycosaminoglycan content of the rabbit flexor digitorum profundus tendon. Connect Tissue Res 7:37–46
30. Mackenzie IC (1974) The effects of frictional stimulation on mouse ear epidermis. I. Cell proliferation. J Invest Dermatol 62:80–85
31. Mackenzie IC (1974) The effects of frictional stimulation on mouse ear epidermis. II. Histologic appearance and cell counts. J Invest Dermatol 63:194–198
32. Wang YN, Sanders JE (2003) How does skin adapt to repetitive mechanical stress to become load tolerant? Med Hypotheses 61:29–35
33. Sonck WA, Cockrell JL, Koepke GH (1970) Effect of liner materials on interface pressures in below-knee prostheses. Arch Phys Med Rehabil 51:666–669
34. Rae JW, Cockrell JL (1971) Interface pressure and stress distribution in prosthetic fitting. Bull Prosthet Res 10-15:64–111
35. Pearson JR, Holmgren G, Marsh L, Oberg K (1973) Pressures in critical regions of the below-knee patellar-tendon-bearing prosthesis. Bull Prosthet Res 10-19:52–76
36. Pearson JR, Grevsten S, Almby B, Marsh L (1974) Pressure variation in the below-knee, patellar teondon bearing suction socket prosthesis. J Biomech 7:487–496
37. Burgess EM, Moore AJ (1977) A study of interface pressures in the below-knee prosthesis (physiological suspension: an interim report). Bull Prosthet Res 10-28:58–70
38. Winarski DJ, Pearson JR (1987) Least-squares matrix correlations between stump stresses and prosthesis loads for below-knee amputees. J Biomech Eng 109:238–246
39. Leavitt LA, Peterson CR, Canzoneri J, Paz R, Muilenburg AL, Rhyne VT (1970) Quantitative method to measure the relationship between prosthetic gait and the forces produced at the stump-socket interface. Am J Phys Med 49:192–203
40. Leavitt LA, Zuniga EN, Calvert JC, Canzoneri J, Peterson CR (1972) Gait analysis and tissue-socket interface pressures in above-knee amputees. South Med J 65:1197–1207
41. Appoldt FA, Bennett L (1967) A preliminary report on dynamic socket pressures. Bull Prosthet Res 10-8:20–55

42. Redhead RG (1979) Total surface bearing self suspending above-knee sockets. Prosthet Orthot Int 3:126–136
43. Bielefeldt A, Schreck HJ (1979) The altered alignment influence on above-knee prosthesis socket pressure distribution. Int Series Biomech 3-A:387–393
44. Steege JW, Schnur DS, Van Vorhis RL, Rovick JS (1987) Finite element analysis as a method of pressure prediction at the below-knee socket interface. In: Proc 10th Annual RESNA Conference. RESNA Press, Washington DC, pp 814–816
45. Sanders JE, Daly CH (1993) Measurement of stresses in three orthogonal directions at the residual limb-prosthetic socket interface. IEEE Trans Rehabil Eng 1:79–85
46. Sanders JE, Zachariah SG, Baker AB, Greve JM, Clinton C (2000) Effects of changes in cadence, prosthetic componentry, and time on interface pressures and shear stresses of three trans-tibial amputees. Clin Biomech 15:684-694
47. Silver-Thorn MB, Steege JW, Childress DS (1992) Measurements of below-knee residual limb/prosthetic socket interface pressures. In: Proc 7th World Congress ISPO, Chicago, IL, 280
48. Torres-Moreno R, Solomonidis SE, Jones D (1992) Load transfer characteristics at the socket interface of above-knee amputees. In: Proc 7th World Congress ISPO, Chicago, IL, 151
49. Van Pijkeren T, Naeff M, Kwee HH (1980) A new method for the measurement of normal pressure between amputation residual limb and socket. Bull Prosthet Res 10-33:31–34
50. Naeff M, Van Pijkeren T (1980) Dynamic pressure measurements at the interface between residual limb and socket – the relationship between pressure distribution, comfort, and brim shape. Bull Prosthet Res 10-33:35–50
51. Mueller SJ, Hettinger T (1954) Die messung der druckverteilung im schaft von prothesen (Measuring the pressure distribution in the socket of the prosthesis). Orthopadie-Technik Heft 9:222–225
52. Lebiedowski M, Kostewicz J (1977) Determination of the pressure exerted by dynamic forces on the skin of the lower-limb stump with prosthesis. Chir Narzadow Ruchu Ortop Pol 42:619–623
53. Krouskop TA, Brown J, Goode B, Winningham D (1987) Interface pressures in above-knee sockets. Arch Phys Med Rehabil 68:713–714
54. Engsberg JR, Springer JN, Harder JA (1992) Quantifying interface pressures in below-knee-amputee sockets. J Assoc Childrens Prosth-Orthot Clin 27:81–88
55. Convery P, Buis AWP (1998) Conventional patellar-tendon-bearing (PTB) socket/stump interface dynamic pressure distributions recorded during the prosthetic stance phase of gait of a trans-tibial amputee. Prosthet Orthot Int 22:193–198
56. Convery P, Buis AWP (1999) Socket/stump interface dynamic pressure distributions recorded during the prosthetic stance phase of gait of a trans-tibial amputee wearing a hydrocast socket. Prosthet Orthot Int 23:107–112
57. Polliack AA, Craig DD, Sieh RC, Landsberger S, McNeal DR (2002) Laboratory and clinical tests of a prototype pressure sensor for clinical assessment of prosthetic socket fit. Prosthet Orthot Int 26:23–34
58. Williams RB, Porter D, Roberts VC, Regan JF (1992) Triaxial force transducer for investigating stresses at the stump/socket interface. Med Biol Eng Comput 30:89–96
59. Sanders JE (1995) Interface mechanics in external prosthetics: review of interface stress measurement techniques. Med Biol Eng Comput 33:509–516

60. Sanders JE, Lam D, Dralle AJ, Okumura R (1997) Interface pressures and shear stresses at thirteen socket sites on two persons with transtibial amputation. J Rehabil Res Dev 34:19-43

61. Armstrong DG, Peters EJ, Athanasiou KA, Lavery LA (1998) Is there a critical level of plantar foot pressure to identify patients at risk for neuropathic foot ulceration? J Foot Ankle Surg 37:303–307

62. Lavery LA, Armstrong DG, Wunderlich RP, Tredwell J, Boulton AJ (2003) Predictive value of foot pressure assessment as part of a population-based diabetes disease management program. Diabetes Care 26:1069–1073

63. Hosein R, Lord M (2000) A study of in-shoe plantar shear in normals. Clin Biomech 15:46–53

64. Lowe LB Jr, van der Leun JC (1968) Suction blisters and dermal-epidermal adherence. J Invest Dermatol 50:308–314

65. Appoldt FA, Bennett L, Contini R (1968) Stump-socket pressure in lower extremity prostheses. J Biomech 1:247–257

66. Sanders JE, Bell DM, Okumura RM, Dralle AJ (1998) Effects of alignment changes on stance phase pressures and shear stresses on trans-tibial amputees: measurements from 13 transducer sites. IEEE Trans Rehabil Eng 6:21–31

67. Sanders JE, Daly CH (1999) Interface pressures and shear stresses: sagittal plane angular alignment effects in three trans-tibial amputee case studies. Prosthet Orthot Int 23:21–29

68. Zhang M, Turner-Smith AR, Roberts VC, Tanner A (1996) Frictional action at lower-limb/prosthetic socket interface. Med Eng Phys 18:207–214

69. Appoldt FA, Bennett L, Contini R (1969) Socket pressure as a function of pressure transducer protrusion. Bull Prosthet Res 10-11:236–249

70. Patterson RP, Fisher SV (1979) The accuracy of electrical transducers for the measurement of pressure applied to the skin. IEEE Trans Biomed Eng 26:450–456

71. Jones D, Paul JP (1978) Analysis of variability in pylon transducer signals. Prosthet Orthot Int 2:161–166

72. Emrich R, Slater K (1998) Comparative analysis of below-knee prosthetic socket liner materials. J Med Eng Technol 22:94–98

73. Covey SJ, Muonio J, Street GM (2000) Flow constraint and loading rate effects on prosthetic liner material and human tissue mechanical response. J Prosthet Orthot 12:15–32

74. Sanders JE, Nicholson BS, Zachariah SG, Cassisi DV, Karchin A, Fergason JR (2004) Testing of elastomeric liners used in limb prosthetics: classification of 15 products by mechanical performance. J Rehabil Res Dev 41:175–186

75. Sanders JE, Zachariah SG, Jacobsen AK, Fergason JR (2005) Changes in interface pressures and shear stresses over time on trans-tibial amputee subjects ambulating with prosthetic limbs: comparison of diurnal and six-month differences. J Biomech 38:(in press)

76. Aukland K, Nicolaysen G (1981) Interstitial fluid volume: local regulatory mechanisms. Physiol Rev 61:556–643

77. Aukland K (1984) Distribution of body fluids: local mechanisms guarding interstitial fluid volume. J Physiol (Paris) 79:395–400

78. Aukland K, Reed RK (1993) Interstitial-lymphatic mechanisms in the control of extracellular fluid volume. Physiol Rev 73:1–78

79. Sanders JE, Fergason JR, Zachariah SG, Jacobsen AK (2002) Interface pressure and shear stress changes with amputee weight loss: case studies from two trans-tibial amputee subjects. Prosthet Orthot Int 26:243–250

80. Sanders JE, Cassisi DV (2001) Mechanical performance of inflatable inserts used in limb prosthetics. J Rehabil Res Dev 38:365–374
81. Silver-Thorn MB, Steege JW, Childress DS (1996) A review of prosthetic interface stress investigations. J Rehabil Res Dev 33:253–266
82. Zachariah SG, Sanders JE (1996) Interface mechanics in lower-limb prosthetics: a review of finite element models. IEEE Trans Rehabil Eng 4:288–302
83. Zhang M, Mak AFT, Roberts VC (1998) Finite element modeling of a residual lower-limb in a prosthetic socket: a survey of the development in the first decade. Med Eng Phys 20:360–373
84. Krouskop TA, Goode BL, Dougherty DR, Hemmen EH (1985) Predicting the loaded shape of an amputees residual limb. In: Proc 8th Annual RESNA Conference. RESNA Press, Washington, DC, pp 225–227
85. Krouskop TA, Muilenberg AL, Doughtery DR, Winningham DJ (1987) Computer-aided design of a prosthetic socket for an above-knee amputee. J Rehabil Res Dev 24:31–38
86. Krouskop TA, Malinauskas M, Williams J, Barry PA, Muilenburg AL, Winningham DJ (1989) A computerized method for the design of above-knee prosthetic sockets. J Prosthet Orthot 1:131–138
87. Steege JW, Schnur DS, Childress DS (1987) Prediction of pressure at the below-knee socket interface by finite element analysis. In: ASME Symposium on the Biomechanics of Normal and Pathological Gait, pp 39–44
88. Steege JW, Childress DS (1988) Finite element prediction of pressure at the below-knee socket interface. In: Report of ISPO Workshop on CAD/CAM in Prosthetics and Orthotics, pp 71–82
89. Steege JW, Childress DS (1988) Finite element modeling of the below-knee socket and limb: phase II. In: Modeling and control issues in biomechanical systems. ASME DSC-12:121–129
90. Steege JW, Silver-Thorn MB, Childress DS (1992) Design of prosthetic sockets using finite element analysis. In: Proc 7th World Congress ISPO, Chicago, IL, 273
91. Steege JW, Childress DS (1995) Analysis of trans-tibial prosthetic gait using the finite element technique. In: Proc 21st Annual Meeting Scientific Symposium AAOP, 13–14
92. Brennan JM, Childress DS (1991) Finite element and experimental investigation of above-knee amputee limb/prosthesis systems: a comparative study. In: Proc ASME, Advances in Bioengineering, BED-20:547–550
93. Quesada P, Skinner HB (1991) Analysis of a below-knee patellar-tendon-bearing prosthesis: a finite element study. J Rehabil Res Dev 28:1–12
94. Mak AFT, Yu YM, Hong ML, Chan C (1992) Finite element models for analyses of stresses within above-knee stumps. In: Proc 7th World Congress ISPO, Chicago, IL, 147
95. Reynolds DP, Lord M (1992) Interface load analysis for computer-aided design of below-knee prosthetic sockets. Med Biol Eng Comput 30:419–426
96. Silver-Thorn MB, Childress DS (1992) Use of a generic, geometric finite element model of the below-knee residual limb and prosthetic socket to predict interface pressures. In: Proc 7th World Congress ISPO, Chicago, IL, 272
97. Silver-Thorn MB, Childress DS (1992) Sensitivity of below-knee residual limb/prosthetic socket interface pressures to variations in socket design. In: Proc 7th World Congress ISPO, Chicago, IL, 148

 98. Silver-Thorn MB, Childress DS (1997) Generic, geometric finite element analysis of the transtibial residual limb and prosthetic socket. J Rehabil Res Dev 34:171–186

 99. Torres-Moreno R, Solomonidis SE, Jones D (1992) Geometrical and mechanical characteristics of the above-knee residual limb. In: Proc 7th World Congress ISPO, Chicago, IL, 149

100. Torres-Moreno R, Solomonidis SE, Jones D (1992) Three-dimensional finite element analysis of the above-knee residual limb. In: Proc 7th World Congress ISPO, 274

101. Sanders JE, Daly CH (1993) Normal and shear stresses on a residual limb in a prosthetic socket during ambulation: comparison of finite element results with experimental measurements. J Rehabil Res Dev 30:191–204

102. Vannah WM, Childress DS (1993) Modeling the mechanics of narrowly contained soft tissues: the effects of specification of Poisson's Ratio. J Rehabil Res Dev 30:205–209

103. Zhang M, Lord M, Turner-Smith AR, Roberts VC (1995) Development of a non-linear finite element modelling of the below-knee prosthetic socket interface. Med Eng Phys 17:559–566

104. Zachariah SG, Sanders JE (2000) Finite element estimates of interface stress in the trans-tibial prosthesis using gap elements are different from those using automated contact. J Biomech 33:895–899

105. Malinauskas M, Krouskop TA, Barry PA (1989) Noninvasive measurement of the stiffness of tissue in the above-knee amputation limb. J Rehabil Res Dev 26:45–52

106. Vannah WM, Childress DS (1996) Indentor tests and finite element modeling of bulk muscular tissues in vivo. J Rehabil Res Dev 33:239–252

107. Pathak AP, Silver-Thorn MB, Thierfelder CA, Prieto TE (1998) A rate-controlled indentor for in vivo analysis of residual limb tissues. IEEE Trans Rehabil Eng 6:12–20

108. Zheng YP, Mak AF, Leung AK (2001) State-of-the-art methods for geometric and biomechanical assessments of residual limbs: a review. J Rehabil Res Dev 38:487–504

109. Duncan JP, Foort J, Mair SG (1974) The replication of limbs and anatomical surface by machining from photogrammetric data. Proc 1974 Symposium Commission V, International Society Photogrammetry Biostereometrics 531–553

110. Fernie GR, Halsall AP, Ruder K (1984) Shape sensing as an educational aid for student prosthetists. Prosthet Orthot Int 8:87–90

111. Fernie GR, Griggs G, Bartlett S, Lunau K (1985) Shape sensing for computer aided below-knee prosthetic socket design. Prosthet Orthot Int 9:12–16

112. Smith DM, Crew A, Hankin A (1985) Silhouetting shape sensor. University of College London, Bioengineering Centre Reports 41–42

113. Oberg K, Kofman J, Karisson A, Lindstrom B, Sigblad G (1989) The CAPOD system – a Scandinavian CAD/CAM system for prosthetic sockets. J Prosthet Orthot 1:139–148

114. Engsberg JR, Clynch GS, Lee AG, Allan JS, Harder JA (1992) A CAD CAM method for custom below-knee sockets. Prosthet Orthot Int 16:183–188

115. Mackie JCH, Jones D, Hughes J (1986) Stump shape identified from multiple silhouettes. In: Proc 5th World Congress ISPO, 303

116. Houston VL, Mason CP, Beattie AC, LaBlance KP, Garbarini M, Lorenze EJ, Thongpop CM (1995) The VA-Cyberware lower limb prosthetics-orthotics optical laser digitizer. J Rehabil Res Dev 32:55–73
117. Schreiner RE, Sanders JE (1995) A silhouetting shape sensor for the residual limb of a below-knee amputee. IEEE Trans Rehabil Eng 3:242–253
118. Commean PK, Smith KE, Vannier MW (1996) Design of a 3-D surface scanner for lower limb prosthetics: a technical note. J Rehabil Res Dev 33:267–278
119. Zachariah SG, Sanders JE, Turkiyyah GM (1996) Automated hexahedral mesh generation from biomedical image data: applications in limb prosthetics. IEEE Trans Rehabil Eng 4:91–102
120. Tremper KK, Shoemaker WC (1981) Transcutaneous oxygen monitoring of critically ill adults, with and without low flow shock. Crit Care Med 9:706–709
121. Dodd HJ, Gaylarde PM, Sarkany I (1985) Skin oxygen monitoring in venous insufficiency of the lower leg. J R Soc Med 78:373–376
122. Gebuhr P, Jorgensen JP, Vollmer-Larsen B, Nielsen SL, Alsbjorn B (1989) Estimation of amputation level with a laser Doppler flowmeter. J Bone Joint Surg Br 71:514–517
123. Adera HM, James K, Castronuovo JJ Jr, Byme M, Deshmukh R, Lohr J (1995) Prediction of amputation wound healing with skin perfusion pressure. J Vasc Surg 21:823–829
124. Meijer JH, Schut GL, Ribbe MW, Goovaerts HG, Nieuwenhuys R, Reulen JP, Schneider H (1989) Method for the measurement of susceptibility to decubitus ulcer formation. Med Biol Eng Comput 27:502–506
125. Meijer JH, Germs PH, Schneider H, Ribbe MW (1994) Susceptibility to decubitus ulcer formation. Arch Phys Med Rehabil 75:318–323
126. van Marum RJ, Meijer JH, Bertelsmann FW, Ribbe MW (1997) Impaired blood flow response following pressure load in diabetic patients with cardiac autonomic neuropathy. Arch Phys Med Rehabil 78:1003–1006
127. Rubin G, Wilson AB (1981) Skeletal attachment of prosthesis. In: Atlas of limb prosthetics – surgical and prosthetic principles Mosby, St. Louis, pp 435–439
128. Hall CW (1974) Developing a permanently attached artificial limb. Bull Prosthet Res 144–157
129. Hall CW (1985) A future prosthetic limb device. J Rehabil Res Dev 22:99–102
130. Branemark R, Branemark PI, Rydevik B, Myers RR (2001) Osseointegration in skeletal reconstruction and rehabilitation: a review. J Rehabil Res Dev 38:175–181
131. Holgers KM, Branemark PI (2001) Immunohistochemical study of clinical skin-penetrating titanium implants for orthopaedic prostheses compared with implants in the craniofacial area. Scand J Plast Reconstr Surg Hand Surg 35:141–148
132. Sullivan J, Uden M, Robinson KP, Sooriakumaran S (2003) Rehabilitation of the trans-femoral amputee with an osseointegrated prosthesis: the United Kingdom experience. Prosthet Orthot Int 27:114–120
133. Von Recum AF (1984) Applications and failure modes of percutaneous devices: a review. J Biomed Mater Res 18:323–336

Perspectives of Numerical Modelling in Pressure Ulcer Research

10

Cees Oomens

Introduction

The primary cause of pressure ulcers is some form of prolonged mechanical load, although environmental and intrinsic factors have an influence on the development. Without the mechanical loading no wound will develop. This means that studying the response of soft biological tissues to mechanical loading is a critical issue and this may be achieved by the use of theoretical models. There is a surprising dearth of published studies on pressure ulcers backed by some form of theoretical analysis. Speculative and intuitive statements on the role of mechanical loads and the influences of shear, pressure and traction on tissue behaviour and on the assumed occlusion of blood vessels are abundant, however, on occasion supported by experimental evidence. One can only guess why this is the case. One reason might be the paucity of bioengineers involved in pressure ulcer research, although it is also true that the level of sophistication of theoretical models has long been far from realistic. However, it is believed that the current prospects are very good, and this is an opportune moment to examine the potential of available theoretical, numerical models as a tool in pressure ulcer research. The objective of this chapter is to show where mechanical modelling can be important or even indispensable. This will include a description of how models were used in the past, what can be expected in the near future and which are the bottlenecks in this research.

Basically there can be two reasons for the development of theoretical models. The first is to use models as a design tool for patient support surfaces in the most general sense, ranging from beds and wheelchairs or wheelchair cushions to prostheses for patients with an amputation. This approach will obviate the need for extensive prototyping and may lead to computer-aided optimization of patient support surfaces. The first section is devoted to modelling that is used for this purpose.

The second reason to use theoretical models is to understand the very complex phenomena in soft tissues such as skin, fat and muscle under prolonged mechanical load. In studies on the aetiology of pressure ulcers these models are indispensable. The second section is devoted to these models.

Models for the Design of Supporting Surfaces

Most of the theoretical models that were developed as design tools for supporting surfaces were devoted to prosthetic sockets for upper- and lower-limb amputees. This work was reviewed recently by Zhang et al. [1] and is discussed in Chap. 9 by Sanders. The present section is limited to supporting surfaces for seated persons in wheelchairs.

Chow and Odell [2] published one of the first finite-element studies with particular reference to this research area. To evaluate the quality of cushions, these authors postulated that it was necessary to predict the complete state of stress and strain inside the soft body tissues of a sitting person. In other words, knowledge of the pressure distribution at the interface was insufficient. Their motivation for this approach was based on the observation that even very high hydrostatic pressures are not damaging to the soft tissues, suggesting that tissue deformation is the critical factor. That is why a finite-element analysis seemed appropriate. Based on measured pressure distributions, Chow and Odell [2] assumed that an axi-symmetric model was sufficient and studied the stress/strain state under different loading conditions with a range of support cushions. The contact properties were modelled by applying a modified cosine pressure distribution at the interface. Their most important conclusion was: "The distortion of tissues is often more severe at internal locations than on the surface of the buttocks".

Todd and Thacker [3] presented a three-dimensional computer model of the human buttocks to understand the risk of developing a pressure ulcer while sitting in a wheelchair. Their objective was to show that a finite-element model could be developed that gave results consistent with experimental data and to relate buttock/cushion interface pressures to internal pressures at the ischium. A finite-element model was developed, based on MR images with a 1-mm resolution. Subjects were placed in supine position in the tube of a whole-body MR system. From transverse cross sections a 3-D image was reconstructed. Bone, soft tissue and cushion properties were modelled. A linear elastic, isotropic model with small deformations was used. For the seated persons the same model was used, but the stiffness values for the tissues were increased to simulate characteristics in the seated position. The load was based on the individual bodyweight of the test persons, with half bodyweight transferred in the seated position. The results were based on displacements, principal stresses and von Mises stresses. The latter parameter appeared to provide a good representation of the areas corresponding to the highest values for tissue deformation. Indeed, von Mises stresses were found near bony prominences, which may explain why in many cases severe ulcers are initiated within the muscle tissues.

Dabnichki et al. [4] attempted to demonstrate that a finite-element model of a buttock can be a valuable tool for evaluation of support surfaces. They were the first group to perform a geometrically nonlinear analysis and employ contact elements to obtain an improved description of the mechanical state at the interface between buttock and cushion. Although some critical remarks can be made with respect to the material laws used for both the soft tissues and the cushion [5], the use of the large deformation theory and contact elements can be considered a considerable step forward in this type of modelling. They used a geometrical model of the buttock comparable to the Chow and Odell model. Frictionless contact and contact with friction were simulated. In the former case, the results suggested a minimal (negative) principal stress near the bony prominence. The highest shear strain was found in the middle of the tissue, although a local maximum was found adjacent to the bony prominence. The case with friction showed only minimal changes near to the bone, but higher compressive stresses were estimated near to the buttock/tissue interface. A softer cushion reduces peak stresses and leads to a change of location for the maximum shear stress.

A logical extension of this model was performed by the present author [6] by employing improved material laws for the soft tissues composite, with distinct properties for skin, fat and muscle layers. For the reference model material properties were used which were obtained from animal experiments. To account for the uncertainty in these data a sensitivity analysis was performed with respect to fat properties and the thickness of individual layers. In addition, variations with cushion properties and different frictional properties of the interface were performed. The major conclusions from previous model studies [4] were confirmed by this study. A remarkable result was that a reduction of the stiffness properties of the cushion led to very high changes in the maximum shear strain in the fat layer. By contrast, the same reduction in cushion stiffness only marginally influenced the high local maximum shear strain in the muscle near the bony prominence. As expected, a softer cushion led to a more equal pressure distribution at the interface with lower peak stresses than with a stiffer cushion. This is an important result, because it confirmed that even though the interface pressure was lower and the shear strains in the fat were lower, the shear strains in the muscle were still at a high risk level. These findings have significant consequences for the design of supporting surfaces.

How realistic is it to assume that mechanical models can really play a role in the future design of supporting surfaces? Finite-element models should satisfy specific demands:

- ▌ They should be realistic, meaning that the geometry, loading history and other boundary conditions have to be realistic.
- ▌ Sufficiently accurate material laws have to be available for the different tissues involved, preferably with information on individual tissue tolerance.
- ▌ As an interactive design tool, the model has to be developed in a limited amount of time.
- ▌ Simulations with the model have to be fast, especially when the model is used in an optimization loop.

At the present time it is possible to develop models with a fairly realistic geometry using loading conditions close to reality. Figure 10.1 shows a solid model of a part of a skeleton and a finite-element model of the buttock region

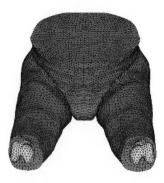 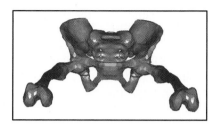

Fig. 10.1. Mesh used for comfort analysis of human sitting on a cushion [7]

and upper limbs of a seated person [7]. This model is based on data of a seated cadaver that was digitized for a large European project (HUMOS I) on human modelling. Starting from this database the meshing of this region took 3 months with a highly sophisticated mesh generator. One single analysis with an explicit code on a medium sized computer (Pentium III) takes approximately 3 days. However, there are reports that with a semi-two-dimensional approach real-time finite-element method comes into reach [8].

Compared with the time it takes to develop mannequins for experimental testing and the costs associated with such experiments, theoretical models of this kind will certainly be competitive. Although the CPU time for the analysis is high for optimization purposes, developments in computer hardware and especially in parallel processing will reduce this problem considerably.

Models to Be Used as a Tool to Understand Aetiology

The alternative approach is to utilize theoretical models to provide an improved understanding of the aetiology of pressure ulcers. This section will include a description of relevant studies on this subject, as well as a comment on future developments.

Sacks et al. [9] provided a simple, but elegant, attempt to understand the inverse relationship between external pressure levels and the risk of developing an ulcer by using a dimensional analysis. The authors assumed that a definable allowable pressure exists that will initiate an ulcer. Moreover, this pressure was assumed to depend on physical properties of the tissue (tissue density ρ, tissue elastic modulus E), time t and the local blood flow Q before the load is applied. Thus a mathematical relationship was formulated, such that:

$$p_s = f(\rho, Q, E, t) \tag{10.1}$$

By using a simple dimension analysis the assumption led to a relationship between the allowable pressure and time:

$$p_s = a + Bt^{-4/3} \tag{10.2}$$

Apart from the constants A and B, which, of course, vary for different types of experiments, the exponent of $-4/3$ of the time in Eq. 10.2 fitted remarkably well to experimental data. An important remark in the paper is the rationale that the formation of pressure ulcers primarily depends on tissue properties, irrespective of the type of loading. These properties change with age and pathology and can make individuals more or less susceptible to pressure ulcers.

In a comparable dimension analysis Sacks [10] demonstrates that experiments on skin blood flow changes can best be presented in dimensionless form of blood flow decrease against tissue strain and not as a relation of blood flow versus pressure. The first presentation allows a comparison between similar groups of patients, while the second method depends on too many geometric variables.

Mak et al. [11] and Zhang et al. [12] explored an idea that had been published earlier by Reddy [13], namely that interstitial fluid flow may play a part in pressure ulcer development. By means of a biphasic poro-elastic analysis these later authors studied the behaviour of skin as a function of time under a prolonged mechanical load. What is clear from the theory is that the interstitial fluid takes up most of the loading just after the external pressure is applied, but with time this fluid diminishes and the load is increasingly carried by the solid matrix. The authors tried to compare their model results with the experimental data from Reswick and Rogers [14]. Although a little premature in view of more recent evidence suggesting the important roles of fixed charge density and charge of ions, causing osmotic swelling effects, this study made clear that the mechanical state of the soft tissues changes with time, even with a constant external load. Keeping in mind that the duration of the load is a risk factor, this must be an important observation.

From the above it should be appreciated that the local tissue deformation is a better predictor of damage leading to a pressure ulcer than the external load or pressure. This becomes more evident when discussing the assumed greater risk of shear than of compression. Shear is supposed to be a higher risk because vessels can be occluded more easily by shear than by compression. However, this discussion was somewhat confused by abuse of terminology. In 1994 Zhang et al. [15] attempted to clarify this confusion with a combined theoretical and experimental analysis. These authors were careful to distinguish clearly between the external load that was applied (which can be a shear force, a compressive force or a combination of both) and the resulting internal stress and strain within the tissue. The best way to illustrate this is by looking at uniaxial compression and simple shear. Consider the uniaxial compression, for which Fig. 10.2a and Fig. 10.2b represent the same object with the same deformation. In the centre point of the specimen the strain tensor of this mechanical system is given by:

$$\underline{\varepsilon} = e_{11}\vec{e}_1\vec{e}_1 + \varepsilon_{22}\vec{e}_2\vec{e}_2 + \varepsilon_{33}\vec{e}_3\vec{e}_3 \text{ with } \varepsilon_{11} = \varepsilon_{33} \tag{10.3}$$

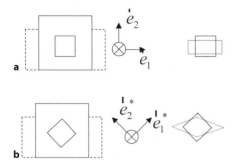

Fig. 10.2 a, b. Schematic drawing of uniaxial compression test. *Solid line,* undeformed configuration; *dotted line,* deformed

If this equation is written in matrix form, with respect to a vector basis $\{\vec{e}_1, \vec{e}_2, \vec{e}_3\}$ this leads to the following strain matrix:

$$\underline{\varepsilon} = \begin{pmatrix} \varepsilon_{11} & 0 & 0 \\ 0 & \varepsilon_{22} & 0 \\ 0 & 0 & \varepsilon_{11} \end{pmatrix} \tag{10.4}$$

If the object is rotated by 45° the matrix representation of the same strain tensor with respect to basis $\{\vec{e}_1^{\,*}, \vec{e}_2^{\,*}, \vec{e}_3^{\,*}\}$ is:

$$\underline{\varepsilon}^* = \frac{1}{2} \begin{pmatrix} \varepsilon_{11} + \varepsilon_{22} & \varepsilon_{22} - \varepsilon_{11} & 0 \\ \varepsilon_{22} - \varepsilon_{11} & \varepsilon_{11} - \varepsilon_{22} & 0 \\ 0 & 0 & 2\varepsilon_{11} \end{pmatrix} \tag{10.5}$$

This means that if a small specimen is cut from the object, like the centre square in Fig. 10.2 a, it stretches in the same way as the macroscopic specimen. However, if a centre square is cut from the object oriented in a way like the square in Fig. 10.2 b it will stretch and shear! Thus, although many might consider that the macroscopic deformation was compressive, it is in fact a combination of compression and shear in nature. For each material point we can find principal strain directions that, if used as a basis, would lead to a matrix like that in Eq. 10.4. We can also find a direction for which the maximum shear strain in a material is reached. In the above example this is an angle of 45° with respect to basis $\{\vec{e}_1, \vec{e}_2, \vec{e}_3\}$. The principal strains and the maximum shear strain are invariants and are mechanical properties that may be suitable to use in damage criteria (depends on the kind of material we look at).

Zhang et al. (1994) examined the maximum shear strain inside the tissue for different external loading conditions, namely, compression, shear, and a combination of the two modes. Their findings may be summarized as:

1. The maximum compressive stress (strain) inside the tissue is determined by the resultant of shear and compression.
2. When an external shear force is applied, the location within the tissue with the highest shear strain will shift in the direction of the load if compared to the location for an external compressive load.

3. The external shear force mainly influences the stress/strain state near the surface, while the compressive load mainly influences this state in the deeper layers.

The aforementioned studies, representing global analyses using fairly simple theoretical models, elucidate some of the confusing discussions on pressure ulcers in the literature. However, to understand the conditions within the tissue more complicated models need to be adopted. This inevitably necessitates the use of micro- or mesoscopic models or a combination of models in a multi-scale approach. One such model, developed at Eindhoven University of Technology in the Netherlands, will be described in the following section.

Multi-scale Modelling of Tissues

The model is based on a number of experimental observations, which will be discussed first. Bouten et al. [17] and Breuls et al. [16] compressed tissue-engineered constructs with well-controlled mechanical loads and related local cell deformation to cell death. From these studies it has become clear that muscle cells are susceptible for deformation, even if transport processes through the construct are not disturbed. It may be that the deformation changes the transport properties of the cell membrane, eventually leading to damage, but it is not caused by a reduced supply of oxygen and nutrients from the environment. From this they concluded that a damage threshold for cells can be defined in relation to deformation of the cells (see Fig. 10.3).

In an alternative approach Bosboom et al. [18, 19] performed animal studies involving the loading of the tibialis anterior muscle of rats with an indenter for 2 h. After 24 h the animals were sacrificed and, by means of histological techniques, damaged muscle cells were localized and quantified. This study was subsequently repeated using T2-weighted MRI (see

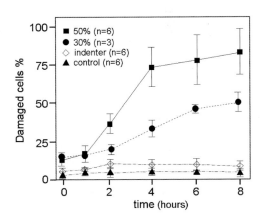

Fig. 10.3. Percentage dead cells as a function of time for different straining regimes (reprinted with permission from [21])

Chaps. 12 and 18). The large variation in damage distributions between samples precluded the adoption of a direct relationship between a deformation index and the resulting damage. To find this relationship it is probably necessary to follow damage development as a function of time, which is possible with MRI. Nonetheless, these studies did indicate that in the initial phases of damage healthy cells were present adjacent to dead cells. It may be postulated that the most vulnerable cells first lose viability, although it may be argued that due to the heterogeneous structure of the tissue, some cells have to carry a much higher load than others.

These two ideas, namely that muscle cells can only withstand a deformation for a limited amount of time and that the inhomogeneous structure of the tissue plays an important role in damage development, were explored theoretically by Breuls et al. [20], using a multi-level finite-element approach. A global macroscopic model of, for example, a skeletal muscle is created by discretizing the geometry in a finite-element mesh. The microstructure at a particular point of the tissue is given by a representative volume element (RVE). In the multi-level finite-element approach, microstructural finite-element models, representing the RVEs, are assigned to each integration point of the macroscopic elements. By using periodic boundary conditions and stress/strain averaging, the global and the microscopic mesh are coupled. In this way it is possible to determine the actual load on individual cells as a result of a typical microstructure and, at the same time, determine how material properties change on a macro scale when cells are dying.

Breuls assumed a damage evolution based on the assumption that if the strain energy density (SED) of a cell exceeds a damage threshold, governed by the adaptive capacity of the cell, a, damage starts to accumulate in the

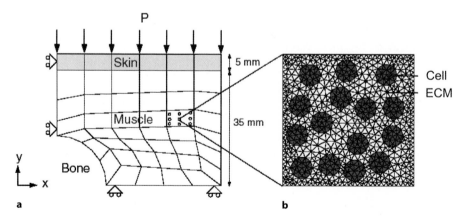

Fig. 10.4. a Macroscopic mesh, representing muscle and skin layers that are compressed against a bony prominence by an external pressure *P*. The nine *circles* in one particular macroscopic element indicate the location of the macroscopic integration points to which the microstructural models are assigned. **b** Microstructural mesh representing a simplified geometry of randomly dispersed cells embedded in extracellular matrix (*ECM*) material (reprinted with permission from [21])

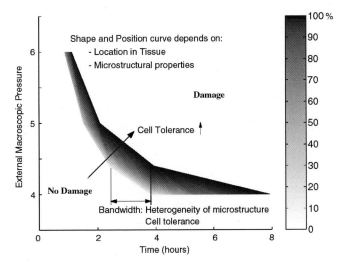

Fig. 10.5. Damage evolution in a particular microstructure at four different external pressures P (4 kPa, 4.4 kPa, 5 kPa and 6 kPa). The vertical axis of each subplot is the external pressure P, while the horizontal axis denotes the time of compression. The *bar* on the right represents the percentage of damaged cells in the microstructure (reprinted with permission from [21])

cell. This adaptive capacity, or tissue tolerance, may change with age or disease. When the accumulated damage becomes higher than a threshold value T_{cell}, the cell will die. It is evident that in a heterogeneous microstructure not all cells "feel" the same SED and, hence, evolution of damage will be different between cells. By fitting the damage evolution of RVEs on the experimental data from cell culture experiments, Breuls et al. were able to determine the parameters and T_{cell} for skeletal muscle cells.

This theory was subsequently applied to a macroscopic muscle and skin layer over a bony prominence, as depicted schematically in Fig. 10.4. The tissue was loaded with a uniformly distributed load at the skin surface. This approach resulted in the observations that damaged areas became evident within the tissue at different points in time.

By performing a number of analyses of this type, a pressure/time risk curve could be produced, as illustrated in Fig. 10.5. Such a curve indicates the importance of cell tolerance, which itself will be influenced by pathology and age, the microstructure of the skeletal muscle and, often ignored, the location in the tissue.

Future Developments

It is difficult to predict the future, but a few trends are visible, which probably will influence developments in the immediate future.

In material science and mechanics of polymers and composites, researchers have acknowledged in the last two or three decades that to really understand and predict the behaviour of materials it is necessary to examine details at the micro-structural level. They realized that the heterogeneity of materials has a profound influence on the way damage initiates and evolves. By understanding the microstructural behaviour it became possible to predict material behaviour and to design new materials on demand. It was also clear that cooperation between different disciplines, including chemistry, mechanical engineering and physics, was necessary to reach this goal. This has led to new theoretical developments, such as non-local continuum mechanics, continuum damage mechanics and multi-level finite-element method, etc.

In biomechanics a comparable development has taken place. By means of studies on cultured cells and by tissue engineering it has become possible to study metabolic processes and damage and adaptation in very well controlled microscopic environments. All kinds of vital imaging techniques are becoming available. At the level of animal experiments and human studies, imaging techniques are also improving, leading to detailed microscopic information that is obtained in an in-vivo set-up. The inhomogeneous structure of all biological materials was cited as a major complication in the past, but was often ignored in the analysis. Currently, the inhomogeneous structure is recognized as an essential feature that has to be included in studies attempting to achieve understanding of damage and adaptation processes in tissues. The aforementioned developments make it possible to adopt such an approach.

From a theoretical point of view phenomenological models at a macroscopic level are no longer sufficient. It is becoming increasingly important to develop models at a microscopic level, including models on the lymph- and microcirculation, detailed models on transport processes of nutrients, small molecules like oxygen and CO_2, models on cell growth and cell death, consumption and synthesis. These will be indispensable to predict the time and location of cell death. Nonetheless it is essential to connect this microstructural research with the macroscopic world of the patient with pressure ulcers. Multi-level type approaches can be a valuable tool for this.

References

1. Zhang M, Mak AFT, Roberts VC (1998) Finite element modelling of a residual lower-limb in a prosthetic socket: a survey of the development in the first decade. Med Eng Phys 20:360–373
2. Chow WW, Odell EI (1978) Deformations and stresses in soft body tissues of a sitting person J Biomech Eng 100:79–87
3. Todd BA, Thacker JG (1994) Three-dimensional computer model of the human buttocks, in vivo. J Rehab Res Dev 31(2):111–119
4. Dabnichki PA, Crocombe AD, Hughes SC (1994) Deformation and stress analysis of supported buttock contact, Part H: J Eng Med 208:9–17
5. Barbenel JC, Lee VSP (1994) Discussion on paper of Dabnichki et al, Part H. J Eng Med 208:263–266

6. Oomens CWJ, Bressers OFJT, Bosboom EMH, Bouten CVC, Bader DL (2003) Can loaded interface characteristics influence strain distributions in muscle adjacent to bony prominences? Comp Meth Biomech Biomed Eng 6(3):171–180

7. Verver MM, Hoof J van, Oomens CWJ, Wismans JSHM, Baaijens FPT (2004) A finite element model of the human buttocks for prediction. Comp Meth Biomech Biomed Eng 7:193–203

8. Linder-Ganz E, Gefen A (2004) Mechanical compression-induced pressure sores in rat hindlimb: muscle stiffness, histology, and computational models. J Appl Physiol 96:2034–2049

9. Sacks AH, O'Neill H, Perkash MD (1985) Skin blood flow changes and tissue deformations produced by cylindrical indentors. J Rehab Res Dev 22(3):1–6

10. Sacks AH (1989) Theoretical prediction of a time-at-pressure curve for avoiding pressure sores. J Rehab Res Dev 26(3):27–34

11. Mak AFT, Huang L, Wang Q (1994) A biphasic analysis of the flow dependent subcutaneous tissue pressure and compaction due to epidermal loadings: issues in pressure sores. J Biomech Eng 116:421–429

12. Zhang JD, Mak AFT, Huang LD (1997) A large deformation biomechanical model for pressure ulcers. J Biomech Eng 119:406–119

13. Reddy NP (1981) Interstitial fluid flow as a factor in decubitus ulcer formation. J Biomech 14:879–881

14. Reswick J, Rogers J (1976) Experience at Rancho Los Amigos Hospital with devices and techniques to prevent pressure sores. In: Kenedi RM, Cowden JM, Scales J (eds) Bed sore biomechanics. Macmillan, London, pp 301–310

15. Zhang M, Lord M, Turner-Smith AR, Roberts VC (1994) Development of a nonlinear finite element modeling of the below-knee prosthetic socket interface. Med Eng Phys 17:559–566

16. Breuls RGM, Bouten CVC, Oomens CWJ, Bader DL, Baaijens FPT (2003) Compression induced cell damage in engineered muscle tissue. Ann Biomed Eng 31(11):1357–1365

17. Bouten CVC, Knight MM, Lee DA, Bader DL (2001) Compressive deformation and damage of muscle cell sub-populations in a model system. Ann Biomed Eng 29(2):153–163

18. Bosboom EMH, Hesselink M., Oomens CWJ, Bouten CVC, Drost MR, Baaijens FPT (2001) Passive transverse mechanical properties of skeletal muscle under in-vivo compression. J Biomech 34 (10):1365–1368

19. Bosboom EMH, Bouten CVC, Oomens CWJ, Straaten HWM van, Baaijens FPT, Kuipers H (2001) Quantification and localisation of damage in rat muscles after controlled loading; a new approach to study the aetiology of pressure sores. Med Eng Phys 23:195–200

20. Breuls RG, Sengers BG, Oomens CWJ, Bouten CVC, Baaijens FPT (2002) A multi-level finite element model to study muscle damage in tissue engineered skeletal muscle. J Biomech Eng 124:198–207

21. Breuls RGM, Oomens CWJ, Bouten CVC, Bader DL, Baaijens FPT (2003) A theoretical analysis of damage evolution in skeletal muscle tissue with reference to pressure ulcer development. J Biomech Eng 125:902–909

Skin Morphology and Its Mechanical Properties Associated with Loading

Satsue Hagisawa, Tatsuo Shimada

Introduction

It is recognized that pressure ulcers develop as a consequence of soft tissue reaction to mechanical loading of localized areas for a prolonged period of time, resulting in ischaemia followed by tissue necrosis. Therefore, in order to prevent the development of pressure ulcers it is essential to reduce the amount and duration of pressure and/or to enhance the tissue tolerance to ischaemia. In this regard, numerous studies have been undertaken in recent decades in the attempt to reduce the amount and duration of interface pressure applied to the skin surface, especially with regard to supporting surfaces. However, not much work has been carried out regarding tissue tolerance in terms of pressure ulcer development and how the structural characteristics of the tissue affect tissue tolerance.

In this chapter, we set out to demonstrate the morphological characteristics of human tissue, especially the skin, to discuss how morphology affects mechanical properties and to highlight the deficiencies in this field of pressure ulcer research.

What Is "Tissue Tolerance"?

What does "tissue tolerance" represent? How can we evaluate "tissue tolerance"? Without answering these questions, how can we verify that all pressure ulcers are preventable?

The tissue tolerance in pressure ulcer development will be defined as a tissue resistance to mechanical stress representing a tissue integrity, where the function and structure are inter-relatively well maintained without adverse sequence. The intensity of tissue resistance is affected by various intrinsic factors (Fig. 11.1). These can be divided into two groups, systemic and local factors, where systemic factors include nutrition [1, 2], mobility/activity [3], oxygen intake and delivery [4], and existing disease/disability, which affect the local tissues' integrity indirectly.

Local factors include nerve control, immunity, metabolism, circulation and tissue structure/composition, all of which affect underlying tissue viability/integrity directly. Ageing [5] and psychological stress [6, 7] may also influence the systemic and local intrinsic factors. Many studies have been

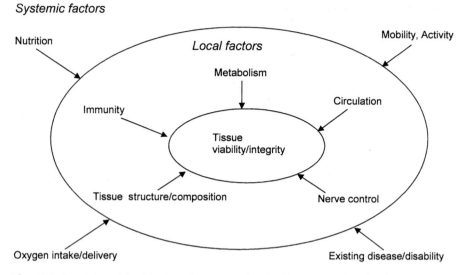

Fig. 11.1. Systemic and local intrinsic factors associated with pressure ulcer development

undertaken to evaluate the tissue viability following ischaemia by measuring skin blood flow [8, 9] and transcutaneous PO_2 ($TcPO_2$) [10, 11], both of which are parameters of function. The circulation is also closely related to metabolism and immunity, participating in tissue tolerance at cellular level. Little work has been undertaken to determine how the tissues react to mechanical forces to protect themselves locally. The cellular enzymes and/or metabolites may be more sensitive indicators of cellular dysfunction and death [12]. Only tentative attempts have been made to seek the potential indicators of pressure ulcer onset through biochemical analysis of sweat during ischaemia [13, 14]. In general, the local tissue metabolism changes in association with the local blood flow under normal conditions; however, it is not certain how this relationship is altered under pathological conditions [15], e.g. multi-organ failure or paralysis. If the relationship is altered, the recovery of blood flow following ischaemia may not be a sign of tissue recovery, as indicated below.

Recently a concept of reperfusion injury has been introduced to explore the mechanism of pressure ulcer development. The reperfusion injury has already been demonstrated in other organs, e.g. brain, liver and heart, in which much of the injury occurs not during the period of hypoxia but rather during the period of reperfusion [16]. During reperfusion, formation of reactive oxygen metabolites, which generate superoxide and hydrogen peroxide, contributes to granulocyte infiltration, microvascular barrier disruption and oedema formation [17, 18]. These products are powerful mediators of endothelial injury and tissue damage and amplify the effects of the initial inflammatory stimulus. The concept that free radicals have a role in ischaemic injury is supported by studies demonstrating that the administration of free radical scavengers inhibits the damage caused by postischaemic reperfusion. Sundin et al. [19] and Houwing et al. [20] investigated the role of reperfusion injury and the effect of free radical scavengers in pigs with regard to pressure ulcer development. They concluded that an inflammatory process is the key mechanism in the development of necrosis in the deeper subcutis and muscle. More basic study is needed to determine how the immune, metabolic and circulatory systems inter-relating in the process of tissue damage-recovery with regard to human pressure ulcer development.

Limitation of Previous Animal Studies on Pressure Ulcers

A number of animal experiments have been undertaken to clarify the development of pressure ulcers histologically, using various animal models. Husain [21], Kosiak [22], Wilms-Kretchmer and Majno [23], and Nola and Vistnes [24] used rats, Groth [25] used rabbits, Kosiak [26] used dogs, and Dinsdale [27] and Daniel et al. [28] used pigs. The results from these studies demonstrate that there is an inverse relationship between the amount of pressure and the duration of time to development of pressure ulcers. Reswick and Rogers [29] demonstrated a similar relationship in human subjects.

However, there are limitations to the extrapolation of results from animal studies to pressure ulcer development in humans. The results with regard to magnitude and duration of pressure before tissue damage occurred are inconsistent and difficult to compare because of the different animal models, different protocols and different parameters measured. In addition, the investigators used mostly healthy, young animals, whereas the susceptible humans are mostly aged and debilitated. In addition, the soft tissue composition of the animal models used (except pigs) differs from that in humans (Table 11.1). The usual laboratory animals with loose skin, e.g. rats and dogs, lack a substantial attachment to the deep fascia, whereas in the pig skin the panniculus carnosus is more intimately connected through a hypodermal fibre network to the deep muscular fascia as well as to the reticular layer of the dermis [30]. Thus, the soft tissue behaviour in animals with loose skin is different from those with fixed skin when the force is applied to the skin. Little work has been done on human tissues with respect to pressure ulcer formation. In addition, human pressure ulcers develop due to localized tissue ischaemia caused by repeatedly applied forces, mostly a combination of compression and shear stress.

One of the difficulties in undertaking the research on pressure ulcer development in human is the issue of ethics; another is that the soft tissue loses its characteristics when it is separated from the living body for the examination. Therefore, it is difficult to create a human pressure ulcer model, especially with regard to loading conditions and clinical status. Thus, the precise mechanisms of pressure ulcer development in humans remain uncertain.

Table 11.1. Differences in characteristics between experimentally generated pressure ulcers in animal models and human pressure ulcers developed

	Animal models of pressure ulcers	Human pressure ulcers
Health condition	Mostly healthy, young adult animals	Mostly elderly, debilitated, or disabled individuals
Pressure application	Mostly wide range of pressure, continuously (recently: determined pressure, repeatedly	Relatively low pressure, repeatedly
Direction of force application	Mostly compression only	Probably compression + shear
Tissue characteristics	Loose-skin (except pig)	Fixed skin

How Does the Skin Respond to Mechanical Loading?

Morphological Architecture in Human Skin

Human tissues function depending on the local tissue need and are controlled in a sophisticated manner with changes in physiology and morphology. Therefore, when discussing morphological changes in relation to pressure ulcer development, we should keep in mind that physiological changes are always present too.

Before discussing the morphological characteristics of skin, we would like to describe how the force is transmitted to the underlying tissues when it is applied to the skin surface.

The underlying soft tissues consist mainly of skin, adiposa tissue and muscle. Because these tissues have different characteristics in respect of linearity, anisotropy and visco-elasticity, it is not easy to identify how differently the individual layers of soft tissues behave when the force is applied to the skin surface and how it is transferred through the soft tissues. In this regard, Le et al. [31] measured pressures at different depths of the tissues overlying the pig trochanter using silicon pressure sensors. They reported that the internal pressure on the weight-bearing bony prominence was several times greater than the surface pressure. However, the sensor they used is somewhat unreliable because of hysteresis and the effect of infusion fluid on local tissue pressure.

Dodd and Gross [32] measured the interface pressure between the skin and an external load, and interstitial fluid pressure over the wing of the ilium of a pig using a wick-in-needle catheter attached to the pressure transducer. They reported that only about 28% of the interface pressure is transferred to the interstitial fluid directly because of the complex geometry of the underlying bone; the load is not purely compressive, as tissues move away from the load and the forces are dissipated to some degree.

The structure of underlying soft tissues also influences the capability of pressure distribution. Sangeorzan et al. [33] investigated the tolerance of skin to mechanical loading over the tibia and over the tibialis anterior muscle in normal volunteers. The results indicated that the applied pressure at which $TcPO_2$ reached 0 was significantly greater for skin over muscle (71 ± 16 mmHg) than for skin over bone (42 ± 8 mmHg). This suggests that a higher pressure is required to interrupt blood supply in skin over muscle than in skin over bone.

In this regard, Todd and Thacker [34] verified a computational three-dimensional model of the human buttock in vivo with magnetic resonance imaging experimentally. The development of a precise model of human soft tissue is needed to examine how the force is transferred to individual tissues and how the individual tissue responds when the force is applied to the surface of the skin.

In this chapter, the mechanical properties of soft tissue are discussed. The focus is on skin as a typical example.

Skin Structure/Physiology

The skin has been called the largest organ of the human body and has many functions; protection from outside injury and invasion, prevention from drying out, regulation of body temperature and release of some body wastes while absorbing nutrients. The structure of the skin is shown in Fig. 11.2.

Morphologically, skin is composed of two layers; a thinner, outer layer known as the epidermis and an inner layer known as the dermis. Because

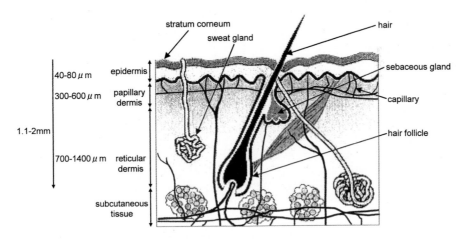

Fig. 11.2. Schematic diagram of skin structure

the epidermis contains keratin, a tough, fibrous protein, and has no blood supply, its nutrition is provided via the papillary layer of the dermis. The exposed surface of the epidermis is illustrated in Fig. 11.3.

The dermis is the connective tissue matrix of the skin, providing structural strength, storing water, and interacting with the epidermis. It consists of papillary and reticular layers containing collagen and elastic fibres, blood vessels, sweat glands, hair follicles and nerves.

The papillary layer, which provides oxygen and nutrition to the epidermis, and the reticular layer are of great importance in maintaining the integrity of the skin and protecting the body from external stimuli. The thickness of the papillary layer varies from site to site (Fig. 11.4); it is thinner in the sacral skin than in the ischial skin of aged individuals post mortem [35]. This suggests that the blood supply and nutritional transport in the sacral skin may be impaired when force sufficient to induce collapse is applied.

The epidermal–dermal junction is an interface between the epidermis and the dermis composed of the basement membrane, which is wavy in shape with finger-like projections into the dermis (Fig. 11.3). It has three major functions: it provides a permeable barrier between the vascular dermis and avascular epidermis; it is thought to influence the epidermal cells during their differentiation, growth, and repair; and it provides adherence of the epidermis to the underlying tissues [36]. In addition, the structure

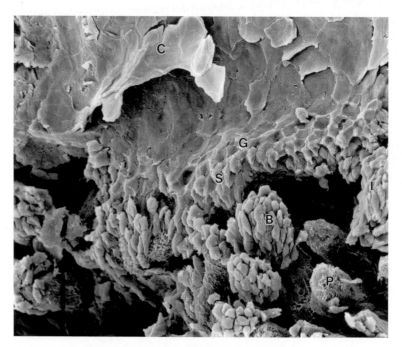

Fig. 11.3. Scanning electron micrograph showing free and lateral surfaces of the human epidermis. Age 73 years, female, sacrum (×560). B stratum basale, C stratum corneum, G stratum granulosum, P dermal papillae, S stratum spinosum

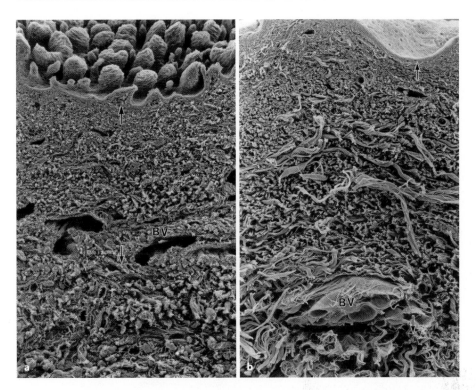

Fig. 11.4 a, b. The papillary layer of the dermis in different body sites. The thickness of the papillary layer allowing tissue fluid transportation is less in the sacrum. *Arrows* show the thickness of the papillary layer. Age 73 years, female (×130). **a** sacrum; **b** gluteus. *BV* Blood vessels

of the epidermal–dermal junction may greatly affect the tissue integrity. The skin capillaries are situated just under the reticulin sheet of the papillary layer of the dermis, providing the oxygen and nutrients to the epidermis. Thus, if the junction becomes flattened, capillary density becomes less and consequently compromises the tissue viability.

The distribution of blood capillaries in the papillary dermis depends upon the local tissue metabolic requirements and thus differs according to site on the body [37], age, and usage [38]. They are densely distributed in the head and neck region in children's skin compared with all other regions except the palm and sole, while they are less dense in the lower limb [39]. This phenomenon is also seen in the adult skin, as confirmed by Xe clearance [40]. A typical example of regional difference is seen in the fingers, where the blood capillaries are densely distributed due to the frequent use.

Capillary distribution in areas susceptible to pressure ulcers in aged post-mortem skin was found to be higher in the sacrum than in the ischial tuberosity (Fig. 11.5) [35].

The lymph vessels are primarily involved with removing proteins, large waste particles, and excess fluids. Most studies on pressure ulcers are inter-

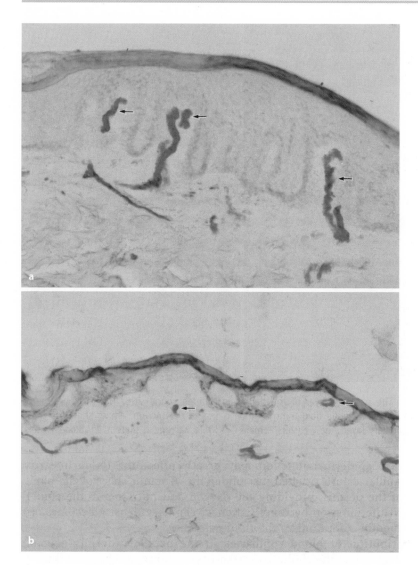

Fig. 11.5 a, b. Blood capillary (*arrows*) distribution in different body sites corresponding to papillae distribution. Age 73 years, female (×100). **a** sacrum; **b** gluteus

ested in blood flow (inflow), but in order to maintain the normal circulation, both inflow and outflow (lymphatic flow), should be well maintained.

The terminal lymphatics, made up of a single layer of endothelial cells, are distributed in the dermis. Several lymphatics join to form collecting lymphatics under the dermis. These join to form larger transporting lymphatics. There are some open junctions and rare intercellular channels in the terminal lymphatics. The surrounding connective perivascular matrix is characterized by regular bundles of collagen and elastic fibres [41]. The terminal lymphatics do not have smooth muscle in the wall. Some of them are collapsed in normal condition and are connected to tissue fibres via anchoring filaments [42, 43]. In contrast, the transporting lymph vessels have smooth muscle, controlling fluid transportation by its contraction. Reddy and Patel [44] attempted to formulate a mathematical model and simulate lymph flow through terminal lymphatics under various physiological conditions.

Lymph flow increases whenever the interstitial fluid pressure rises above its normal level. Miller and Seale [45] investigated lymph clearance during compressive loading on the hind limb of mongrel dogs and reported that a pressure of 60 mmHg can initiate lymph vessel closure. They also suggested that it is more likely that the terminal lymph vessels would collapse before the collecting lymph vessels as they are smaller and closer to the site of pressure application. Krouskop [7] reported that the lymphatic propulsion is dependent on lymphatic smooth muscle sensitive to hypoxia. However, not much attention has been paid to how the lymph flow affects the viability in the impending tissues with respect to pressure ulcer development.

The defence system of the body against external stimuli – Langerhans' cells in the epidermis and the immune system participating in the body's immune response – is related to tissue integrity. If the barrier is disrupted, both a cytokine response and an increase in Langerhans' cell density are induced [46].

Little attention has been paid to how this defence system is associated with pressure ulcer formation. Recently Sundin et al. [19] investigated the role of allopurinol and deferoxamine, both acting to prevent free radical formation or to scavenge free radicals. They attempted to explore pressure ulcer pathogenesis using pigs, in which 150 mmHg of pressure was applied to the scapulae repeatedly. As a conclusion, it was demonstrated that deferoxamine could significantly reduce cutaneous and skeletal muscle necrosis compared with allopurinol. Similarly, research was undertaken by Houwing et al. [20] to test the hypothesis that pressure ulcers are the results of inflammation caused by ischaemia and reperfusion, and that the pressure damage can be reduced by prophylactic administration of vitamin E as a free radical scavenger. A constant force (100 N) was applied to the trochanteric region of the pig for 2 h. Immediately after release of pressure, no pressure damage in the muscle was visible microscopically, whereas 2 h after, there was severe influx of granulocytes and the myocytes had completely disappeared, showing muscle necrosis. There was a significant increase in hydrogen peroxide after pressure release. After pre-treatment with vitamin E, however, there was no increase in hydrogen peroxide and the tissue damage was significantly less.

Mechanical Properties of the Skin

The skin is a visco-elastic material showing unique mechanical properties primarily reflecting the characteristics of the network of collagen and elastic fibres that support tensile loads (Fig. 11.6).

Therefore, if the structure/composition of the skin has been changed, it is assumed that the mechanical properties of the skin are also altered.

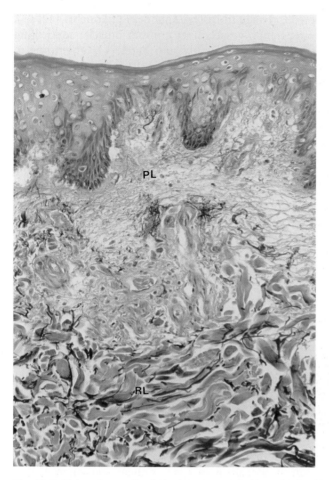

Fig. 11.6. Light micrograph of the human sacral skin stained with both aldehyde-fuchsin and light green. In the dermis, elastic fibres (*purple*) are in close proximity to collagen fibres (*green*). Both types of fibres are much denser and much larger in the reticular layer (*RL*) than in the papillary layer (*PL*). Age 79 years, male (×280)

In the relaxed state, the collagen fibres are unoriented, convoluted structures separated from each other by tissue fluid and ground substance [47]. As skin is stretched along one or both of the axes within its plane, collagen fibres become straightened and then begin to align with the applied force. When the skin is fully stretched, tissue fluid and ground substance between the collagen fibres is displaced. A stress–strain curve for skin is characterized by three components – low modulus, linearity and yield – and by failure when the load is increased [47].

The behaviour of the soft tissues, and thus the nature of the recovery, will depend on the rate and time of loading as well as the magnitude. Short-term loading generally produces elastic deformation with minimum

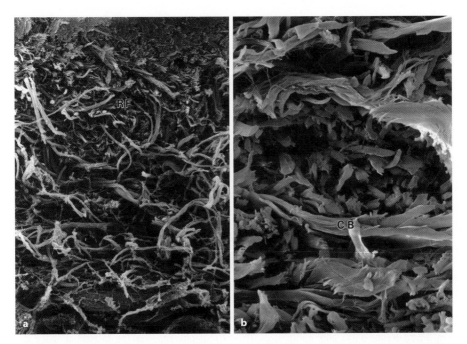

Fig. 11.7. Higher magnification views of the cut surface of the papillary (a) and the reticular (b) dermis. Delicate reticulin fibrils (*RF*) with small diameter are seen in the papillary layer. In the reticular layer, collagen bundles (*CB*) consisting of collagen fibrils form a feltwork. Age 79 years, male (×1,400)

creep and rapid elastic recovery, whereas long-term loading results in marked creep and requires significant time for complete tissue recovery.

When the force is applied, initially elastic fibres are thought to be stretched, while collagen fibres change their geometrical configuration before they play a part in load resistance. If the force applied is extensive, the collagen fibres will not return to their original alignment even after the force is removed [47].

Collagen, elastic fibres and proteoglycans play a key role in determining the mechanical properties acting to maintain tissue shape, transmit/absorb loads, and recover from deformation. Collagen is the major structural component existing in a variety of diameters and geometries (Fig. 11.7)

Collagen fibres are made up of fibrils. The molecules of the fibrils are arranged in a staggered array with quarter-length overlap between adjacent molecules via cross-links that provide stress-bearing networks. In the absence of cross-links, connective tissue would not be able to support tensile loads. The type and extent of cross-link may be a critical factor affecting mechanical properties. The collagen fibres consist of bundles of fibrils, 0.6–1.8 μm in diameter in the papillary layer, and 6–10 μm in the reticular layer, that are responsible for preventing tensile and shear failure.

The collagen fibrils in the skin are composed primarily of collagen types I and III. The diameter of collagen type I, 80–120 nm, is greater than that of

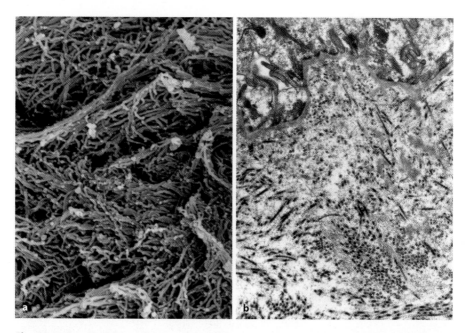

Fig. 11.8. Scanning (**a**) and transmission (**b**) micrographs showing the interstitial space between reticulin fibrils of the dermal papillae. It allows transportation of tissue fluid and metabolites. Age 84 years, female, sacrum (**a** ×20,600; **b** ×14,300)

type III, 40–60 nm. The most superficial surface of the papillary layer is made up of a continuous thin sheet of reticulin fibrils (type III), showing finger-like configuration, a delicate network and regular arrangement of the dermal papillae. The reticulin fibrils are interwoven in slightly loose networks with 30- to 60-nm spaces through which the tissue fluid and other substances pass [48]. This space plays an important role in maintaining viability of the tissues by enabling exchange nutrients and metabolites (Fig. 11.8).

Type I collagen fibrils are mainly found in the reticular layer of the dermis. This layer is composed of a dense meshwork of large-diameter collagen fibres showing a feltwork appearance, accompanied by elastic fibres (Fig. 11.7).

Collagen fibril diameter distribution is a function of both the applied load and its duration. The mechanical properties of a connective tissue are strongly correlated with the collagen fibril diameter distribution [49].

The mechanical properties of elastic fibres can be compared with a rubber-like state. The ultimate tensile stress of elastic fibres amounts to only several percent of that of collagen fibres [50]. Therefore, elastic fibres are weaker, softer, and more extensible than collagen fibres.

Elastic fibre networks dominate the low-strain mechanical response in tissues where energy and shape recovery are critical parameters [50]. The diameter of elastic fibres is approximately 1–10 μm; each fibre is made up of microfibrils of 10-12 nm in diameter. The fibres are connected via cross-

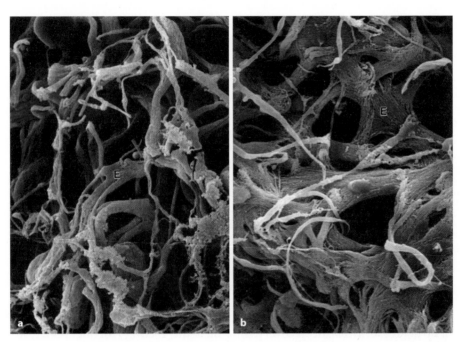

Fig. 11.9 a, b. Elastic bundles (*E*) distributed in the human papillary layer. Thick elastic bundles are densely distributed in the ischial skin. Elastic fibres were exposed with a treatment of 6N NaOH solution at 60 °C to enable three-dimensional visualization. Age 87 years, female (×6,500). **a** sacrum; **b** ischium

links, similar to collagen. The distribution of elastic fibres in the areas of the skin prone to pressure ulcers has been examined microscopically by Hagisawa et al. [35]. Thick elastic fibres (5–10 μm) are densely distributed in the ischial skin, where extension of the skin is needed associated with various body movements, in contrast with the sacral skin, where thinner, less dense elastic fibres (2–3 μm) are seen (Fig. 11.9). This difference may greatly contribute to tissue recovery from deformation in the ischial skin, in which the blood restoration may also be facilitated following ischaemia.

Proteoglycans consists of a protein core to which glycosaminoglycan side chains are attached, composing the bulk of the interfibrillar matrix, including hyaluronic acid, chondroitin sulphate and dermatan sulphate. Proteoglycans are involved in resisting compressive forces and facilitation of the response to stress at the fibrillar level [50].

Factors Affecting Tissue Integrity

When the structure/composition of the skin has been changed by various factors, the mechanical properties leading to tissue integrity may also be altered. However, little work has been undertaken to demonstrate how it is altered. In this chapter, ageing, loss of autonomic nerve control and moisture are described as affecting factors.

Age-associated changes in skin are manifested in all regions of the body. Many of the structural alterations correlate with mechanical, biochemical, and physiological changes associated with advancing age. The epidermis becomes thinner and flatter, and the epidermal–dermal junction is flattened with loss of rete pegs, resulting in decreased attachment strength and interface communication. Age-associated changes also increase the chance of skin breakdown when force is applied tangentially, thus making blisters or tear-type injury more likely [51].

The quality of collagen fibres changes in aged skin, affecting the tensile strength. The collagen fibres may appear looser and fibre bundles may be disrupted by tangled fibrils, or the collagen may be densely packed in some areas with loss of ground substance [52], resulting in less potential for spaces between the fibres. The number of intramolecular cross-links become less soluble and the size of the collagen fibres increase with advancing age; thus, there is exaggerated tensile strength and decreased extensibility [53].

The elastin fibres are also altered with ageing. They become frayed, porous and matted together [54], leading to loss or delay of resiliency and recuperability after stretching. Daly and Odland [55] revealed an age-dependent decrease in elastic recovery, in which the recovery of the skin to its initial resting place after mechanical depression in young adults was complete within a few minutes while in the elderly a full recovery or reconstitution often required over 24 h.

There are decreased numbers of capillary loops in the papillary dermis, corresponding to the loss of dermal papillae with advancing age. The remaining capillaries are shorter and tend to have relatively greater proportions of thickened basement membrane [54].

A number of studies have reported an age-associated diminution in the inflammatory response; thus the elderly will not experience the early warnings and will tend to fail to take appropriate action. The number of Langerhans' cells (LC) has been reported to decline in aged skin by approximately 50% from young adulthood to senescence [56]. This loss impairs the cell-mediated immune response. The effect of ageing on epidermal LC and on their response to a single ultraviolet (UV) exposure has been studied using skin biopsy specimens of healthy adults [56]. The data demonstrated an age-associated loss of epidermal LC and slowing of LC response to UV irradiation. A similar result was obtained in the study indicating a lower percentage of LC in the sacral epidermis of elderly patients with pressure ulcers than in age-matched elderly controls [57]. These structural changes associated with ageing probably contribute to reduction in tissue tolerance of external stimuli, including pressure.

Loss of autonomic nerve control, frequently seen in patients with spinal cord injury, generates loss of vasomotor control and muscle pumping action, subsequently leading to alteration in skin structure. Quantitative and qualitative changes in skin collagen synthesis and catabolism below the level of injury can lead to reduction of the skin's ability to resist mechanical insult.

Rodriguez and Claus-Walker [58] reported that the amino acid content and the activity of the enzyme lysyl hydroxylase were lower in the insensitive skin than in the sensitive skin of individuals with spinal cord injuries. The hydroxylation of lysine is an important first step in collagen cross-link formation. Decreased formation of hydrolysine will decrease cross-link formation and will result in structurally weaker collagen. Klein et al. [59] reported that 2–3 months after denervation followed by disuse, the newly synthesized collagen in adult rats had fewer cross-links, and was therefore probably biomechanically weaker, than the original collagen.

Rodriguez et al. [60] reported the excretion of collagen metabolites increased after injury, reaching a peak between 3 and 6 months, then declined gradually, reaching control values about a year after injury. Stover et al. [61] reported that type III collagen, distributed in a fine network in the papillary layer of the dermis, is less prevalent in the upper dermis, while type I collagen is more prevalent in the reticular dermis in the denervated skin of patients with spinal cord injury. This suggests skin thickening and clumping of collagen, flattening of rete pegs and hypertrophy of sweat glands and erector pilae muscle. Thickening skin associated with increase of collagen I may decrease the space available for tissue fluid transportation in the dermis, leading to reduced tissue viability.

When a region is disused, for example the paralysed area in patients with spinal cord injury, the affected tissue is alive but with a lower oxygen and nutrient supply, leading to alteration of skin structure. The epidermal–dermal junction becomes flattened, distribution of blood capillaries in the skin is scattered and arterio-venous shunt develops [62, 63]. If the shunt is developed, the blood flows via the "by-pass" route, not through the capillaries that supply nutrients to the tissue. Therefore, a threat to tissue viability is more likely, although observation suggests that skin blood flow is well maintained. Lymph flow is also impaired by paralysis. The lymph vessels of the skin of paraplegic patients with thromboembolic disease showed a dilated lumen surrounded by rarefied perivascular connective matrix characterized by dissociation and disruption of collagen and elastic fibres. Also the endothelial wall was generally attenuated and indented, and numerous open junctions along the endothelial cells were observed [41]. These alterations appear to be responsible for an impairment of interstitial fluid exchange, leading to reduced removal of tissue catabolites in paraplegics.

The mechanical tissue integrity of the skin is a result of the balance of solid structures (collagen, elastic fibres, etc.) and liquid components (lipids, water) [64]. The stratum corneum provides impermeability and resistance to mechanical insults. If the gross biophysical properties are altered due to environmental factors, e.g. humidity, the membrane's biological performance can be affected. When the skin is allowed to transmit moisture without excessive hydration, the mechanical integrity of the stratum corneum is maintained. The normal moisture content of stratum corneum is between 10 and 20% [65].

The tensile strength of the stratum corneum is reduced when it is wet. It has been demonstrated that the lower the frictional force, the greater the amount of work required to rupture the epidermis. The frictional force on the skin depends on the amount of moisture at the skin surface. It has been reported that the breaking strength decreases with increasing relative humidity (RH) up to 90% RH [66]. Skin with such reduced strength may also be more prone to mechanical insult due to shear stress or abrasion.

Incontinence is frequently noted as a contributing factor in pressure ulcer development. It is a major cause of moisture, local skin irritation and secondary infection. Urine, stool, perspiration and wound drainage contain substances other than moisture that may irritate the skin. It is unclear what causes increased susceptibility to skin injury: moisture only, as described earlier [68]; substances contained in urine and faeces, e.g. ammonia; or combination of these two factors. Allman et al. [67] reported that there was no association of urinary incontinence with pressure ulcers when patients with catheters were excluded, whereas faecal incontinence may be a more important risk factor. Berlowitz and Wilking [68] also studied risk factors for pressure ulcers, in which neither urinary nor faecal incontinence was associated with ulcer development. Overall, incontinence may be one of the contributing factors, but its possible relevance as an independent predictor remains unclear.

The precise relationship of cause-effect, e.g. in incontinent patients with diapers who develop pressure ulcers, should be clarified.

Effect of Repetitive Loading on Skin Structure/Composition

Loading stimulation also changes the skin's structure and composition leading to changes in the mechanical properties of the skin when it is repeated, depending on the degree and duration of pressure and how frequently it is applied to the skin. The site, the patient's age and the direction of loading are also important.

There are a number of published studies examining histologically, in animal models, how mechanical loading produces tissue damage [21, 26, 27]. However, at that time, not much attention was paid to how the tissue recovers following ischaemic insult. For example, if the loading stress is below the threshold, the tissue will recover completely. If the stress is the same order as threshold level, some compensation mechanism will take place within the tissue to maintain the tissue integrity or, if the stress is repeated, adaptation of the tissue will result. If the stress is severe and beyond the threshold, tissue damage or degeneration will be apparent. When the equilibrium between breakdown and regeneration cannot be maintained because of excessive duration or magnitude of force, catabolic processes overcome reparative mechanisms and the net result is tissue breakdown.

With the aim of preventing the destructive process, Sanders et al. [36] have attempted to address skin adaptation to mechanical stress by increasing load tolerance in rehabilitation practice. For example, spinal cord-injured patients, when the spine is becoming stable, begin a wheelchair-sitting tolerance program. Sitting is limited to 30–60 min initially and increased periodically if hyperaemia resolves within 30 min [69].

Similarly, the ambulating protocol for a person with below-knee amputation is begun as early as 1–2 days postoperatively to stimulate wound healing and expose the antero-distal region of their residual limbs to high compressive and shear stress due to interaction with the prosthetic socket. Such protocols have been followed empirically for patients during the rehabilitation period.

Based on an extensive literature review, Sanders et al. [70] conducted animal experiments using the hind limb of the pig. Cyclic compressive and shear stress at 106.7 ± 4.7 kPa and 22.6 ± 5.9 kPa in the first session to 229.4 ± 4.2 kPa and 53.0 ± 0.8 kPa in the final session were applied at a frequency of 1 Hz for 1 h/day, 5 days/week for 4 weeks. Qualitative morphological analysis demonstrated that collagen fibril diameters were greater and fibril densities significantly lower in loaded skin than in control skin. Wang and Sanders [71] hypothesise that the adaptation occurs by forming new collagen fibrils with larger diameters as opposed to increasing diameters of existing fibrils. Such studies have been initiated only recently more extensive investigations are required.

Initial Damage Occurring in the Susceptible Areas

Whether the initial damage leading to pressure ulcers occurs at the surface of the skin or in muscle is controversial. Animal studies seem to indicate that pressure ulcers start from the muscle, because muscle is considerably less tolerant to ischaemia due to high metabolic need [24, 25, 28]. In contrast, clinical observation indicates that human pressure ulcers start from the skin [72]. Both may be true in certain situations. If an unconscious or immobilized person is left on the operating table for prolonged period of time [73], force is exerted perpendicularly (compression only), supporting the hypothesis that pressure ulcers start from muscle. However, in a conscious person or one with limited mobilization, force is exerted not only perpendicularly but also tangentially (compression and shear), supporting the hypothesis that pressure ulcers start from the skin. No reliable conclusion has yet been reached. There are unanswered questions: for example, if it is assumed that all human pressure ulcers develop from muscle, how can it be explained that some stage I pressure ulcers are resolved by effective pressure relief. Since muscle fibres, once damaged, cannot regenerate, fibrous tissues like collagen will replace the area, appearing as an irregular surface of the skin. In order to clarify these questions, more comprehensive research on the mechanism of pressure ulcer development is needed.

Only a few studies using histological methods are available for understanding of human pressure ulcers [48, 74–77]. Witkowski and Parish [74], who attempted to investigate human pressure ulcer development extensively, reported that the initial changes were found in the papillary dermis, where the capillaries and venules were greatly dilated showing blanchable erythema with intact skin. This change is completely reversible if adequate pressure relief is given. The next stage of pressure ulcers, which is called non-blanchable erythema, shows the consistent feature of red blood cell engorgement of the capillaries and venules, followed by perivascular and later diffuse haemorrhage; however, the epidermis still appears normal. The vessels in the reticular dermis may also be engorged with red blood cells. Some vessels show fibrin thrombi and degeneration of the eccrine sweat glands, and subcutaneous fat is more often seen. In addition, the sebaceous glands begin to show evidence of degeneration, There is loss of cell membranes and an inflammatory infiltrate.

Barnett [75] examined surgically excised human tissue samples in which a pressure ulcer was present and developed a diagrammatic representation of how a pressure ulcer develops and heals. At an early stage, thinning of the epidermis, death of the papillary layer and loss of elasticity and strength of collagen are characterised, probably due to impairment of blood/nutrient supply and lymph flow in the papillary layer of the dermis although the skin surface remains intact. At the next stage, equivalent to stage II pressure ulcer in the NPUAP classification, one finds breakdown of the epidermis ultimately resulting in an open ulcer and death of collagen leading to loss of integrity and thrombosed blood vessels.

Moore et al. [76] conducted a study using the edge of pressure ulcer tissues excised for flap surgery. They reported that irregularly sized and

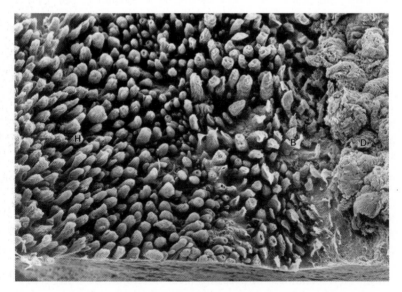

Fig. 11.10. Outer surface of the papillary dermis in the sacrum. Numerous dermal papillae with a finger-like profile are visible in the healthy (*H*) and boundary (*B*) areas. No papillae are seen in the damaged (*D*) area of stage II pressure ulcer. Age 84 years, female (×100)

shaped rete pegs were observed from the outer margin of the pressure ulcer through a transition zone of atypical rete pegs and finally disappear at the junction with granulation tissue.

Similar morphological findings were reported by Arao et al. [48], who carried out a post-mortem examination of the skin tissue of the sacrum of a subject who had stage II pressure ulcers, using light microscopy and transmission and scanning electron microscopy (Fig. 11.10).

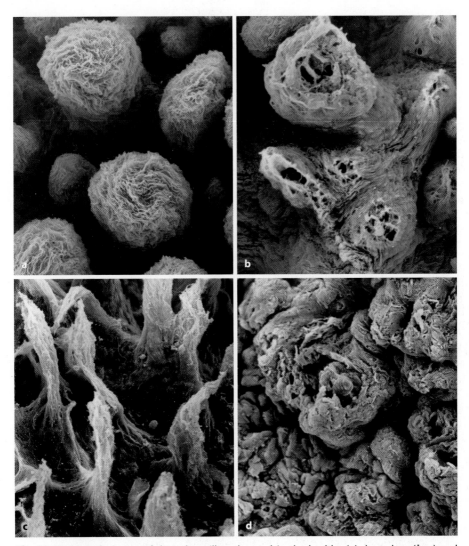

Fig. 11.11. Magnified view of dermal papillae observed in the healthy (**a**), boundary (**b**, **c**) and damaged (**d**) areas resulting from stage II pressure ulcer. The papillae in the healthy area all show a finger-like profile and are regularly arranged. In some papillae of the boundary area the top is broken (**b**), and others show atrophic changes (**c**). In the damaged area an irregular contour with no papillae is shown. Age 84 years, female (**a**, **b**, **c** ×700; **d** ×200)

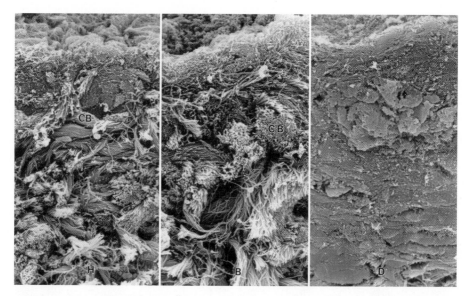

Fig. 11.12. Cut surface of the papillary layer showing the bundles of collagen fibrils (*CB*). These bundles are larger in the boundary area (*B*) than in the healthy area (*H*). In the damaged area (*D*) resulting from stage II pressure ulcers, the fibrils are densely packed and individual fibrils cannot be identified. Age 84 years, female (×3,300)

It was found that the atrophic, irregularly shaped dermal papillae – partially broken, with foramina – were characterised in the boundary zone between healthy and damaged areas (Fig. 11.11).

In addition, a relatively dense network of collagen fibres in the papillary layers was observed, in contrast with the healthy area, where collagen fibres were scarce (Fig. 11.12).

In the area damaged by pressure ulcer, no epidermis and no dermal papillae were observed, and the fibrous elements of the dermis were exposed to the surface (Fig. 11.11). These findings suggested that the morphological changes of the papillae observed in the boundary area impairs tissue viability of the epidermis and papillary by inhibiting nutritive blood supply and by accumulating metabolites which predispose to tissue damage.

Shimamura and Watanabe [77] examined 23 tissue samples of the sacrum in mostly elderly humans with pressure ulcers post mortem. They reported that the earliest sign of tissue damage occurs in the superficial layers and subsequently extends towards the deeper layers. They assumed that the damage in the subcutaneous tissue and deep fascia may extend more easily since there is no structural diffusion barrier in those tissues. In this regard, the meshwork of collagen and elastic fibres of the papillary and reticular layers may play an important role in preventing the transmission of external pressure to deeper tissues.

Further Studies

Studies of the following nature would be beneficial:

1. More systematic and comprehensive animal studies are needed to enhance our understanding of the whole mechanism of tissue damage-recovery following loading. The results of previous animal studies are not comparable; therefore, the protocols of future experiments should be similar. For example, studies should use the same kind of animal (e.g. pig) or in-vitro model, the same indentor shape and loading system, the same site for indentation, and continuous loading of predetermined pressure and duration, examined using physiological, biochemical and immunohistological techniques. Once the threshold curve between magnitude and duration of pressure has been established, then the effect of repetitive loading can be investigated.

2. Characterization of the altered mechanical properties of the skin accompanying altered structure/composition in susceptible individuals, for example the elderly, patients with spinal cord injury and those with disuse syndrome. In addition, characterization of the altered mechanical properties of the skin due to repetitive loading.

3. Qualitative and quantitative analysis of tissue viability using more sensitive morphological tools, for example immunohistochemical analysis or non-invasive techniques (e.g. magnetic resonance imaging) that provide such information.

4. In-vitro investigation using a vital soft tissue model, that needs to be established, to clarify how the force is transferred to the individual layers of the soft tissue and how a given layer behaves differently when the force is applied to the skin.

One of the reasons why the aetiology of pressure ulcers has been investigated so little over the past decades is a lack of involvement of basic medical scientists or biologists in pressure ulcer research. In order to facilitate these studies, a multidisciplinary approach is needed involving biologists, basic medical scientists, bioengineers, clinicans, and other medical care specialists. This approach would provide significant advances in the pathogenesis of pressure ulcer.

References

1. Osborne S (1987) A quality circle investigation. Nurs Times Feb 18:73–76
2. Goode HF, Burns E, Walker BE (1992) Vitamin C depletion and pressure sores in elderly patients with femoral neck fracture. BMJ 305(17):925–927
3. Exton-Smith AN, Sherwin RW (1961) The prevention of pressure sores: Significance of spontaneous bodily movements. Lancet II:1124–1126
4. Defloor T (1999) The risk of pressure sores: A conceptual scheme. J Clin Nurs 8:206–216

5. Allman RM (1989) Pressure ulcers among the elderly. N Engl J Med 320(13): 850–853
6. Anderson TP, Andberg MM (1979) Psychosocial factors associated with pressure sores. Arch Phys Med Rehabil 60:341–346
7. Krouskop TA (1983) A synthesis of the factors that contribute to pressure sore formation. Med Hypotheses 11(2):255–267
8. Schubert V, Fagrell B (1991) Evaluation of the dynamic cutaneous post-ischemic hyperemia and thermal responses in elderly subjects and in an area at risk for pressure sores. Clin Physiol 11:169–182
9. Hagisawa S, Ferguson-Pell M, Cardi M, Miller SD (1994) Assessment of skin blood content and oxygenation in spinal cord injured subjects during reactive hyperemia. J Rehabil Res Dev 31(1):1–14
10. Bader DL (1990) The recovery characteristics of soft tissues following repeated loading. J Rehabil Res Dev 27:141–150
11. Bogie KM, Nuseibeh I, Bader DL (1992) Transcutaneous gas tension in the sacrum during the acute phase of spinal injury. Proc Inst Mech Eng [H] 206(1):1–6
12. Holloway GA (1984) Physiological causes of skin breakdown, In National Symposium on the Care, Treatment and Prevention of Decubitus Ulcers. Conference Proceedings, Virginia, pp 13–16
13. Ferguson-Pell M, Hagisawa S (1988) Biochemical changes in sweat following prolonged ischemia. J Rehabil Res Dev 25(3):57–62
14. Polliack AA, Taylor R, Bader DL (1991) Sweat analysis of soft tissue under load. Annual Report 18, Oxford Orthopaedic Engineering Centre, pp 19–24
15. Hyman WA, Artigue RS (1977) Oxygen and lactic acid transport in skeletal muscle effect of reactive hyperemia. Ann Biomed Eng 5:260–272
16. McCord JM (1985) Oxygen- free radicals in postischemic tissue injury. N Engl J Med 312(3):159–163
17. Gute DC, Ishida T, Yarimizu K, Korthuis RJ (1988) Inflammatory responses to ischemia and reperfusion in skeletal muscle. Mol Cell Biochem 179:169–187
18. Cotran RS, Kumar V, Collins T (1999) Acute and chronic inflammation. In: Pathologic basis of disease, 6th edn. Saunders, Philadelphia, pp 50–88
19. Sundin BM, Hussein MA, Glasofer S, El-Falaky MH, Abdel-Aleem SM, Sachse RE, Klitzman B (2000) The role of allopurinol and deferoxamine in preventing pressure ulcers in pigs. Plast Reconstr Surg 105:1408–1421
20. Houwing R, Overgoor M, Kon M, Jansen G, Asbeck ACV, Haalboom JRE (2000) Pressure-induced skin lesions in pigs: reperfusion injury and the effects of vitamin E. J Wound Care 9(1):36–40
21. Husain T (1953) An experimental study of some pressure effects on tissues with reference to the bed-sore problem. J Pathol Bacteriol 66:347–358
22. Kosiak M (1961) Etiology of decubitus ulcers. Arch Phys Med Rehabil 42:19–29
23. Wilms-Kretschmer K, Majno G (1969) Ischemia of the skin. Am J Pathol 54(3):327–343
24. Nola GT, Vistnes LM (1980) Differential response of skin and muscle in the experimental production of pressure sores. Plast Reconstr Surg 66(5):728–733
25. Groth KE (1942) Klinische Beobachtungen und Experimentelle Studien über die Entstehung des Decubitus. Acta Chir Scand 87[Suppl 76]:1–203
26. Kosiak M (1959) Etiology and pathology of ischemic ulcers. Arch Phys Med Rehabil 40:62–68

27. Dinsdale SM (1973) Decubitus ulcers in swine: Light and electron microscopy study of pathogenesis. Arch Phys Med Rehabil 55:51–56, 74

28. Daniel RK, Priest LD, Wheatley DC (1981) Etiologic factors in pressure sores: An experimental model. Arch Phys Med Rehabil 62:492–498

29. Reswick JB, Rogers JE (1976) Experience at Rancho Los Amigos Hospital with devices and techniques to prevent pressure sores. In: Kenedi RM, Cowden JM, Scales JT (eds) Bedsore biomechanics. University Park Press, London, pp 301–310

30. Rose EH, Vistnes LM, Ksander GA (1977) The panniculus carnosus in the domestic pig. Plast Reconstr Surg 59(1):94–97

31. Le KM, Madsen BL, Barth PW, Ksander GA, Angell JB. Vistnes LM (1984) An in-depth look at pressure sores using monolithic silicon pressure sensors. Plast Reconstr Surg 74(6):745–754

32. Dodd KT, Gross DR (1991) Three-dimensional tissue deformation in subcutaneous tissues overlying bony prominences may help to explain external load transfer to the interstitium J Biomechanics 24(1):11–19

33. Sangeorzan BJ, Harrington RM, Wyss CD, Czerniecki JM, Matsen FA (1989) Circulatory and mechanical response of skin to loading. J Orthop Res 7:425–431

34. Todd BA, Thacker JG (1994) Three-dimensional computer model of the human buttocks, in vivo. J Rehabil Res Dev 31(2):111–119

35. Hagisawa S, Shimada T, Arao H, Asada Y (2001) Morphological architecture and distribution of blood capillaries and elastic fibres in the human skin. J Tissue Viability 11(2):59–63

36. Sanders JE, Goldstein BS, Leotta DF (1995) Skin response to mechanical stress: adaptation rather than breakdown – a review of the literature. J Rehabil Res Dev 32(3):214–226

37. Pasyk KA, Thomas SV, Hassett CA, Cherry GW, Faller R (1989) Regional differences in capillary density of the normal human dermis. Plast Reconstr Surg 83(6):939–947

38. Ryan TJ (1983) Cutaneous circulation, In: Goldsmith LA (ed) Biochemistry and physiology of the skin., Oxford University Press, New York, pp 828–831

39. Liu X, Zhang Y, Liao J (1998) Regional differences in density of children's skin – an enzyme histochemical and stereological study, Zhonghua Zheng Xing Shao Wai Ke Za Zhi 14(6):448–451

40. Tsuchida Y (1987) Regional differences in the skin blood flow at various sites of the body studied by Xenon 133. Plast Reconstr Surg 80(5):705–710

41. Scelsi R, Scelsi L, Bocchi R, Lotta S (1995) Morphological changes in the skin microlymphatics in recently injured paraplegic patients with ilio-femoral venous thrombosis. Paraplegia 33:472–475

42. Reddy NP (1990) Effects of mechanical stresses on lymph and interstitial fluid flows, In: Bader DL (ed) Pressure sores: clinical practice and scientific approach. Macmillan Scientific & Medical, London, pp 203–220

43. Shimada T, Morita T, Oya M.(1991) Structures and architectures of lymphatic capillaries: Morphological differences from blood capillaries. Jpn Soc Electron Microsc 26(1):66–71

44. Reddy NP, Patel K (1995) A mathematical model of flow through the terminal lymphatics. Med Eng Phys 17(2):134–140

45. Miller GE, Seale J (1981) Lymphatic clearance during compressive loading, Lymphology 14:161–166

46. Ghadially R (1998) Aging and the epidermal permeability barrier: implications for contact dermatitis. Am J Contact Dermatitis 9(3):162–169

47. Gibson T, Kenedi RM, Craik JE (1965) The mobile micro-architecture of dermal collagen. Br J Surg 52:764–770
48. Arao H, Obata M, Shimada T, Hagisawa S (1998) Morphological characteristics of the dermal papillae in the development of pressure sores. J Tissue Viability 8(3):17–23
49. Parry DAD, Barnes GRG, Craig AS (1978) A comparison of the size distribution of collagen fibrils in connective tissues as a function of age and a possible relation between fibril size distribution and mechanical properties. Proc R Soc Biol Sci 203:305–321
50. Silver FH, Kato YP, Ohno M, Wasserman AJ (1992) Analysis of mammalian connective tissue: relationship between hierarchical structure and mechanical properties. J Long-Term Effects Med Implants 2(2,3):165–198
51. Richey M, Richey HK, Fenske NA (1988) Aging-related skin changes: development and clinical meaning. Geriatrics 43(4):49–64
52. Lavker RM, Zheng PS, Dong G (1986) Morphology of aged skin. Dermatol Clin 4(3):379–389
53. Fenske NA, Conard CB (1988) Aging skin. Am Fam Physician 37(2):219–230
54. Smith L (1989) Histopathologic characteristics and ultrastructure of aging skin. CUTIS 43:414–423
55. Daly CH, Odland GF (1979) Age-related changes in the mechanical properties of human skin. J Invest Dermatol 73:84–87
56. Gilchrest BA, Murphy GF, Soter NA (1982) Effect of chronologic aging and ultraviolet irradiation on Langerhans cells in human epidermis. J Invest Dermatol 79(2):85–88
57. Kohn S, Kohn D, Schiller D (1990) Epidermal Langerhans' cells in elderly patients with decubital ulcers. J Dermatol 17:724–728
58. Rodriguez GP, Claus-Walker J (1988) Biochemical changes in skin composition in spinal cord injury: a possible contribution to decubitus ulcers. Paraplegia 26:302–309
59. Klein L, Dawson MH, Heiple KG (1977) Turnover of collagen in the adult rat after denervation. J Bone Joint Surg 159-A(8):1065–1067
60. Rodriguez GP, Claus-Walker J, Kent MC, Garza HM (1989) Collagen metabolite excretion as a predictor of bone- and skin-related complications in spinal cord injury. Arch Phys Med Rehabil 70:442–444
61. Stover SL (1987) Arthritis related interests in spinal cord injury J Rheumatol 14[Suppl 15]:82–88
62. Tanaka K (1963) Structural changes in the capillary of the skin in chronic spinal cord injured patients examined with vital microscopy. Scientific Report of National Hakone Sanatorium, Japan, pp 222–231 (in Japanese)
63. Van Den Hoogen F, Brawn LA, Sherriff S, Watson N, Ward JD (1986) Arteriovenous shunting in quadriplegia. Paraplegia 24:282–286
64. Fischer TW, Wigger-Alberti W, Elsner P (2001) Assessment of 'dry skin': Current bioengineering methods and test designs. Skin Pharmacol Appl Skin Physiol 14:183–195
65. Blank IH (1953) Further observation on factors which influence the water content of stratum corneum. I Invest Dermatol 259–269
66. Wildnauer RH, Bothwell JW, Douglass AB (1971) Stratum corneum biomechanical properties. I. Influence of relative humidity on normal and extracted human stratum corneum. J Invest Dermatol 56(1):72–78

67. Allman RM, Laprade CA, Noel LB, Walker JM, Moorer CA, Dear MR, Smith CR (1986) Pressure sores among hospitalized patients. Ann Int Med 195:337–342

68. Berlowitz DR, Wilking SVB (1989) Risk factors for pressure sores: A comparison of cross-sectional and cohort-derived data. J Am Geriatr Soc 37:1043–1050

69. Yarkony GM (1993) Aging skin, pressure ulcers and spinal cord injury, In: Whitenock GG et al (eds) Aging with spinal cord injury. Demos, New York, pp 39–52

70. Sanders JE, Goldstein BS (2001) Collagen fibril diameters increase and fibril densities decrease in skin subjected to repetitive compressive and shear stresses. J Biomechanics 34:1581–1587

71. Wang YH, Sanders JE (2003) How does skin adapt to repetitive mechanical stress to become load tolerant? Med Hypotheses 61(1):29–35

72. Shea JD (1975) Pressure sores classification and management. Clin Orthop 112:89–100

73. Vermillion C (1990) Operating room acquired pressure ulcers. Decubitus 3(1):26–30

74. Witkowski JA, Parish LC (1982) Histopathology of the decubitus ulcer. J Am Acad Dermatol 6:1014–1021

75. Barnett SE (1987) Histology of the human pressure sore. CARE – Science and Practice 5:13–18

76. Moore JC, Ray AK, Shakespeare PG (1993) Ultrastructure of human dermis and wounds. Br J Plast Surg 46:460–465

77. Shimamura K, Watanabe H (2001) Histological study of pressure ulcers from cadaver sacral skin with special reference to the site of initial pathological changes and the progress of the tissue damage. Jpn J P U 3(3):305–314 (English abstract)

Compression-Induced Tissue Damage: Animal Models

12

Anke Stekelenburg, Cees Oomens, Dan Bader

Introduction

To gain insight into the aetiology of pressure ulcers, different kinds of studies have been performed in the past 50 years: from experimental studies, using animal models and humans, to theoretical and numerical studies. In this chapter animal studies on the aetiology of pressure ulcers and on factors that influence the development of pressure ulcers are described, particularly studies performed in the past decade. A clear trend is visible in studies performed in recent years. They focus less on deriving pressure/time curves and more on practical aspects like the influence of temperature, medicine, nutrition and the method of pressure relief.

To be able to investigate the role of tissue (re)perfusion and lymph flow as well as the interaction between tissue layers in bulk tissue, animal experiments are needed. However, the number of animal experiments is fortunately being reduced by the recent trend towards in-vitro model systems such as tissue-engineered skin or muscle for studies on the effect of mechanical loading on tissues. In-vitro models are, however, never conclusive with respect to the results because in-vitro cultures behave differently from animals or humans. Furthermore, new technologies which are non-invasive, such as MRI, also reduce the number of animals needed.

General Requirements

The aetiology of pressure ulcers has been the topic of numerous studies for over half a century. Many animal models have been developed in that time, but it has proven very difficult to develop a suitable animal model for ubiquitous investigation. This can be illustrated by three seminal studies. Groth [1] studied the effect of constant local pressure on the gluteal muscle of rabbits, Husain [2] attached a pressure cuff to the legs of rats and guinea pigs, and Kosiak [3] applied external pressure over the femoral trochanter and ischial tuberosity of dogs. These studies contributed much to the present state of knowledge related to the aetiology of pressure ulcers. Kosiak's work was reported to be "the cornerstone of modern pressure ulcer research" [4]. However, the clinical relevance to human pressure ulcers was limited because the skin of rabbits and dogs differs anatomically and physiologically from human skin.

Animals can be conveniently divided into two broad groups, those with loose skin and those with fixed skin, based on anatomic, embryologic, and physiologic characteristics. Since 1970, the animals most used for pressure ulcer research are swine (fixed skin) and rats (loose skin). A major exception was a study using greyhounds [5]. These dogs are particularly susceptible to the development of pressure ulcers, because of their angular conformation, short hair, and thin skin. Therefore, they can serve as an appropriate model to study pressure ulcers.

The use of swine has long been considered acceptable for pressure ulcer research primarily because of the similarity of skin structure and cardiovascular system in swine and humans. For example, swine have a relatively fixed skin and there are further similarities to the human when considering the soft tissue coverage of bony protuberances. The possibility of inducing model conditions such as radiation damage, paraplegia, and diabetes in both domestic and miniature swine has allowed for the modulation of these parameters to simulate clinical situations in humans. The most common relevant site used to create pressure-induced damage in animal model has typically involved the greater femoral trochanters [4, 6–9].

However, the use of a large animal model precludes the possibility of conducting a large number of individual experiments. By contrast, the rat represents a common small animal model offering the advantages of low initial cost and maintenance [10, 11]. It is thus highly efficient from a financial standpoint and well suited for extensive experimental trials. As an example, Salcido and colleagues [11–13] developed a fuzzy rat animal model for production of pressure ulcers. In contrast to the normal rat, this breed of rat is essentially hypotrichotic and, therefore, does not require depilation or prior treatment of the skin, which might contribute to the formation of damage artefacts. Another major reason for their selection of the rat was that more is known about the pharmacological effects on absorption, distribution, and metabolism of drugs in rats than in any other species. Rats were also used in the research of Bosboom et al. [14]. One of the goals of their research was to reconstruct the loaded muscle underneath the compressed skin using magnetic resonance imaging (MRI) and finite-element (FE) modelling, and that required a small animal.

The advantages and disadvantages of using swine or rats as an animal model in pressure ulcer research are summarised in Table 12.1. When studying skin damage and superficial wounds, it is obvious that swine as an animal model is more suitable because of the similarities in skin between pig and human. Many studies, however, have shown that damage caused by application of pressure can also start at deeper levels (muscle tissue) and extend to the surface. For studying muscle damage, and the influence of possible predisposing factors such as (re)perfusion on damage evolution, rats can be used as an animal model as well.

To study the aetiology of pressure ulcers using animal models various methods/interventions are required, such as anaesthesia, fixation and/or skin indentation. The methods most commonly used entail sedation or anaesthesia of animals during pressure application. It is, however, undesirable to

Table 12.1. Advantages and disadvantages of using swine or rats as animal model in pressure ulcer research

Animal model	Advantages	Disadvantages
Swine	Skin properties comparable to human skin; relatively fixed skin; cardiovascular system comparable to that of human; susceptible to conditions such as diabetes and paraplegia; large surface areas for pressure application	Large animal: reduced possibility of large scale experiments, relatively expensive, require large experimental set-ups
Rat	Small animal: easy to handle, well suited for large-scale experiments, relatively inexpensive; a lot is known about effects of drugs in rats	Loose skin; skin properties not comparable to those of human skin

anaesthetise animals for prolonged periods and on more than one occasion. Furthermore, the physiological consequences of anaesthesia may compromise the true effects of pressure on unanaesthetised animals. Hyodo and colleagues [7] developed a technique that avoids the need for animal anaesthesia. This method used a specially designed pressure applicator which was secured into the bone (the greater trochanter of a pig) and compressed the skin with a spring-loaded disk (Fig. 12.1 d). Peirce et al. [10] also developed a model in which the animal was not anaesthetised during periods of skin ischaemia and reperfusion. They produced injury by applying and removing a permanent magnet to a dorsal region of rat skin under which a ferromagnetic steel plate was implanted (Fig. 12.1 e). These methods do not require anaesthesia during pressure application; however, they allow free movement of the animal, which prevents the use of some techniques, e.g. MRI.

Pressure ulcers are a continuing clinical problem for the spinal cord-injured subject. This has resulted in a number of pressure ulcer-related studies involving paraplegic animals. For example, Groth [1] applied pressure to the gluteus muscle of both normal and spinal cord-transected rabbits. His conclusion was that pressure necrosis occurred in paralysed animals in a comparable manner as in controls. Dinsdale [15] analysed the effects of pressure in the production of pressure ulcers for both normal and paralysed swine. He also found a similarity in the pathological changes present in normal swine and in swine that had been paraplegic for 8 days. It has been suggested by Daniel et al. [4] that in order to examine realistic effects associated with paraplegic animals, a period of time is required in order for the animal weight to increase twofold and manifest extensive atrophy of muscle and subcutaneous tissue. Indeed, after a 6-week period, the paraplegic swine exhibited a pressure–time response which was similar to that in normal swine, as illustrated in Fig. 12.2.

However, damage in the former animal model occurred over a shorter time scale [16]. These findings were attributed to impaired mobility and sensation and incontinence in paraplegic swine leading to skin maceration, and the atrophy of soft tissues resulting in an effective increase in interface pressures at bony prominences. However the invasive procedures involving spinal cord transection, performed by Daniel and colleagues, caused bowel and urinary dysfunction and increased rates of both complications and morbidity. In an attempt to reduce the complications and mortality associated with the previous models, Hyodo et al. [7] developed a pig model in which monoplegia was created by surgical resection of unilateral lumbar nerve roots in the spinal canal and applied pressure to the denervated skin over the trochanteric area. Muscle atrophy in the denervated limb was obvious within 7 days after denervation. No bladder and bowel dysfunction occurred throughout the experimental period. Hyodo and colleagues began pressure application 1–2 weeks after transection.

Pressure-Delivery Systems

Different methods for the application of pressure to induce pressure-induced damage have been developed. The early study by Groth [1] utilised a balance beam, whereas more recent studies involve advanced computer-controlled surface pressure-delivery systems [9, 13].

For the simple balanced beam, as illustrated in Fig. 12.1 a, weights applied to one arm caused the other arm, which consisted of circular discs, to apply pressure. There was no reported measurement of applied or transmitted pressure. Dinsdale [15] also used a mechanical arm. Weights were added to a spindle at one end of a beam, and a metal applicator applied the force. Applied pressure was measured with a strain gauge before and after each experiment. An alternative method employed by Husain [2], involved the application of a cuff to the limb of an animal. This effectively produces a hydrostatic pressure. As illustrated in Fig. 12.1 b, Kosiak [6] applied pressure by means of inverted 20-cc syringes driven by compressed air. He reported a 10% variation in pressure measured between the compressed air system and the point of pressure application. Tissue pressure was measured by means of a hydraulic needle transducer.

Associated with the application of constant pressure, several authors have described monitoring systems for applied pressures and other parameters, such as perfusion and temperature. Daniel et al. [4] developed an electro-mechanical system for pressure application. It was composed of a computer-controlled servomotor whose rotational output was converted to a linear driven indenter by means of a mechanical interface. A force transducer was mounted in line with the indenter to provide feedback control.

In the computer-controlled surface pressure delivery systems of Salcido et al. [11] and Sundin et al. [17] both the force and the pressure-induced reduction of cutaneous blood perfusion using a fibre-optic laser Doppler

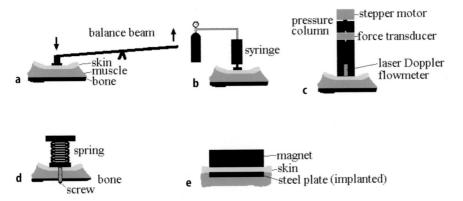

Fig. 12.1 a–e. Schematic drawings of indenter systems. **a** balance beam used by Groth [1]; **b** inverted syringes driven by compressed air used by Kosiak [6]; **c** pressure column used by Salcido et al. [11]; **d** pressure applicator secured into bone used by Reger et al. [20] and Hyodo et al. [7]; **e** magnet compressing skin used by Peirce et al. [10]

flowmeter were measured. Goldstein and Sanders [8] and Houwing et al. [9] also used computer-controlled devices. The former study involved the application of a constant normal force to the skin and, simultaneously, a cyclic shear force. The apparatus involved was a load applicator device positioned on a universal joint and hydraulic lift. A normal force was applied by lowering the hydraulic lift and a shaker motor and power amplifier were used to deliver cyclic shear forces. To enable measurement of skin temperature, a thermistor probe was placed in the pressure applicators in the devices used by Houwing et al. [9].

An important part of the pressure-delivery systems is the pressure applicator itself. Investigators have been using a range of pressure applicators, precluding the direct comparison of results. Pressure is most often applied by an indenter, but pressure cuffs [2], magnets [10] and air bladders [17] have also been used. The size of the used indenter is generally matched to the site of indentation and the size of the animal. Thus Goldstein and Sanders [8], Hyodo et al. [7] and Houwing et al. [9], who applied pressure to the skin above the greater femoral trochanter of pigs, used animals of different sizes, with weights of 6, 18 and 30 kg, respectively, and associated indenter sizes of 7×8 mm, 30 and 50 mm diameter.

Relationship Between Pressure and Time

The objectives of many studies have involved the establishment of threshold values for external loads that will predict the onset of tissue damage. These values can be derived either by analysing (retrospectively) clinical cases or by using animal models. Reswick and Rogers [18] developed a pressure/time curve (Fig. 12.2) that has been used as a clinical guideline

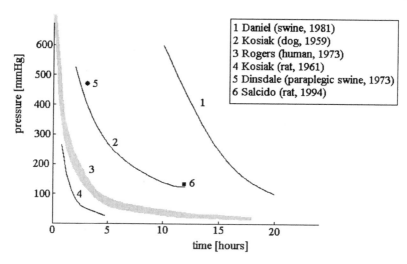

Fig. 12.2. Risk curves with regard to pressure ulcers. Time/pressure combinations above the curve result in tissue breakdown

clue in the early 1970's. They monitored the skin–cushion interface pressures in 800 volunteer normal human subjects and patients.

In the animal experiments soft tissues are loaded, generally by compressing the soft tissues between an indenter and the underlying bone, while the magnitude and the duration of the compressive loads are varied. Groth [1] was the first to publish an extensive systematic study on the primary causes of pressure ulcers using histological techniques. He examined the load-induced evolution of damage by indenting the gluteus muscles of rabbits with a range of forces and application periods. After a period of observation, typically a few days, the animals were killed and post-mortem analysis and histological examination were performed. The findings suggested that all loads cause degenerative changes, but there is a point where these changes become irreversible. Groth defined the threshold level as the point where changes became macroscopically visible and thus was able to define a pressure/time curve. Above this level, permanent damage would occur; below it, any damage was defined as reversible.

Husain [2] also performed pressure experiments with varying degree and duration of pressure. He attached a pressure cuff to the legs of rats and guinea pigs. Using a hydrostatic form of pressure, a threshold pressure of 100 mmHg (13.3 kPa) applied for 2 h was observed to produce definite microscopic changes in the leg muscles of rats. Furthermore, Husain suggested that a low pressure maintained for long periods of time induces more extensive tissue damage than high pressures for short periods. With the guinea pig model, cuff pressures of 100, 200 and 300 mmHg (13.3, 26.7 and 40 kPa) were applied for up to 3 h. Tissue changes, such as oedema, vascular congestion, cellular infiltration and muscle degeneration, were first observed at a pressure of 200 mmHg applied for 2 h.

Using a canine model, Kosiak [6] applied pressures of different intensities for various durations over two locations, namely the femoral trochanter and ischial tuberosity. After release of pressure, oedema and cellular infiltration were observed immediately and persisted for 1–2 days. Kosiak also reported that intense pressures of short duration are as injurious to tissues as low pressures applied for longer periods, as indicated in Fig. 12.2. In a later experiment on a rat model [3], Kosiak applied a constant load and equal amounts of intermittent loads and reported a higher susceptibility of tissue to the constant load. Although no changes were noted in the animals that were subjected to pressures of 35 mmHg (4.7 kPa) for periods up to 4 h, the application of 70 mmHg (9.3 kPa) produced changes after 2 h. By contrast, the application of pressures up to 190 mmHg (25.3 kPa) for 1 h did not produce any noticeable microscopic change in the tissue.

Several investigations have been published since those seminal studies. For example, Lindan [19] compressed rabbit ears and found that pressures of 90 mmHg (12 kPa) applied for a period of 13 h resulted in tissue necrosis. Dinsdale et al. [15] applied pressures to the posterior superior iliac of normal and paraplegic swine. He also found an inverse relationship between the magnitude of pressure and the duration of pressure in the production of pressure ulcers. It is of interest to note that for paraplegic swine no ulcerations occurred when pressure was less than 480 mmHg (64 kPa) applied for 3 h. In 1981, Daniel and colleagues [4] experimentally produced pressure ulcers in swine. The animals were subjected to localised pressures ranging from 30 mmHg to 1000 mmHg (4–133.3 kPa) for periods between 2 h and 18 h. The indenter was placed over the greater femoral trochanter. With their results, the investigators were also able to plot a critical pressure/time curve for pressure ulcers in swine (Fig. 12.2). In their fuzzy rat model, Salcido et al. [11] applied pressure for a 6-h period on each of two consecutive days. This resulted in tissue damage at a pressure of 145 mmHg (19.3 kPa).

Although animal experiments have the advantage over clinical studies of being defined and more controllable, a large variation exists in the threshold values for tissue damage found in the different studies. This variation arises from diversity in experimental conditions, animal models, loading methods and regions/locations of load application. A means of overcoming the diversity in animal models and interpreting the differences between the results could be to relate the applied external load to the local loads inside the tissues. These local loads determine the tissue state and hence the occurrence of tissue damage (Fig. 12.3) [21].

Bosboom [21] compared the maximum shear strain distributions in the tissue, calculated using FE modelling, and the amount and location of initial tissue damage in the skeletal muscle beneath the indented skin. The first results (Fig. 12.4) showed that the shear strain distribution showed some coincidence with the area of tissue damage, but more measurements and calculations are needed (and are being performed by the authors: see "Future Perspectives").

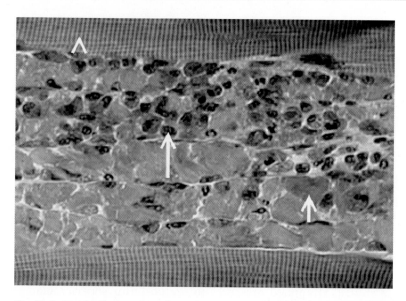

Fig. 12.3. Longitudinal section of muscle, showing the typical cross-striated appearance of skeletal muscle (*arrowhead*), loss of cross-striation of muscle fibres in the damaged area (*short arrow*) and the infiltration of mononuclear cells (*long arrow*). Reproduced with permission from Bosboom [21]

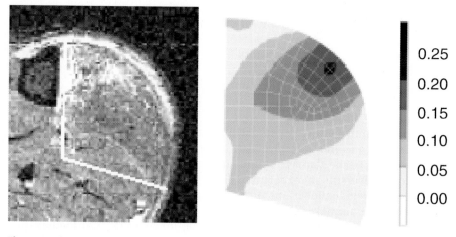

Fig. 12.4. Comparison of the area of muscle damage in a transverse MR image with maximum shear strain distribution for the reference model. Adapted from [21]

Sacks [22] calculated a theoretical pressure versus time curve for the onset of pressure ulcers which was based upon the use of dimensional analysis. He assumed that there is a definable pressure that will initiate a pressure ulcer, and that it will depend primarily upon the physical properties of the tissue in question (tissue density and elastic modulus) and the blood flow through it, as well as the duration of exposure. Comparison with available data from humans, dogs and swine indicated that this approach agreed well with experimental data.

Influence of Shear Forces

A number of animal models have been developed to study the influence of pressure, but relatively few have examined the influence of shear forces. Of these, Reichel [23] was probably the first to point out the danger of shear stress. From anatomical observations he concluded that shear occludes blood vessels more easily than normal stress on its own. This led to the work of Dinsdale [24], who combined the application of normal loads and friction on pig skin and measured their effects on blood flow. This combined loading was found to be more effective in blood flow cessation. However, it was postulated that friction-induced ulceration was not caused by ischaemia, but was a direct result of tearing apart of the top layers of skin, in particular the stratum corneum.

Goldstein et al. [8] also studied the influence of shear forces. They applied different normal and shear forces for relatively short periods to the greater femoral trochanter and the tibialis anterior of swine. Shear forces between 1 and 5 N and normal forces between 2 and 15 N were applied. The results confirmed the clinical observations that shear forces injure skin and body wall tissues and that there is a more rapid onset of damage at increased shear forces. In addition, it was noted that tissue breakdown occurred at a normal force of 14 N in the presence of a 2.5-N shear force. However, when the shear force was increased to 4 N, tissue breakdown occurred at a normal force of only 7 N. These data also confirmed previous studies that shear force alone did not induce tissue breakdown [25].

Ischaemia–Reperfusion Injury

Ischaemia–reperfusion (I/R) injury can be a factor in the formation of pressure ulcers. Clinical observations of pressure ulcers showed that ulcers typically occur after, rather than during, a period in which pressure is applied to the body. I/R injury can be defined as cellular injury resulting from the reperfusion by blood of tissue areas that had been previously exposed to an ischaemic insult. Reperfusion injury to skeletal muscle is characterised by a number of features, including muscle necrosis, endothelial cell swelling and release of intracellular enzymes and proteins [27, 28] Reperfusion injury is mediated through free radicals. Production of oxygen free radicals may initiate a cascade of biochemical events that can significantly contribute to or result in the production of pressure ulcers [9, 10]. Under normal circumstances oxygen free radicals are buffered by free radical scavengers, such as reduced glutathione. However, in tissues undergoing oxidative stress, there is a decrease in the levels of these enzymes. As a consequence, during reperfusion the oxygen free radicals are buffered to a lesser degree and this is reflected in an increase in concentration of hydrogen peroxide [26, 28, 29].

Several recent studies have examined the effects of reperfusion on the formation of pressure ulcers in animal models. Peirce et al. [10] induced I/R injury by implanting a ferromagnetic steel plate in the dorsal region of rat skin and then applying and removing a permanent magnet over the region. The application of the magnet compressed the skin and reduced blood flow, thus causing ischaemia, while removal of the magnet allowed reperfusion of blood to the ischaemic region. A pressure of 50 mmHg (6.7 kPa) was chosen as representative of a clinically relevant interface pressure. Different numbers of I/R cycles were applied to the skin tissues, each cycle consisting of 2 h of ischaemia and 0.5 h of reperfusion. The results indicated that five I/R cycles, equivalent to a total ischaemic period of 10 h, were more damaging to the skin than one continuous compression-induced ischaemic period of 10 h. The extent of the damage was indicated by an increase in both necrotic area and the degree of leucocyte extravasation in the I/R group compared with the ischaemia-alone group. Houwing and colleagues [9] also studied the influence of ischaemia and reperfusion. A pressure of 375 mmHg (50 kPa) was applied for 2 h on the skin above the greater femoral trochanters of 8-week-old pigs. Specimens taken immediately after cessation of pressure application showed no histopathological signs. Early signs of damage in the muscles and subcutaneous tissue under the pressure device appeared only after a reperfusion period in excess of 1 h. The observed damage distal to the pressure applicator was identical to the damage immediately below the applicator, suggesting that the process followed a vascular pattern and was a result of ischaemia. Thus it was concluded that although pressure resulted in damage, the observed damage was not a direct result of pressure per se.

Several substances are thought to prevent free radical formation or to scavenge free radicals once they are formed. These substances include superoxide dismutase, catalase and allopurinol, which function at the enzymatic level, and dimethylsulfoxide, deferoxamine and vitamin E, which function non-enzymatically [28]. Houwing et al. [9] investigated the effect of one such scavenger, vitamin E. The study showed that pre-treatment with 500 mg of vitamin E prevented damage caused by pressure to a large degree. Although vitamin E does not prevent oxidative stress during the application of pressure, as reflected in the decrease in reduced glutathione and total glutathione, it does prevent the excess production of oxygen free radicals and hydrogen peroxide during reperfusion.

The role of allopurinol and deferoxamine was examined by Sundin et al. [17]. They applied pressure to the scapulae of pigs in a 4-h cycle, consisting of 210 min of an applied pressure of 150 mmHg (20 kPa) followed by zero pressure for 30 min. This cycle was repeated continuously for 48 h. Both biochemical markers improved cutaneous blood flow and tissue oxygenation, but only deferoxamine significantly reduced necrosis of cutaneous and skeletal muscle tissues. Indeed, a significant decrease in the extent of muscle infarction was evident in the deferoxamine group compared with the control group. According to the authors, the protective effect of deferoxamine can be explained in several ways. Deferoxamine has a relatively low molecular weight, which facilitates its entry into cells. In addition, deferoxamine has a high binding affinity for iron, which, under ischaemic conditions, becomes more available. By binding iron, deferoxamine inhibits the formation of the hydroxyl radical (OH) from superoxide radicals (O_2). Salcido et al. [12] tested the effect of a potent anti-inflammatory agent, ibuprofen, on the development of pressure ulcers. Their hypothesis was that transcutaneous pressure intervention, resulting in the production of experimental pressure ulcers, may be mechanistically similar to the vascular damage resulting from burns injury, which has shown to be responsive to ibuprofen intervention. The effect of ibuprofen intervention before, during and after the application of pressure [145 mmHg (19.3 kPa) for five consecutive daily pressure sessions, each of 6 h duration] to the fuzzy rat model was examined. However, their results suggested that ibuprofen intervention was not effective in reducing the incidence or severity of pressure ulcers and might, in some cases, have been detrimental.

Another known way to diminish reperfusion injury is gradual reperfusion of the ischaemic tissues. Ünal and colleagues [30] investigated the effect of gradual increase in blood flow on I/R injury of the skeletal muscle. They induced ischaemia by applying clamps to the femoral vessels of rats. Three groups of rats were used:

- A control group: no ischaemia was induced.
- A conventional clamp release group: 150 min ischaemia was followed by immediate release of the clamps.
- A gradual clamp release group: 150 min ischaemia was followed by gradual release of the clamps (blood flow velocity recovered in 120 s).

Histological examination was performed and malonyldialdehyde (MDA) and myeloperoxidase (MPO) levels were measured (Fig. 12.5). MPO is a sign of neutrophil accumulation and MDA is a by-product of radical-induced lipid disintegration.

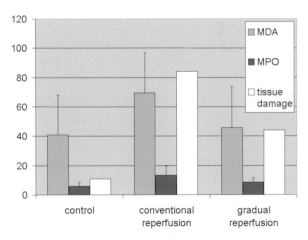

Fig. 12.5. Mean tissue myeloperoxidase levels (*MPO*; units per gram protein), mean malonyldialdehyde levels (*MDA*; nanomoles per gram) and histopathological tissue injury scores (percent tissue damage) for the three different groups

Inflammatory cell infiltration and loss of striation of the muscle were noticeably less in the gradual-reperfusion group than in the conventional-reperfusion group. The tissue MPO and MDA values of the conventional group were significantly greater than those of the gradual group. The investigators demonstrated that gradual reperfusion decreases neutrophil accumulation, superoxide radical occurrence, and tissue infarction in the rat hind limb model.

Influence of Temperature

Since the work of Groth, Kosiak and others, it has become clear that tissue breakdown is a multi-dimensional process. Besides pressure, factors that (may) have influence include shear, friction, moisture, age, nutrition, physiological abnormalities, sensory loss, mobility, and temperature.

The role of temperature in the causation of pressure ulcers has been examined in only a few studies. It is, however, known that, in general, an increase of 1°C in skin temperature results in an approximately 13% increase in tissue metabolic requirements [31]. The heightened need for nutrients and oxygen cannot be fulfilled, however, because of tissue compression or in tissues which are subjected to pressure-induced ischaemia. Studies indicating an increase in local skin temperature caused by both pressure application [32] and the insulating effect of specific foam cushions and mattresses [33] appear to affirm temperature as an important factor in pressure ulcer development.

Kokate et al. [34] described a porcine model for the creation and assessment of temperature-modulated pressure-induced damage to tissues. A device was developed which was capable of applying both pressure and temperature. Applied pressure was 100 mmHg (13.3 kPa) and applied temperatures were 25, 35, 40 and 45 °C, the latter temperature representing a commonly accepted upper limit for thermal therapies applied to skin, such as water beds. The local application of 100 mmHg for 5 h resulted:

▌ At 25°C in no damage
▌ At 35°C in moderate muscle damage
▌ At 40°C in partial epidermal necrosis and moderate muscle damage
▌ At 45°C in full-thickness epidermal necrosis, moderate dermal and subdermal damage and severe muscle damage.

Kokate and colleagues concluded that these results motivated the conjecture that lower applied temperature could be protective to soft tissue. In a subsequent study [35], temperatures of 25, 27, 30 and 32°C were applied. The findings confirmed that at lower temperature of the skin and the underlying tissues exposed to the increased pressures, less severe tissue damage resulted in all the soft tissue layers.

Increased temperature results not only in increased tissue metabolism and oxygen consumption but also in increased perfusion. Patel et al. [36] examined the combined effect of increased temperature and surface pressure on tissue perfusion and deformation. A heater, designed to raise the skin surface temperature locally, was attached to the pressure applicator. Skin displacement was measured by a linear variable differential transformer. A range of pressures between 3.7 and 73 mmHg (0.5 and 9.7 kPa) were applied at two different temperatures, $T = 28\,°C$ (no heating) and $T = 36\,°C$. The major conclusions of this study were that there was a significant increase in perfusion, measured by a laser Doppler flowmeter, with increased temperature at surface pressures below 18 mmHg (2.4 kPa), probably due to local auto-regulatory mechanisms. No increase in perfusion was seen at higher pressures, most likely because of mechanical occlusion of vessels induced by high surface pressure. In addition, increased temperature caused skin to become stiffer in response to increased surface pressure. At constant pressures, heated skin did not deform as much as unheated skin.

Results and Future Perspectives

The main animal model studies are summarised in Table 12.2. A number of aspects have been considered. For example, some studies have focused on the aetiology of pressure ulcers [9, 10, 14], while others have examined the influence of medicine and nutrition [11, 17] or the effects of temperature [34, 35].

The table also includes details of the pressures applied and the duration of application for the different studies. The considerable variation, reflecting the range of animals used, their size and the test site, precludes a direct interstudy comparison. It also confirms the importance of deriving a parameter that is independent of geometry, such as local internal stress, which can be calculated using FE modelling.

In all previous animal studies histological examination was used for the evaluation of the tissue. This has two main drawbacks. First, tissue histology is a destructive methodology. It therefore precludes follow-up studies to investigate the evolution of tissue damage with time, which is particularly appropriate when studying mechanisms associated with reperfusion damage. In addition, histology is labour-intensive, and thus hampers experiments on a larger scale. MRI is considered a promising alternative, since it is non-destructive and, although inherently expensive, less time consuming. In the study of Bosboom [21] the ability of MRI to assess local muscle damage after prolonged transverse loading was investigated. A pressure of 1875 mmHg (250 kPa) was applied for 2 h and analysis was performed 24 h after its completion. Histological examination was used as the gold standard and data were compared with in vivo MR images. Damage in histological slices was indicated manually from evidence of loss of cross-striation of the muscle fibres and/or the infiltration of inflammatory cells. When a muscle fibre was damaged at least every 30 μm, a mark was placed in the centre of the damaged fibre (bottom images, Fig. 12.6).

Table 12.2. Studies performed during the last decade on tissue damage due to mechanical loading. Pressures given in mmHg (7.5 mmHg ≡ 1 kPa)

(First) author	Animal	Applied pressure/time	Damage	Focus on
Swaim [5]	Dog ($n=15$)	Cast for 14 days (0.03 N/mm^2)	Skin damage	Pressure wounds
Salcido [11]	Rat ($n=65$)	145 mmHg/6 h, five daily sessions	Damage in all layers	Effect of ibuprofen
Hyodo [7]	Pig ($n=9$)	800 mmHg/48 h	Full-thickness ulcers	Pressure ulcers, spinal cord injury
Kokate [34]	Pig ($n=16$)	100 mmHg/5 h	Damage in all layers	Pressure, temperature
Iaizzo [35]	Pig ($n=6$)	100 mmHg/2,5 and 10 h	Damage in all layers	Pressure, temperature (cooling)
Goldstein [8]	Pig ($n=8$)	675 mmHg/40 min+shear stress, 20 daily sessions	Skin breakdown	Repetitive mechanical stress
Peirce [10]	Rat ($n=52$)	50 mmHg/10 h	Skin ulcer (pressure was only applied to skin)	Ischaemia, reperfusion
Houwing [9]	Pig ($n=6$)	375 mmHg/2 h	Damage in muscle and subcutaneous tissue	Reperfusion, vitamin E
Sundin [17]	Pig ($n=18$)	150 mmHg/5 h	Damage in all layers	Effect of allopurinol, deferoxamine
Bosboom [21]	Rat ($n=5$)	1875 mmHg/2 h	Muscle damage	Deformation (using MRI)

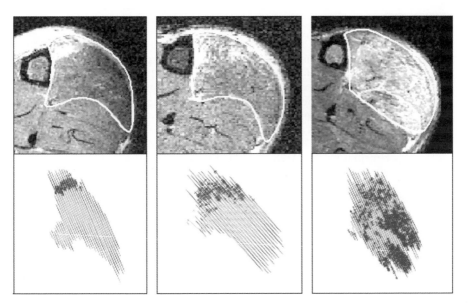

Fig. 12.6. Damage in transverse histological slices (below) and MR images located at the middle of the indenter

In T2-weighted MR images, increased signal intensity reflects tissue damage. Increased signal intensity on T2-weighted MR images can reflect a range of pathologies, including oedema, necrosis, inflammation and fatty infiltration [37]. The two analyses are illustrated for three animals in Fig. 12.6. It can be seen that the location of damage in the MR image coincided well with that determined from transverse histological slices.

The hypothesis that prolonged cell deformation is the primary trigger for the onset of tissue damage related to pressure ulcers was subsequently investigated by comparing the maximum shear strain distributions in the tissue, using FE modelling, and the amount and location of initial tissue damage. The shear strain distribution showed some coincidence with the area of muscle damage but not enough to confirm, or reject, the hypothesis at that stage. By modifying the experimental set-up used by Bosboom the present authors will attempt to create more reproducible tissue damage. Ultimately the aim is to establish a clear understanding of the influence of both tissue deformation and reperfusion on the development of pressure ulcers.

To be able to simultaneously collect MR data and apply pressure to the muscle, we are developing a MR-compatible loading apparatus. A large variety of imaging techniques have been developed that can be applied to assess structure, function and metabolism of skeletal muscle (extensively described in Chap. 18). Tagging MRI can be used to measure local tissue deformation (necessary for the FE model), perfusion MRI offers the possibility of measuring tissue perfusion, and with MR spectroscopy information on the biochemical status of tissue can be obtained.

References

1. Groth KE (1942) Klinische Beobachtungen und experimentelle Studien über die Entstehung des Dekubitus. Acta Chir Scand 87 [Suppl 76]:198–200
2. Husain T (1953) An experimental study of some pressure effects on tissues, with reference to the bed-sore problem. J Pathol Bacteriol 66: 347–358
3. Kosiak M (1961) Etiology of decubitus ulcers. Arch Phys Med Rehabil 42:19–29
4. Daniel RK, Priest DL, Wheatley DC (1981) Etiologic factors in pressure sores: an experimental model. Arch Phys Med Rehabil 62(10):492–498
5. Swaim SF, Bradley DM, Vaughn DM, Powers RD, Hoffman CE (1993) The greyhound dog as a model for studying pressure ulcers. Decubitus 6(2):32–35, 38–40
6. Kosiak M (1959) Etiology and pathology of ischemic ulcers. Arch Phys Med Rehabil 40:62–69
7. Hyodo A, Reger SI, Negami S, Kambic H, Reyes E Browne EZ (1995) Evaluation of a pressure sore model using monoplegic pigs. Plast Reconstr Surg 96(2):421–428
8. Goldstein B, Sanders J (1998) Skin response to repetitive mechanical stress: a new experimental model in pig. Arch Phys Med Rehabil 79(3):265–272
9. Houwing R, Overgoor M, Kon M, Jansen G, Asbeck BS, Haalboom JRE (2000) Pressure-induced skin lesions in pigs: reperfusion injury and the effects of vitamin E. J Wound Care 9(1): 36–40
10. Peirce SM, Skalak TC, Rodeheaver GT (2000) Ischemia-reperfusion injury in chronic pressure ulcer formation: a skin model in the rat. Wound Repair Regen 8(1):68–76
11. Salcido R, Donofrio JC, Fisher SB, LeGrand EK, Dickey K, Carney JM, Schosser R, Liang R (1994) Histopathology of pressure ulcers as a result of sequential computer-controlled pressure sessions in a fuzzy rat model. Adv Wound Care 7(5):23–24, 26, 28 passim
12. Salcido R, Fisher SB, Donofrio JC, Bieschke M, Knapp C, Liang R, LeGrand EK, Carney JM (1995) An animal model and computer-controlled surface pressure delivery system for the production of pressure ulcers. J Rehabil Res Dev 32(2):149–161
13. Salcido R, Donofrio JC, Fisher SB, LeGrand EK, Carney JM, Schosser R, Rodgers J, Liang R (1995) Evaluation of ibuprofen for pressure ulcer prevention: application of a rat pressure ulcer model. Adv Wound Care 8(4):30–32, 34, 38–40 passim
14. Bosboom EMH, Bouten CVC, Oomens CWJ, van Straaten HWM, Baaijens FPT, Kuipers H (2001) Quantification and localisation of damage in rat muscles after controlled loading; a new approach to study the aetiology of pressure sores. Med Eng Phys 23(3):195–200
15. Dinsdale SM (1973) Decubitus ulcers in swine: light and electron microscopy study of pathogenesis. Arch Phys Med Rehabil 54(2):51–56 passim
16. Daniel RK, Wheatley DC, Priest DL (1985) Pressure sores and paraplegics: an experimental model. Ann Plast Surg 15:41–49
17. Sundin BM, Hussein MA, Glasofer S, El-Falaky MH, Abdel-Aleem SM, Sachse RE, Klitzman B (2000) The role of allupurinol and deferoxamine in preventing pressure ulcers in pigs. Plast Reconstr Surg 105 (4):1408–1421

18. Reswick JB, Rogers JE (1976) Experience at Rancho Los Amigos Hospital with devices and techniques to prevent pressure sores. In: Kenedi RM, Cowden JM, Scales JT (eds) Bedsore Biomechanics. Macmillan, London, pp 301–310

19. Lindan O (1961) Etiology of decubitus ulcers: an experimental study. Arch Phys Med Rehabil 42:774–783

20. Reger S, Negami S, Reyes E, McGovern T, Navarro R (1990) Effect of DC electrical stimulation on pressure sore healing in pigs. RESNA Conference, Washington, DC, p 379

21. Bosboom EMH (2001) Deformation as a trigger for pressure sore related muscle damage, PhD thesis, TUE, Netherlands, ISBN 90-386-2962-1

22. Sacks AH (1989) Theoretical prediction of a time-at-pressure curve for avoiding pressure sores. J Rehabil Res Dev 26(3):27–34

23. Reichel SM (1958) Shearing force as a factor in decubitus ulcers in paraplegics. JAMA 166:762–763

24. Dinsdale SM (1974) Decubitus ulcers: role of pressure and friction in causation. Arch Phys Med Rehabil 55(4):147–152

25. Bennett L, Kavner D, Lee BK, Trainor FA (1979) Shear vs pressure as causative factors in skin blood flow occlusion. Arch Phys Med Rehabil 60(7):309–314

26. McCord JM(1985) Oxygen-derived free radicals in postischemic tissue injury. N Engl J Med 312(3):159–163 Review

27. Kukreja RC, Janin Y (1997) Reperfusion injury: basic concepts and protection strategies. J Thromb Thrombolysis 4(1):7–24

28. Russell RC, Roth AC, Kucan JO, Zook EG (1989) Reperfusion injury and oxygen free radicals: a review. J Reconstr Microsurg 5(1):79–84

29. Parks DA, Granger DN (1988) Ischemia-reperfusion injury: a radical view. Hepatology 8(3):680–682

30. Ünal S, Ozmen S, Demir Y, Yavuzer R, LatIfoglu O, Atabay K, Oguz M (2001) The effect of gradually increased blood flow on ischemia-reperfusion injury. Ann Plast Surg 7(4) 412–416

31. Brown AC, Brengelmann G Energy metabolism. In: Ruch RC, Patton HD (eds) Physiology and biophysics, 20th edn. Saunders, London, pp 1030–1049

32. Mahanty SD, Roemer RB (1979) Thermal response of skin to application of localized pressure. Arch Phys Med Rehabil 60(12):584–590

33. Fisher SV, Szymke TE, Apte SY, Kosiak M (1978) Wheelchair cushion effect on skin temperature. Arch Phys Med Rehabil 59(2):68–72

34. Kokate JY, Leland KJ, Held AM, Hansen GL, Kveen GL, Johnson BA, Wilke MS, Sparrow EM, Iaizzo P (1995) Temperature-modulated pressure ulcers: a porcine model. Arch Phys Med Rehabil 76(7):666–673

35. Iaizzo P, Kveen GL, Kokate JY, Leland KJ, Hansen GL, Sparrow EM (1995) Prevention of pressure ulcers by focal cooling: histological assessment in a porcine model. Wounds 7(5):161–169

36. Patel S, Knapp CF, Donofrio JC, Salcido R (1999) Temperature effects on surface pressure-induced changes in rat skin perfusion: implications in pressure ulcer development. J Rehabil Res Dev 36(3):189–201

37. Fleckenstein JL (1996) Skeletal muscle evaluated by MRI. In Grant DM, Harris RK (eds) Encyclopedia of nuclear magnetic resonance. ,Wiley, Chichester, pp 4430–4436

38. Barczk CA, Barnett RI, Jarczynski Childs E, Bosley LM (1997) Fourth national pressure ulcer prevalence survey. Adv Wound Care 10:18–26

39. Bosboom EMH, Bouten CVC, Oomens CWJ, Baaijens FPT, Nicolay K (2001) High-resolution MRI to assess skeletal muscle damage after prolonged transverse loading. J Appl Phys 95:2235–2240
40. Herrman EC, Knapp CF, Donofrio JC, Salcido R (1999) Skin perfusion responses to surface pressure-induced ischemia: implication for the developing pressure ulcer. J Rehabil Res Dev 36(2):109–120
41. Nola GT, Vistnes LM (1980) Differential response of skin and muscle in the experimental production of pressure sores. Plast Reconstr Surg 66(5):728–733

The Role of Oxidative Stress in the Development and Persistence of Pressure Ulcers

13

RICHARD TAYLOR, TIM JAMES

Introduction

Pressure ulcers are a major drain on health resources and can cause severe ill health or disruption to life, and much work has been done to establish the factors leading to their development. A clear understanding of the aetiology of pressure ulcers remains elusive because of the multiple factors thought to contribute. However, many of the risk factors, such as age, nutritional status, heart failure and impaired mobility, can be shown to contribute to different extents to the biochemical changes leading to pressure ulcers [1–3]. Major causative factors are thought to be ischaemia causing impaired tissue perfusion, and ischaemia–reperfusion injury in which there are cycles of ischaemia and reperfusion causing a characteristic form of tissue injury. Key components of tissue injury by these mechanisms are various reactive oxygen or nitrogen species. The body has natural defences against these, with the outcome depending on the ability to prevent or minimise damage. Reactive oxygen and nitrogen molecules are also involved in inflammatory processes that occur in pressure ulcers. In this chapter we review the nature of oxidative stress and its potential to contribute to tissue breakdown and formation of pressure ulcers. We review information that has been obtained through the analysis of clinical materials, such as sweat and wound fluid, providing clues that link oxidative stress to chronic wounds.

Oxidative Stress

Oxidative processes are fundamental to biological reactions and in any living organism there is a constant production of what are collectively described as reactive oxygen species (ROS). The nature of ROS has been reviewed in detail [4–6]. ROS include free radicals, atoms or molecules containing one or more unpaired electrons [7]. Free radicals are unstable and are highly reactive. To control inappropriate oxidation and ensure continued biological function, antioxidant mechanisms have evolved [8].

Oxidative stress occurs when there is either an increased production of oxidative species or when there is a depletion of antioxidants [5]. In both situations the balance will favour oxidation. Structural changes to bio-molecules including DNA, proteins and lipids can occur. If the structural change leads to loss of normal biological function, as is often the case, pathological changes to the organism may ensue.

When free radicals were discovered and linked to human disease processes it was questioned whether they arose as a consequence of pathological processes or were part of them. However, as methods to investigate and monitor ROS have developed it is now known that oxidative species are involved in a wide range of pathological processes, including cancer, cardiovascular disease, rheumatoid arthritis and diabetes mellitus [5].

ROS is a collective term used to describe both radical and non-radical derivatives of oxygen. Oxygen radicals include superoxide, hydroxyl, peroxyl and hydroperoxyl radicals. Non-radicals include hydrogen peroxide, ozone, hypochlorous acid and peroxynitrite. ROS interact with each other, and one radical will react with another molecule or radical to produce a further radical of greater, equivalent or lesser reactivity [4].

The superoxide radical, $O_2^{\cdot-}$, is a free radical that arises when an additional electron is added to the outer orbital of oxygen. The most important source of superoxide is the mitochondrial electron transport system, particularly in the ubiquinone–cytochrome b reaction. Superoxide can also be produced in mitochondria from the NADH dehydrogenase reaction. At physiological oxygen levels the electron transport system can leak between 1 and 3% of the oxygen being reduced in the mitochondria and the rate of leakage will increase with a higher oxygen tension. The rate of ROS production can be influenced by the cell's energy substrate availability and energy utilisation through effects on the rate of influx of electrons and the proton gradient [9]. ROS can also be produced by peroxisomes. Oxidative reactions within these organelles generate hydrogen peroxide (H_2O_2), which can in turn generate free radicals. Under circumstances of high peroxisomal activity such as ischaemia–reperfusion injury, H_2O_2 leakage from peroxisomes may occur [10]. Production of superoxide is also mediated by enzymes such as NADPH oxidase or xanthine oxidase.

The other major sources of superoxide and H_2O_2 are phagocytic cells [11], such as neutrophils, and sensitised monocytes and macrophages. There is activation of NADPH oxidase and increased oxygen consumption, termed the 'oxidative burst', accompanying the generation of free radicals [12].

NADPH oxidase has a key role in signalling cascades. NADPH oxidase in activated neutrophils and macrophages can be induced by cytokines or bacterial products [13]. It produces large quantities of superoxide, which is released and can cause local tissue damage. Through their myeloperoxidase activity these cells can produce hypochlorous acid [14]. NADPH oxidase is also present in non-phagocytic cells such as fibroblasts, smooth muscle cells, endothelial cells and chondrocytes and can generate ROS, which can regulate intracellular signalling cascades [15–19].

ROS can also be generated by xanthine oxidase (XO). The enzyme is generated by proteolytic cleavage of xanthine dehydrogenase. Normally XO is not a major mechanism of ROS production [20] but may make a signifi-

cant contribution in conditions such as ischaemia [21] or ischaemia–reperfusion [22].

The superoxide radical can undergo a dismutation, a reaction in which the
same species is simultaneously oxidised and reduced, to produce hydrogen
peroxide. H_2O_2 is also generated by enzymes, including xanthine, urate and
D-amino acid oxidases. H_2O_2 is relatively unreactive, but it has a relatively
long half-life, can cross membranes easily and can react with transition metals, particularly iron and copper, to form the hydroxyl radical. The reaction
with ferrous ions is known as the Fenton reaction. The ferric ions produced
can react with reducing agents such as ascorbate or superoxide to regenerate
ferrous ions, which can react with more hydrogen peroxide. In this process,
known as the iron-catalysed Haber-Weiss reaction, superoxide and hydrogen
peroxide generate the highly reactive hydroxyl radical [5]:

$$H_2O_2 + O_2^{\cdot-} \rightarrow OH^{\cdot} + O_2 + OH^-$$

Therefore, hydrogen peroxide and subsequently hydroxyl radicals (OH),
mediated by iron, can exert their oxidative effects in neighbouring cells
through the passage of hydrogen peroxide across their membranes. Copper
transport and storage is tightly controlled to minimise free copper concentrations. It has a tendency to complex with macromolecular structures
such as proteins, DNA and carbohydrates and once complexed can undergo
redox cycling and act as a locus for site-specific radical formation [23].
Such metal-catalysed formation of OH can cause a cascade of lipid radical
formation with oxidation of lipids resulting in damage to the lipid bilayers
of membranes. Oxidatively modified proteins are recognised by the cell
and are rapidly destroyed by intracellular proteolytic systems. Over-activa-
tion of these systems may lead to cellular damage and may be linked to
the activation of apoptosis [24]. Copper, superoxide and hydrogen peroxide
have been implicated in damage to DNA [25].

Peroxyl and alkoxyl radicals arise from the decomposition of organic
peroxides (ROOH). Peroxyl radicals can also arise when carbon-centred
radicals are produced in aerobic conditions. Hypochlorous acid, an extremely damaging species, is generated from the enzyme myeloperoxidase,
an enzyme found in activated neutrophils.

Oxygen centred radicals are not the only damaging radicals. Both nitro-
gen-centred [26] and sulphur-centred [27] families of radicals exist. Nitric
oxide (NO) is a free radical as it has an unpaired electron but it can act as
a pro-oxidant or antioxidant. NO is generated enzymically by nitric oxide
synthases (NOS). As a pro-oxidant it can form several reactive nitrogen
species (RNS) such as peroxynitrite ($ONOO^-$), nitrosonium cation (NO^+)
and nitroxyl anion (NO^-) [28]. Peroxynitrite, formed by reaction of NO
with superoxide, is able to oxidise lipids; aromatic amino acids, affecting
protein structure; and sulphur-containing amino acids, leading to glutathione depletion, lipid peroxidation and depletion of antioxidants. Peroxynitrite has a relatively long half-life, i.e. an increased period in which to
react. NO-related radicals have been heavily investigated because of their

multiple physiological roles [29] and it is known that excessive production can result in cell injury [30]. NOS exists in three isoforms. The type 2 isoform (iNOS) is inducible by cytokines, lipopolysaccharides and immunological factors [31]. Expression of NOS type 2 is affected by transcription factors such as NF-kappa B, which is activated by ROS among other factors [32]. NF-κB also upregulates the transcription of leucocyte adhesion molecules such as ICAM-1 and VCAM-1 and cytokines such as TNF-α, IL-1, and IL-6, which have important regulatory roles in inflammation [33, 34].

Antioxidants

Antioxidants have been defined as "any substance that, when present in low concentrations compared with those of an oxidisable substrate, significantly delays or prevents oxidation of that substrate" [35]. Antioxidants act by a range of mechanisms outlined in Table 13.1.

There are enzymatic reactions and non enzymatic antioxidants. Some are extracellular, and within cells there are antioxidants in the cytoplasm and in specific organelles. It is likely that the various antioxidant defences are linked in an antioxidant network [36].

The dismutation of the superoxide radical to H_2O_2 is accelerated by the superoxide dismutase (SOD) family of enzymes [36, 37]. Superoxide generally cannot cross biological membranes. Therefore, to detoxify the superoxide radical at the site of production, distinct cytosolic, mitochondrial and

Table 13.1. Important antioxidants and their mode of action

Mode of action	Examples
Enzymatic removal of reactive species	Superoxide dismutase Catalase Glutathione peroxidase Glutathione reductase
Transition metal ion binding	Transferrin Caeruloplasmin Haptoglobin
Sacrificial antioxidants	Vitamin C Vitamin E (tocopherol) Carotenes Lycopenes Ubiquinol Glutathione Uric acid Bilirubin

extracellular SOD enzymes exist. These SODs have either Cu(II)/Zn(II) or Mn(III)/Fe(III) at their active site. Their importance is demonstrated by the many disease states that arise from deficiencies of SOD [39]. The CuZn form is located predominantly in the cytoplasm. The mitochondrial form, MnSOD, is important for regulating the significant quantities of ROS generated in the organelle [40]. Numerous studies have shown that MnSOD can be induced to protect against pro-oxidant insults, and overexpression of MnSOD has been shown to protect against pro-apoptotic stimuli and ischaemic damage. It can also undergo oxidative inactivation which may lead to increased intramitochondrial ROS and to mitochondrial dysfunction and cell death [41]. The SOD isoenzymes may be induced under cytokine co-ordination in addition to direct responses to oxidants [38].

Catalase, a haem enzyme present mainly in peroxisomes, breaks down hydrogen peroxide to water and oxygen. This is an important mechanism for dealing with H_2O_2 generated by the oxidative enzymes in this organelle.

Glutathione peroxidase, a selenium-containing enzyme, converts H_2O_2 to water in the cytoplasm and mitochondria and can also remove lipid peroxides, consuming reduced glutathione, which is regenerated by glutathione reductase [42]. Glutathione S-transferase can remove oxidised substrates by reaction with reduced glutathione. Glutathione is present in cells in millimolar quantities and is a general small molecule antioxidant [35]. It is an important protector of the thiol groups found in the active sites of many enzymes. Its production is inducible by oxidative stress and glutathione depletion [43]. The enzymatic antioxidants are predominantly intracellular. There are no enzymes to remove specifically the most damaging hydroxyl radical, but the reactions leading to its production are tightly controlled.

Proteins can act as antioxidants [7] by binding the metal ions capable of driving the Fenton reaction. Ferric ion binding proteins include transferrin and lactoferrin. Similarly, copper ions in blood are bound by the transport protein caeruloplasmin, but the latter can also bind ferric iron, removing it from Fenton reactions [44]. Iron-containing molecules that accelerate lipid peroxidation, such as haemoglobin and haem, have a diminished ability to catalyse this reaction if bound to haptoglobin and haemopexin, and these proteins are therefore considered antioxidants. Albumin has one thiol group per molecule capable of ROS scavenging and is present in high concentrations in blood [12].

There are numerous low-molecular-weight components that act as antioxidants by virtue of their own vulnerability to oxidants [5]. The major diet-derived "sacrificial" antioxidants are vitamin C (ascorbate) in the aqueous compartment and vitamin E (α-tocopherol) in the lipid compartment, with both functioning extracellularly and intracellularly. Vitamin E reacts with lipid peroxyl radicals and is itself regenerated by reaction with reduced vitamin C, which is consumed and must be replaced from dietary intake. In mitochondria vitamin E radicals can be removed by oxidation with ubiquinol, which is regenerated in the electron transport chain [35]. Dietary intake of potential antioxidants such as vitamin C, vitamin E, carotenoids and ubiquinol is important for maintaining antioxidant systems [45]. Dehydroascorbate, the oxidised form of ascorbate, can be reduced enzymically or non-enzymically to ascorbate by glutathione and by dihydrolipoate [46].

Two low-molecular-weight antioxidant molecules produced in-vivo are uric acid and bilirubin. In many extracellular fluids they represent a significant proportion of the total antioxidant pool. Uric acid is oxidised to allantoin and bilirubin to biliverdin [35].

The Skin, Antioxidants and Oxidative Stress

Most work undertaken to study antioxidants and ROS with respect to skin relate to identifying the mechanism of UV-radiation-mediated damage and the link to skin ageing and skin cancer [47–49]. However the data generated from these investigations provide interesting baseline data for any research into other pathological skin conditions, including chronic wounds.

In the stratum corneum a-tocopherol is suggested to be a critical antioxidant that becomes depleted upon exposure to UV radiation [50]. The low levels of hydrophilic antioxidants, such as ascorbate, in the stratum corneum capable of recycling oxidised tocopherol may prevent the restoration of defences that is observed in other tissues. Two notable factors have been derived from studies of the stratum corneum. First there is a gradient of antioxidants from low concentrations found in the uppermost tissue exposed to the environment to higher concentrations in the deeper tissue. Secondly the antioxidant levels of skin can be enhanced through topical application of agents including vitamin E acetate and vitamin C [51, 52].

The antioxidant defences of deeper skin beneath the stratum corneum have also been determined and it has been found that hydrophilic, lipophilic and enzymic antioxidants are present at higher levels in the epidermis than in the dermis [53]. Ascorbate, urate and glutathione were more than four times higher, ubiquinol 10 was nine times higher and catalase was seven times higher, emphasising the importance of the epidermis as a biological barrier to oxidative damage.

ROS can be generated by the bacterial flora of human skin. Mechanical injury, abnormal humidity, immunodeficiency or metabolic disorders can result in increased bacterial infection which could result in increased bacterial ROS production. This could act synergistically with ROS from host phagocyte cells to increase the generation of pro-inflammatory agents causing tissue damage [54, 55]. Damage to the integrity of the skin by mechanical injury or maceration is known to increase susceptibility to tissue damage [1].

As skin ages, significant changes occur to its antioxidant composition, and these effects are dependent on whether the skin is exposed to the UV radiation of sunlight. Chronological (intrinsic) ageing affects skin in a similar manner to other organs, with photoageing superimposed upon this. Intrinsic ageing and photoageing have partly overlapping biochemical and molecular mechanisms. Pressure ulcers occur in skin that is intrinsically aged rather than photoaged.

Table 13.2. Antioxidant changes occurring in naturally aged skin (derived from 20)

	Epidermis	Dermis
Enzymatic antioxidants		
Superoxide dismutase	Similar	Similar
Glutathione peroxidase	Similar	Similar
Glutathione reductase	Increased	–
Catalase	Increased	Decreased
Non-enzymatic antioxidants		
α-Tocopherol	Decreased	Similar
Ascorbate	Decreased	Decreased
Glutathione	Decreased	Decreased
Uric acid	Similar	Similar

Table 13.2 summarises the changes that occur in this process from a recent study [56]. Data from normal subjects measuring cysteine/cystine and glutathione/glutathione disulphide ratios suggest that there is a slow linear increase in oxidative events within the body throughout life, but with the capacity of the glutathione antioxidant system maintained until age 45, followed by a relatively rapid decline [57]. Such findings may be of significance for the development of pressure ulcers in the elderly [58]. In a normally healing wound, tissue concentrations of enzymatic and non-enzymatic antioxidants fall during healing as part of the healing process [59]. It is possible that the failure of the host to respond appropriately to ROS signals, particularly due to the ageing process, leads to vulnerability to oxidative stress. The thiol/disulphide redox state of plasma becomes more oxidative with ageing and, as redox signalling mechanisms can respond to this as well as to ROS, the sensitivity of cells to redox signalling may change systematically with this age-related pro-oxidative shift [9].

In a study of aged rats [60] where tirilazad, an antioxidant analogue of vitamin E, was used to enhance the antioxidant levels during tissue repair an interesting observation was made in older animals. Enhancement of antioxidant levels in the early phase of the tissue repair impaired the healing process whereas later enhancement accelerated healing. Therefore, suggestions that antioxidants could be used to enhance healing need to be considered carefully.

It would appear that a physiologically significant contribution to lipophilic antioxidants of skin upper layers and surface is derived from sebaceous gland secretions [61]. The contribution of sweat to skin antioxidants has not been comprehensively studied.

The Metabolically Compromised Patient

Patients who develop pressure ulcers are suffering illness [62], likely to be catabolic and are therefore metabolically compromised. In addition to requirements for energy and protein substrates [63] which contribute to maintenance of the immune system [64], several components of the antioxidant defence system are either themselves micronutrients, such as vitamin C and vitamin E, or are required for activity, such as copper, zinc and manganese in SOD enzymes [65]. Under conditions of metabolic stress the intake of these micronutrients may be particularly important for maintaining or restoring tissue viability. Numerous studies have highlighted both generalised and specific nutritional deficiencies in patients with pressure ulcers. Little information is available to comment on whether these factors were present during development of the pressure ulcer or whether they arose as a consequence.

The antioxidant ascorbic acid has received much attention with respect to pressure ulcers [66, 67]. Despite the long-noted susceptibility of these patients to ascorbate deficiency it remains a significant problem. In a recent study where plasma ascorbate was measured in pressure ulcer patients [68] it was observed that the mean serum concentration of 4.2 ± 3.4 µg/ml in patients with pressure ulcers was significantly lower than in matched controls, mean 7.4 ± 5.4 µg/ml, which was in turn lower than in a reference population, at 10.9 ± 1.9 µg/ml. A study of serum vitamins A, C and E in subjects with chronic spinal cord injury living in the community, with and without pressure ulcers, showed 16–37% had serum concentrations below the reference range for each vitamin [69]. Higher vitamin A was associated with being less impaired, having better function and not having had a pressure ulcer in the past 12 months. In this study patient outcome measures were not related to vitamin C concentration. Further work remains to be done to establish a causal relationship between vitamin levels and healing or rehabilitation outcomes. The randomised controlled trials conducted to date evaluating the effectiveness of enteral or parenteral nutrition on the prevention and treatment of pressure ulcers are insufficient to be conclusive [70, 71]. No study has comprehensively assessed the antioxidant status of patients with pressure ulcers [71].

Zinc is important for both tissue repair and activation of antioxidant enzymes [72]. It can prevent transition metal-mediated oxidation of proteins and may protect against further cell injury resulting from such reactions. A study of copper and zinc in patients with skin disorders [73] demonstrates a problem associated with the laboratory tools available to assess nutritional status. In patients with pressure ulcers the zinc concentration was observed to be significantly lower than in a control group. However, this may not reflect nutritional deficiency. The serum zinc level is known to fall as part of an acute-phase response [74] which may simply be due to redistribution. This is an example of the weakness of present laboratory measures and why nutritional assessment can be poor. No study has shown improved wound healing in patients supplemented with zinc who were not zinc deficient.

Ischaemia–Reperfusion Injury

In ischaemia there is impaired tissue perfusion with inadequate delivery of oxygen and other substrates and impaired removal of metabolic products. Unrelieved tissue ischaemia will result in cell death through necrosis. After a period of ischaemia tissues may or may not fully recover following reperfusion, depending on the period of ischaemia and the tissue in question. Some tissues are more tolerant of ischaemia than others. Paradoxically, reperfusion results in injury that was not apparent during the ischaemic period. The hypothesis of ischaemia–reperfusion injury (IRI) proposes that reperfusion can activate damaging processes through reactions of re-introduced oxygen that generate ROS [75]. The mechanism of IRI is similar in most tissues and organs [76] and is considered to involve ROS produced by two major sources, the enzyme XO and phagocytic cells, most notably neutrophils. ROS are thought to be central to the development of IRI, exceeding the free radical-scavenging capacity of the tissues. Work in various tissues has shown this leads to inflammation through the activation of endothelial cells which release cytokines and express adhesion molecules that recruit circulating leucocytes. The adherent leucocytes can themselves release ROS and other toxic agents that cause further localised tissue damage. Monocytes and macrophages are also recruited and there is endothelial cell swelling with reduction in arteriolar diameter, restricted blood flow in the microcirculation and increased permeability of the vasculature to injurious substances [77–80].

During ischaemia the enzyme xanthine dehydrogenase is converted to XO. This generates ROS when oxygen is re-introduced and is a key mechanism for generation of ROS in IRI. The behaviour of skin tissue to ischaemia and IRI has been studied in animal experiments [81, 82]. Upon reperfusion the oxygen returning to tissue is utilised by XO to produce superoxide and hydrogen peroxide (Fig. 13.1).

In patients with chronic venous leg ulcers the hypoxanthine level in wound fluid was higher than in plasma, and wound fluid total antioxidant

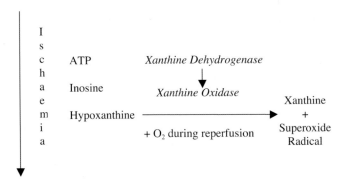

Fig. 13.1. Purine metabolism during ischaemia–reperfusion

capacity was inversely related to hypoxanthine, suggesting a hypoxic wound environment with increased consumption of antioxidants [83]. The evidence to support the involvement of XO in ischaemia–reperfusion (IR)-induced tissue damage includes the fact that XO inhibitors, such as allopurinol, decreased necrosis and biochemical evidence of tissue damage [81]. Immunohistochemical and biochemical findings demonstrate that in ischaemia–reperfusion injury ROS, particularly superoxide and peroxynitrite, cause endothelial and tissue injury, neutrophil and other phagocyte activation, damage to membrane lipids, ion channels and transporters, and DNA strand breakage [84].

Nitric oxide appears to promote IRI in some tissues through reaction with superoxide to produce peroxynitrite, although whether this occurs in human leucocytes is unclear [85, 86]. Inhibitors of NO synthesis protect against immune-complex-induced vascular injury in animals [87] and limit neutrophil accumulation and vascular protein leakage in skeletal tissue [88]. Peroxynitrite involvement is implicated by the observation that oxygen free radical scavengers are as effective as NO synthase inhibitors in reducing tissue injury in IR models [89].

Antioxidants act in a complementary manner to regulate and counter the functional changes resulting from ROS reactions. Mitochondrial MnSOD appears to be particularly important for countering ROS in cardiac tissue [90]. Extracellular SOD has a major role in the protection of extracellular spaces from superoxide damage, particularly from activated phagocytes such as in IRI, and enhances arterial relaxation by protecting NO from inactivation [91].

ROS can induce the expression of neutrophil adhesion molecules on the surface of endothelial cells [92] and can activate neutrophils [93–95], which are themselves synergistic with ROS in the processes leading to tissue damage [76]. Activated neutrophils secrete myeloperoxidase, which catalyses the formation of hypochlorous acid (HOCl) from H_2O_2 and chloride ions. HOCl is a powerful oxidising and chlorinating agent that can react with primary amines in proteins and peptides affecting function and structure. Neutrophils adhere to the walls of post-capillary venules [96] after no-flow or low-flow ischaemia [97], or can become trapped in the capillary bed [98]. Leucocyte adhesion in partial ischaemia may be partly due to low shear rates that increase leucocyte adhesion in postcapillary venules [99]. Tissue oedema may contribute to neutrophil trapping in the capillary bed [100].

Key findings in reperfusion damage are the interaction of ROS-activated neutrophils with vascular endothelium through changes to adhesion molecules such as selectins and β-2 integrins. This is a complex process, modulated by macrophages and lymphocytes, which is not well understood. Antioxidants limit the ROS-mediated activation of the signal transduction pathways regulated by NF-kappa B and MAPK that determine the fate of the cell [90].

Evidence that neutrophil-derived ROS contribute to reperfusion injury comes in part from studies showing reduced effects using neutrophil-depleted blood [101, 102]. The damage is also ameliorated when adhesion of neutrophils is inhibited. Other cell signalling and regulatory processes are also involved in the development of IRI [103]. Complement activation can contribute to the recruitment of neutrophils and macrophages [103], to produce cytokines, chemokines and adhesion molecules, and may also have a role in regulation of apoptosis. Recent work in murine renal tissue suggests that complement activation can also modulate IR damage by neutrophil-independent as well as neutrophil-dependent pathways [104].

Necrosis occurs in response to severe injury. Cell swelling, including mitochondrial swelling, occurs with plasma membrane rupture and release of cellular contents. This can cause injury or death to surrounding cells [105]. It is accompanied by a rapid fall in ATP and is a relatively passive process.

Apoptosis is a form of cell death that can be triggered by external or internal stresses and is tightly regulated within the cell. It is a mechanism for the removal of cells that are damaged, and for cell replacement and tissue remodelling. It is accompanied by characteristic changes to phospholipids on the external surface of the cell membrane, mitochondrial depolarisation, formation of apoptotic bodies, cell shrinkage, nuclear fragmentation and condensation of nuclear DNA. A major regulatory mechanism for apoptosis is activation by caspases [106]. These are proteases found in the cytoplasm, the intermembrane space of mitochondria and the nucleus [107]. They contain thiol groups that are sensitive to oxidation or reaction with a reactive nitrogen radical to produce an S-nitrosylated form. Oxidants such as H_2O_2 or quinones have been shown to cause apoptosis at low concentrations and necrosis at higher concentrations [108, 109]). Neutrophils become apoptotic after the respiratory burst, with ROS thought to be involved in the induction of apoptosis [110, 111].

Apoptosis can be triggered by inflammatory processes mediated for example by TNF-a or Fas [112] and by UV radiation or certain drugs [113]. This is associated with NADPH oxidase activity, superoxide generation and caspase activation [114]. Cell surface receptors such as Fas or TNF-R respond to external signals and cause the assembly of death-inducing signalling complexes, which activates an initiator caspase such as procaspase-8. The activated caspase 8 triggers effector caspases such as procaspase-3, with the activated caspase-3 causing proteolysis leading to cell death [115].

The action of ROS in the mitochondria is thought to be a major mechanism for the initiation of apoptosis [116]. Superoxide generated in mitochondria is converted to H_2O_2 by Mn-SOD and in the cytoplasm by Cu/Zn-SOD. Apoptosis can be triggered by mitochondrial dysfunction leading to release of cytochrome c and the formation of a complex in the cytoplasm known as the apoptosome, which causes caspase-9 activation, leading to caspase-3 activation and induction of apoptosis [117].

Lipid peroxidation is well known to occur in conditions of oxidative stress from excessive production of ROS and depletion of reduced glutathione. Lipid free radicals may be able to attack nuclear chromatin directly, leading to apoptosis. Their production may also lead to loss of membrane integrity and function, leading to cell necrosis. Reduced glutathione is likely to be important for regulating these processes [118].

Apoptosis can also be activated by mechanisms not requiring caspase activation, such as that involving apoptosis-inducing factor (AIF) [119, 120]. Poly(ADP-ribose) polymerase-1 (PARP) is highly expressed in the nucleus and has a role in repairing DNA. This requires ATP and NAD^+. In conditions of oxidative stress, PARP activity increases substantially, depleting ATP and NAD^+. Cell necrosis ensues if extreme ATP and NAD^+ depletion occurs. PARP activity is able to direct the cell to apoptosis by rapid signalling from the nucleus to the mitochondria, causing mitochondrial depolarisation and release of AIF. The AIF migrates to the nucleus where it induces the apoptotic lysis of chromatin and cell death. AIF also causes mitochondrial cytochrome c release and caspase activation, features of caspase-dependent apoptosis [119, 120].

NO also has a major role in cell death [121], being able to induce and protect against apoptosis and also to drive an apoptotic response to a necrotic response. NO has been shown to be essential for TNF-a-mediated apoptosis, but in other circumstances can inhibit it [122]. Low concentrations of NO can be associated with inhibition of apoptosis. NO appears to be involved in several of the recognised processes by which apoptosis can be induced. These include the Fas death receptor [123], production of peroxynitrite [124], reduction of ATP production in the mitochondrion [125] and inhibition of antioxidant enzymes [126].

Nuclear gene transcription factors p53, NF-kappa B and AP-1 can be activated by H_2O_2, which may lead to upregulation of death proteins or production of inhibitors of proteins required for cell survival. Single-strand cleavage of DNA is characteristic of apoptosis. Iron and copper are closely associated with chromatin in the nucleus and may be responsible for generating hydroxyl radical from superoxide or H_2O_2 that can cause DNA cleavage [118, 127]. However it is not clear what the role of ROS is in direct DNA degradation [128].

There are tightly regulated mechanisms for controlling apoptosis that involve modulation of ROS and cell redox state. Reduced glutathione (GSH) removes H_2O_2 in cytoplasm and mitochondria and catalase removes H_2O_2 in peroxisomes. The glutathione is normally 95% reduced, giving the cell a buffer against oxidative stress. Depletion of GSH has been shown to be associated with the onset of apoptosis [129] and can make cells more susceptible to apoptosis [130]. The decrease in GSH has been shown to be due to increased efflux from the cell, possibly through a specific membrane channel [131]. Caspases can be inactivated by oxidation of their thiol groups at a cysteine residue in the active site, preventing the activation of apoptosis at various stages [132]. This may lead to necrosis rather than apoptosis. A large fall in intramitochondrial ATP may also result in necrosis rather than apoptosis [133].

There are several mechanisms by which NO can protect against apoptosis. Many of these involve S-nitrosylation of proteins, which is clearly a key regulatory mechanism in apoptosis. Many proteins, such as ion channels, G proteins and transcription factors and several of the caspases, can be modified in this way. NO can also S-nitrosylate other signalling proteins known to be involved in apoptosis, such as NF-kappa B [134], AP-1 [135]

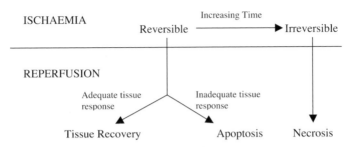

Fig. 13.2. General consequences of ischaemia–reperfusion

and gene transcription factor p53 [136]. NO can also stimulate cGMP production, which is able to inhibit apoptosis by a mechanism as yet unclear. In mitochondria NO inactivates cytochrome c oxidase [137], and inhibits complexes I and II. Inhibition of complex I and cytochrome c oxidase causes increased superoxide production and decreased ATP production. NO is also thought to have a role in regulating the opening of the mitochondrial permeability transition pore [138], leading to cytochrome c release, the formation of the apoptosome and caspase-9 activation, leading to caspase-3 activation and induction of apoptosis.

Apoptosis can also be inhibited by expression of Bcl-2, with evidence that it operates through modulation of GSH concentration or redistribution within the cell, especially to the nucleus [139, 140], changing the nuclear redox potential and DNA binding of transcription factors such as p53, NF-kappa B and AP-1 [141]. Bcl-2 can regulate the signalling pathway controlling the permeability of the mitochondrial membrane and release of cytochrome c and other apoptogenic proteins [142]. The mechanism by which IR insults result in cell death and injury may be linked to the mitochondrial permeability transition pore formed from a complex of mitochondrial membrane proteins [143, 144]. It is thought that in certain situations, which include low ATP and high intracellular calcium, the pore is opened, allowing diffusion of low-molecular-weight substances across the inner membrane and leading to cell necrosis. In apoptosis, binding of the pro-apoptotic proteins such as Bax to the complex occurs. This regulates the opening of the pore and the release of apoptogenic proteins from the intermembrane space into the cytosol [144].

Cell death following reperfusion is thought to occur through apoptosis (Fig. 13.2), whereas cell death following ischaemia is by necrosis.

Development of Pressure Ulcers and Impaired Healing

Wound healing generally follows a sequence through defined stages of coagulation, inflammation, cell proliferation and matrix repair, re-epithelialisation and remodelling [145]. In the inflammatory phase local blood vessels dilate, capillary permeability increases, and complement is activated.

Leucocytes and macrophages migrate to the wound to destroy invading pathogens and degrade damaged extracellular matrix. The stages of healing overlap and are inter-related, with growth factors, cytokines and chemokines as essential regulators. Failure of adequate healing in one part of the process can influence other stages. For example, venous ulcers in individuals with diabetes can fail to progress beyond the inflammatory stage [146], and in chronic wounds cell proliferation is impaired, with hyperproliferation of the extracellular matrix but inadequate epithelial cell growth. It is accepted that ROS and RNS have essential roles in the progression of the normal healing process. For example NO has important regulatory functions [147]. ROS generation and release by activated neutrophils is an essential component of the mechanism for removing damaged tissue and countering bacterial colonisation in the inflammatory phase of wound healing. Superoxide can stimulate fibroblast chemotaxis [148]. H_2O_2 can stimulate neutrophil chemotaxis [149] and is a signalling intermediate in the induction of metalloprotease 1 in cultured human fibroblasts [150]. Furthermore, it is becoming evident that tissue and cellular redox status have a direct fundamental role in regulating wound healing [151, 152]. Very low concentrations of ROS, well below the concentrations known to cause tissue damage, can regulate cellular signalling and can be generated in the cell types present in wounds by an array of NADPH oxidases [153]. It is likely that such ROS signalling is relevant to many of the processes in wound healing progression. It can influence platelet aggregation and recruitment, the activity of PDGF, neutrophil adhesion to endothelium, and TNF-a, IL-1-β and IL-6 function. ROS can influence re-epithelialisation through induction of smooth muscle cell proliferation and migration, induction of matrix metalloproteases (MMPs) and modulation of EGF activity. Development of granulation tissue is influenced by a ROS-dependent increase in FGF-2 receptor affinity and angiogenesis is stimulated by ROS-dependent induction of VEGF [153].

However, excessive oxidative processes can disrupt healing progression, by direct tissue damage and over-stimulation of inflammatory processes. For example, excessive stimulation of NADPH oxidase by cytokines can lead to overexpression of cell adhesion molecules [154]. XO activation in reoxygenated human vascular endothelial cells generates superoxide free radicals which further react with iron to form the reactive hydroxyl radical, which in turn causes cell death [155]. H_2O_2 overproduction caused overexpression of matrix metalloprotease 1 in cultured human fibroblasts [156]. Many factors have the potential to impair the progression of wounds to healing, summarised in Table 13.3. Individuals with one or more of these factors, as is common in the elderly, may be particularly prone to the development of chronic wounds. Pressure ulcers in such patients often fail to heal due to a combination of the factors listed in the table. ROS are contributory in many instances.

Healing of the epidermis normally involves migration of keratinocytes from the wound edge which undergo proliferation, differentiation and apoptosis. A recent study of re-epithelialisation in patients with diabetic or varicose ulcers found that inadequate epithelialisation or defects in apopto-

Table 13.3. Factors contributing to impaired wound healing

Factor	Comments
Age	Compromised immune function; impaired cell replication: increased likelihood of blood vessel disease
Nutrition	Systemic (generalised malnutrition) or local (impaired delivery to wound)
Concurrent pathology	Anaemia; diabetes; vascular disease (venous or arterial or both)
Infection	Bacterial; fungal; viral
Medication	Glucocorticoids; cytostatics; immuno-suppressive; penicillamine; anticoagulants
Physical factors	Pressure; friction
Psychological/social	

tic cell death were not the primary causes of failure to heal [157]. Histology of biopsies showed hyperproliferative stem cells and actively proliferating keratinocytes at the ulcer margin. These did not progress to the differentiated cells characteristic of actively healing wounds. Staining for bcl2, bax, caspase-3 and DNA breaks showed evidence of cell turnover but no major changes in apoptosis from controls. Despite the presence of hyperproliferative keratinocytes, healing of the ulcers was slow, suggesting that the problems actually lie with distorted organisation of the wound bed. In these patients it may have been caused by infection and impaired nutritional supply, which impairs keratinocyte migration. ROS may be implicated in impairment of earlier stages of healing in the wound bed in these diabetic and varicose ulcers through inflammatory processes, with an imbalance of ROS and antioxidant processes. Failure of pressure ulcers to heal may also involve impairment of healing progress by ROS generated by these and other processes, such as IRI.

Leucocyte proteases, enzymes capable of protein digestion, have multiple physiological roles and their appropriate, timely production is essential for normal wound repair [158]. Many proteases exist, and they are classified into distinct families of enzymes that include serine proteases, acid proteases and MMPs [159]. Chronic wound fluid is highly proteolytic [160] and the presence of inappropriately elevated levels of proteases is thought to contribute to poor healing [161]. Wound fluid collected from pressure ulcers has proteolytic activity similar to that of fluid collected from chronic venous ulcers and approximately 30 times higher than observed in fluid collected from acute wounds. Most of the proteolytic activity is due to MMPs, particularly MMP-2 and MMP-9.

It is possible that an inappropriate increase in the activity of proteases could be due to inactivation of the naturally occurring inhibitors of MMPs, tissue inhibitors of metalloprotease (TIMPs). Hypochlorite produced by the action of myeloperoxidase on H_2O_2 can generate chloramines, which can inactivate TIMPs and other antiproteases [161]. The TIMPs are produced during wound repair [162]. Neutrophils have been shown to release collagenase in an inactive form which is activated by hypochlorous acid, also generated by neutrophils [163]. Inappropriate regulation of this oxidative activation could lead to excessive breakdown of extracellular collagen. Very large numbers of neutrophils have been found in chronic pressure ulcer granulation tissue, supporting their role in the persistence of pressure ulcers [164].

Studies measuring transcutaneous gas pressures [165] and lactate in sweat [166, 167] provide evidence that tissue loading results in conditions of both hypoxia and acidosis, both of which favour neutrophil adhesion. On tissue loading in normal subjects when tcPO$_2$ fell below a threshold of 60% of basal tcPO$_2$ the sweat lactate was found to increase in proportion to any further fall in tcPO$_2$, giving biochemical evidence of ischaemia and hypoxia [168]. Hypoxia and high lactate are characteristic of healing wounds, and lactate remains elevated even when oxygen tension increases [169]. In the context of wound healing significant amounts of lactate are also produced in association with ROS in the oxidative burst, and it has been proposed that lactate per se has a regulatory role in wound healing. Lactate production lowers cellular NAD^+ concentration, which down-regulates ADP ribosylation reactions. This has the effect of stimulating collagen synthesis and increasing the release of vascular endothelial growth factor (VEGF), which stimulates growth of new blood vessels [170, 171]. However, the angiogenic effect is inhibited by clinical hypoxia and wound re-oxygenation is required for optimal collagen synthesis.

Neutrophils are recruited to tissue through chemotactic factors that include cytokines generated during ischaemia. ROS are also considered important chemotactic molecules [173]. When the neutrophils enter the ischaemic tissue they adhere through neutrophil-endothelial interactions that are modulated through expression of cell surface molecules such as the integrins and selectins [174]. This ensures an effective inflammatory response.

IRI is now accepted as a significant factor in the development and persistence of pressure ulcers and other chronic skin lesions such as diabetic ulcers and venous ulcers [175–177]. It has become clear that simple ischaemia does not account as adequately for the injury process observed [175, 176] and that IRI and ischaemia generate different patterns of injury [177].

Evidence to support a role for ischaemia–reperfusion in human skin subjected to cycles of pressure loading has come from analysis of sweat. A high-performance liquid chromatography method was used to measure xanthine, hypoxanthine and uric acid in sweat (see chapter 8). The concentration of these metabolites was observed to increase in relation to pressure loading and relief. This suggests significant ATP degradation during ischaemia.

There have been several experimental models using mechanical devices to generate pressure-induced injury. Some have used a single application of pressure giving a model of ischaemia. Others have used IR cycles with various applied pressures and durations [175, 178]. A recent murine model claiming to be clinically relevant to IRI generated visual and histological changes similar to those observed in humans [176]. Tissue damage was proportional to the number of IR cycles, the duration of ischaemia and the IR cycle frequency. Significantly, IR cycles were more damaging than a single ischaemic period of equal duration, demonstrating the importance of the reperfusion phases and the role of free radical generation in the evolution of tissue injury. This model has been used to investigate the role of neutrophils as contributors to tissue damage [179]. Inhibition of the A2A-adenosine receptor on activated neutrophils, which are involved in leucocyte adhesion and release of ROS, improved tissue perfusion by reducing inflammation. There was a 65% reduction in necrosis, suggesting that inhibition of neutrophil-mediated damage could have potential as a therapeutic agent in prevention of pressure ulcers. A mouse model also using implanted magnets to produce cyclical cutaneous IRI yielded similar findings [180]. Leucocyte infiltration is so closely associated with IRI that it was used as one of the indices of IRI in validating this model. Tissue injury was related to IRI cycling and the duration of ischaemia. Apoptotic activity increased significantly. iNOS mRNA expression was greatly increased, suggesting a critical role for iNOS and NO in cell signalling in IRI, particularly in the early stages of tissue injury [181], although its precise role in pressure ulcers remains to be elucidated.

Examination of tissue after 2 h of pressure-induced ischaemia and reperfusion in a porcine model with a computer-controlled pressure device showed characteristic inflammatory changes in the subcutis and underlying muscle with neutrophil adherence to capillary endothelium [182]. Pressure alone caused a significant decrease in blood total and reduced glutathione, implicating oxidative stress. After pressure release the blood H_2O_2 rose, suggesting a decreased antioxidant reserve. Pre-treatment with vitamin E for 14 days did not prevent the pressure-induced decrease in glutathione but it abolished the rise in H_2O_2 on reperfusion and significantly reduced the tissue damage evident on histological examination. These observations in this relatively small study suggest that IRI is implicated in the early signs of pressure-induced tissue injury and that antioxidant therapy may be beneficial, for example, before extensive surgery in the elderly.

In another porcine model [183], cyclical pressure of 210 min ischaemia followed by 30 min reperfusion, applied to the scapulae over 2 days, was used to produce pressure injuries. Allopurinol, a XO inhibitor, administered orally for 2 days before the IR period, and desferrioxamine, an iron-binding agent administered by injection 2 h before the procedure, were both able to improve blood flow and tissue oxygenation. However, only desferrioxamine reduced tissue necrosis. These observations suggest that free iron was even more damaging than XO activated by IRI. The removal of excess iron from the wound bed by chelation has shown promise as an approach to improved wound healing [184].

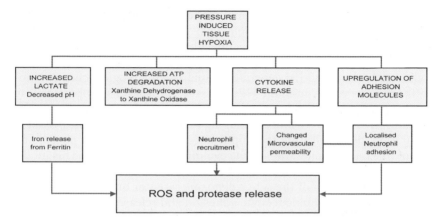

Fig. 13.3. Biochemical factors contributing to the release of reactive oxygen species in hypoxic tissues

Figure 13.3 presents a hypothesis of the biochemical and physiological processes that combine to produce a pressure ulcer.

Approaches to Wound Healing Therapy Involving Redox Status and ROS

Recombinant growth factors, such as PDGF, have been applied to wounds with some success [145]. It may be that the wound bed milieu is not suitable for their action. Proteases in wound fluid can degrade them, as has been shown with fluid from chronic wounds in cell culture experiments. Tissue hypoxia can inhibit the action of growth factors. Recent research suggests several additional approaches. Regulation of wound oxygen tension and lactate concentration could stimulate cell signalling for growth [153]. Amelioration of hypoxia would allow collagen maturation and new vessel growth [170]. Reducing the damaging effect of excessive neutrophil activation could allow healing to progress [176], assuming the wound bed has been prepared adequately for new tissue [164]. Antioxidant therapy [183] and iron chelation [184] have shown potential as effective therapies.

References

1. Lyder CH (2002) Pressure ulcer prevention and management. Annu Rev Nurs Res 20:35–61
2. Ferguson M, Cook A, Rimmasch H, Bender S, Voss A (2000) Pressure ulcer management: the importance of nutrition. Medsurg Nurs 9:163–175
3. Schubert V (1991) Hypotension as a risk factor for the development of pressure sores in elderly subjects. Age Ageing 20:255–261

4. Halliwell B, Gutteridge JMC (1999) Chemistry of biologically important radicals In: Free radicals in biology and medicine, 3rd edn. Oxford University Press, Oxford, pp 246–350
5. Vervaart P, Knight KR (1996) Oxidative stress and the cell. Clin Biochem Rev 17:3–16
6. Halliwell B and Gutteridge JMC (1999) The chemistry of free radicals and related 'reactive species'. In: Free radicals in biology and medicine, 3rd edn. Oxford University Press, Oxford, pp 36–104
7. Gutteridge JMC (1995) Lipid peroxidation and antioxidants as biomarkers of tissue damage. Clin Chem 41:1819–1828
8. Buettner GR (1993) The pecking order of free radicals and antioxidants: lipid peroxidation, α-tocopherol and ascorbate. Arch Biochem Biophys 300:535–543
9. Dröge W (2002) Free radicals in the physiological control of cell function. Physiol Rev 82:47–95
10. McCord JM (1985) Oxygen-derived free radicals in post-ischemic tissue injury N Engl J Med 312:159–163
11. Halliwell B (1987) Oxidants and human disease: some concepts. FASEB J 1:358–364
12. Babior BM (2000) Phagocytes and oxidative stress. Am J Med 109:33–44
13. Bonizzi G, Piette J, Merlville MP, Bours V (2000) Cell type-specific role for reactive oxygen species in nuclear factor NF-kappaB activation by interleukin-1. Biochem Pharmacol 59:7–11
14. Hampton MB, Kettle AJ, Winterbourn CC (1998) Inside the neutrophil phagosome: oxidants, myeloperoxidase, and bacterial killing. Blood 92:3007–3017
15. Jones SA, Wood JD, Coffey MJ, Jones OT (1994) The functional expression of p47-phox and p67-phox may contribute to the generation of superoxide by an NADPH oxidase-like system in human fibroblasts. FEBS Lett 355:178–182
16. Meier B, Radeke HH, Selle S, Younes M, Siesh, Resch K, Habermehl GG (1989) Human fibroblasts release reactive oxygen species in response to interleukin-1 or tumor necrosis factor-alpha. Biochem J 263:539–545
17. Suzuki YG, Ford GD (1999) Redox regulation of signal transduction in cardiac and smooth muscle. J Mol Cell Cardiol 31:345–353
18. Zweier JL, Broderick R, Kuppusamy P, Thompson-Gorman S, Lutty GA (1994) Determination of the mechanism of free radical generation in human aortic endothelial cells exposed to anoxia and reoxygenation. J Biol Chem 269:24156–24162
19. Lo YY, Cruz TF (1995) Involvement of reactive oxygen species in cytokine and growth factor induction of c-fos expression in chondrocytes. J Biol Chem 270:11727–11730
20. Chance B, Sies H, Boveris A (1979) Hydroperoxide metabolism in mammalian organs. Physiol Rev 59:527–605
21. Rees R, Smith D, Li TD, Cashmer B, Garner W, Punch J, Smith DJ Jr (1994) The role of xanthine oxidase and xanthine dehydrogenase in skin ischemia. J Surg Res 56:162–167
22. Granger DN (1988) Role of xanthine oxidase and granulocytes in ischaemia-reperfusion injury. Am J Physiol Heart Circ Physiol 255:H1269–H1275
23. Chevion M (1988) A site-specific mechanism for free radical induced biological damage: the essential role of redox-active transition metals. Free Radic Biol Med 5:27–37
24. Thornberry NA and Lazebnik Y (1998) Caspases: enemies within. Science 281:1312–1316

25. Halliwell B and Haruoma OI (1992) DNA damage by oxygen derived species: its mechanism, and measurement using chromatographic techniques. In: Scandalios JG (ed) Molecular biology of free radical scavenging systems. Cold Spring Harbor Laboratory Press, New York, pp 47–68
26. Drew B, Leeuwenburgh C (2002) Aging and the role of reactive nitrogen species. Ann NY Acad Sci 959:66–81
27. Wardman P, von Sonntag C (1995) Kinetic factors that control the fate of thiyl radicals in cells. Methods Enzymol 251; 31–45
28. Stamler JS, Single D, Loscalzo J (1992) Biochemistry of nitric oxide and its redox-activated forms. Science 258:1898–1902
29. Vallance P, Collier J (1994) Biology and clinical relevance of nitric oxide. BMJ 309:453–457
30. Snyder SH. (1995) Nitric oxide. No endothelial NO. Nature 377:196–197
31. Bogdan C (2001) Nitric oxide and the immune response. Nat Immunol 2:907–916
32. Forstermann U, Kleinert H (1995) Nitric oxide synthase: expression and expressional control of the three isoforms. Naunyn Schmiedebergs Arch Pharmacol 352:351–364
33. Roy S, Sen CK, Packer L (1999) Determination of cell-cell adhesion in response to oxidants and antioxidants. In: Methods in enzymology: oxidants and antioxidants. Academic, San Diego, pp 395–401
34. Sellak H, Franzini E, Hakim J, Pasquier C (1994) Reactive oxygen species rapidly increase endothelial ICAM-1 ability to bind neutrophils without detectable upregulation. Blood 83:2669–2677
35. Halliwell B and Gutteridge JMC (1999) Chapter 3. Antioxidant defences. In: Free radicals in biology and medicine, 3rd edn. Oxford University Press, Oxford, pp 105–245
36. Marczin N, El-Habashi N, Hoare GS, Bundy RE, Yacoub M (2003) Antioxidants in myocardial ischemia-reperfusion injury: therapeutic potential and basic mechanisms. Arch Biochem Biophys 420:222–236
37. Fridovich I (1995) Superoxide radical and superoxide dismutase. Annu Rev Biochem 64:97–112
38. Stralin P, Marklund SL (1994) Effects of oxidative stress on expression of extracellular superoxide dismutase, CuZn superoxide dismutase and Mn superoxide dismutase in human dermal fibroblasts. Biochem J 298:347–352
39. Noor R, Mittal S, Iqbal J (2002) Superoxide dismutase-applications and relevance to human diseases. Med Sci Monit 8:210–215
40. Inoue M, Sato EF, Nishikawa M, Park AM, Kira Y, Imada I, Utsumi K (2003) Mitochondrial generation of reactive oxygen species and its role in aerobic life. Curr Med Chem 10:2495–2505
41. Macmillan-Crow LA, Cruthirds DL (2001) Manganese superoxide dismutase in disease. Free Radic Res 34:325–336
42. Fridovich I, Freeman B (1986) Antioxidant defenses in the lung. Annu Rev Physiol 48:693–702
43. Shi MM, Kugelman A, Iwamoto T, Tian L, Forman HJ (1994) Quinone induced oxidative stress elevates glutathione and induces gamma glutamylcysteine synthetase activity in rat lung epithelial L2 cells. J Biol Chem 269:26512–26517
44. Dreosti IE (1991) The physiological biochemistry and antioxidant activity of the trace elements copper, manganese, selenium and zinc. Clin Biochem Revs 12:127–129

45. Evans P, Halliwell B (2001) Micronutrients: oxidant/antioxidant status. Br J Nutr 85 Suppl 2:S67–74
46. Guo Q, Packer L (2000) Ascorbate-dependent recycling of the vitamin E homologue Trolox by dihydrolipoate and glutathione in murine skin homogenates. Free Rad Biol Med 29:368–374
47. Podda M, Grundmann-Kollmann M (2001) Low molecular weight antioxidants and their role in skin ageing. Clin Exp Dermatol 26:578–582
48. Pinnell SR (2003) Cutaneous photodamage, oxidative stress, and topical antioxidant protection. J Am Acad Dermatol 48:1–19
49. Trouba KJ, Hamadeh HK, Amin RP, Germolec DR (2002) Oxidative stress and its role in skin disease. Antioxid Redox Signal 4:665–673
50. Thiele JJ, Schroeter C, Hsieh SN, Podda M, Packer L (2001) The antioxidant network of the stratum corneum. In: Thiele J, Elsner P (eds) Current problems in dermatology, vol 29: Oxidants and antioxidants in cutaneous biology. Karger, Basle, pp 26–42
51. Dreher F, Maibach H (2001) Protective effects of topical antioxidants in humans. In: Thiele J, Elsner P (eds) Current problems in dermatology, vol 29: Oxidants and antioxidants in cutaneous biology. Karger, Basle, pp 157–164
52. Nabi Z, Travakkol A, Dobke M, Polefka TG (2001) Bioconversion of vitamin E acetate in human skin. In: Thiele J, Elsner P (eds) Current problems in dermatology, vol 29: Oxidants and antioxidants in cutaneous biology. Karger, Basle, pp 175–186
53. Shindo Y, Witt E, Han D, Epstein W, Packer L (1994) Enzymic and non-enzymic antioxidants in epidermis and dermis of human skin. J Invest Dermatol 102:122–124
54. Ginsburg I (1998) Could synergistic interactions among reactive oxygen species, proteinases, membrane-perforating enzymes, hydrolases, microbial hemolysins and cytokines be the main cause of tissue damage in infectious and inflammatory conditions? Med Hypotheses 51:337–346
55. Ginsburg I (2002) The role of bacteriolysis in the pathophysiology of inflammation, infection and post-infectious sequelae. APMIS 110:753–770
56. Rhie G, Shin MH, Seo JY, Choi WW, Cho KH, Kim KH, Park KC, Eun HC, Chung JH (2001) Aging- and photoaging-dependent changes of enzymic and nonenzymic antioxidants in the epidermis and dermis of human skin in vivo. J Invest Dermatol 117:1212–1217
57. Jones DP, Mody VC Jr, Carlson JL, Lynn MJ, Sternberg P Jr (2002) Redox analysis of human plasma allows separation of pro-oxidant events of aging from decline in antioxidant defenses. Free Radic Biol Med 33:1290–1300
58. Casimiro C, Garcia-de-Lorenzo A, Usan L (2002) Prevalence of decubitus ulcer and associated risk factors in an institutionalized Spanish elderly population. Nutrition 18:408–414
59. Shukla A, Rasik AM, Patnaik GK (1997) Depletion of reduced glutathione, ascorbic acid, vitamin E and antioxidant defence enzymes in a healing cutaneous wound. Free Radic Res 26:93–101
60. Khodr B, Khalil Z (2001) Modulation of inflammation by reactive oxygen species: implications for aging and tissue repair. Free Radic Biol Med 30:1–8
61. Thiele JJ, Weber SU, Packer L (1999) Sebaceous gland secretion is a major physiologic route of vitamin E delivery to skin. J Invest Dermatol 113:1006–1010
62. Bliss MR (1998) Pressure injuries: causes and prevention. Hosp Med 59:841–844
63. Aquilani R, Boschi F, Contardi A, Pistarini C, Achilli MP, Fizzotti G, Moroni S, Catapano M, Verri M, Pastoris O (2001) Energy expenditure and nutri-

tional adequacy of rehabilitation paraplegics with asymptomatic bacteria and pressure sores. Spinal Cord 39:437–441

64. Cruse JM, Lewis RE, Dilioglou S, Roe DL, Wallace WF, Chen RS (2000) Review of immune function, healing of pressure ulcers, and nutritional status in patients with spinal cord injury. J Spinal Cord Med 23:129–135

65. Evans P, Halliwell B (2001) Micronutrients: oxidant/antioxidant status. Br J Nutr 85 [Suppl 2]:S67–S74

66. Taylor TV, Rimmer S, Day B, Butcher J, Dymock IW (1974) Ascorbic acid supplementation in the treatment of pressure-sores. Lancet 2:544–546

67. Burr RG, Rajan KT (1972) Leucocyte ascorbic acid and pressure sores in paraplegia Br J Nutr 28(2):275–281

68. Selvaag E, Bohmer T, Benkestock K (2002) Reduced serum concentrations of riboflavine and ascorbic acid, and blood thiamine pyrophosphate and pyridoxal-5-phosphate in geriatric patients with and without pressure sores. J Nutr Health Aging 6:75–77

69. Moussavi RM, Garza HM, Eisele SG, Rodriguez G, Rintala DH (2003) Serum levels of vitamins A, C, and E in persons with chronic spinal cord injury living in the community. Arch Phys Med Rehabil 84(7):1061–1067

70. Langer G, Schloemer G, Knerr A, Kuss O, Behrens J (2003) Nutritional interventions for preventing and treating pressure ulcers. Cochrane Database Syst Rev 4:CD003216

71. Thomas DR (2001) Improving outcome of pressure ulcers with nutritional interventions: a review of the evidence. Nutrition 17:121–125

72. Powell SR (2000) The antioxidant properties of zinc. J Nutr 130:1447S–1454S

73. Tasaki M, Hanada K, Hashimoto I (1993) Analyses of serum copper and zinc levels and copper/zinc ratios in skin diseases. J Dermatol 20:21–24

74. Kruse-Jarres JD (1998) Zinc. In: Clinical Laboratory Diagnostics. English edition. T-H Books, Frankfurt 347–349

75. McCord JM (1987) Oxygen-derived radicals: a link between reperfusion injury and inflammation. Fed Proc 46:2402–2406

76. Granger DN, Korthuis RJ (1995) Physiological mechanisms of postischaemic tissue injury. Annu Rev Physiol 57:311–332

77. Harris A, Skalak TC (1996) Effects of leukocyte plugging in skeletal muscle ischemia-reperfusion injury. Am J Physiol 271:H2653–2660

78. Pretto EA (1991) Reperfusion injury in the liver. Transplant Proc 23:1912–1914

79. Hourmant M, Vasse N, le Mauff B, Soulillou JP (1997) The role of adhesion molecules in ischemia-reperfusion injury of renal transplants. Nephrol Dial Transplant 12:2485–2487

80. Suval WD, Duran WN, Boric MP, Hobson RW, Berendsen PB, Ritter AB (1987) Microvascular transport and endothelial cell alterations preceding skeletal muscle damage in ischemia and reperfusion injury. Am J Surg 154:211–218

81. Punch J, Rees R, Cashmer B, Wilkins E, Smith DJ, Till GO 1992) Xanthine oxidase: its role in the no-reflow phenomenon. Surgery 111:169–170

82. Mellow CG, Knight KR, Angel MF, Coe SA, O'Brien BM (1992) The biochemical basis of secondary ischemia. J Surg Res 52:226–227

83. James TJ, Cherry GW, Taylor RP (2003) Analysis of purines in wound fluid and plasma from patients with chronic venous ulceration. Proc. 13th Annual Meeting European Tissue Repair Society. Amsterdam, 21–23 Sep 2003; abstract P.011, p 109

84. Salvemini D, Cuzzocrea S (2002) Superoxide, superoxide dismutase and ischemic injury. Curr Opin Investig Drugs 3:886–895
85. Su Z, Ishida H, Fukuyama N, Todorov R, Genka C, Nakazawa H (1998) Peroxynitrite is not a major mediator of endothelial cell injury by activated neutrophils in vitro. Cardiovasc Res 39:485–491
86. Goode HF, Webster NR, Howdlr PR, Walker BE (1994) Nitric oxide production by human peripheral blood polymorphonuclear leucocytes. Clin Sci (Colch) 86:411–415
87. Mulligan MS, Hevel JM, Marletta MA, Ward PA (1991) Tissue injury caused by deposition of immune complexes is L-arginine-dependent. Proc Natl Acad Sci USA 88:6338–6342
88. Seekamp A, Mulligan MS, Till GO, Ward PA (1993) Requirements for neutrophil products and L-arginine in ischemia-reperfusion injury. Am J Pathol 142:1–10
89. Beckman JS, Crow JP (1993) Pathological implications of nitric oxide, superoxide and peroxynitrite formation. Biochem Soc Trans 21:330–334
90. Marczin N, El-Habashi N, Hoare GS, Bundy RE, Yacoub M (2003) Antioxidants in myocardial ischemia-reperfusion injury: therapeutic potential and basic mechanisms. Arch Biochem Biophys 420:222–236
91. Stralin P, Marklund SL (1994) Effects of oxidative stress on expression of extracellular superoxide dismutase, CuZn superoxide dismutase and Mn superoxide dismutase in human dermal fibroblasts. Biochem J 298:347–352
92. Lo SK, Janakidevi K, Lai L, Malik AB (1993) Hydrogen peroxide-induced increase in endothelial cell adhesiveness is dependent on ICAM-1 activation. Am J Physiol 264:L406–412
93. Patel KM, Zimmerman GA, Prescott SM, McEver RP, McIntyre TM (1991) Oxygen radicals induce human endothelial cells to express GMP–140 and bind neutrophils. J Cell Biol 112:749–759
94. Suzuki M, Inauen W, Kvietys PR, Grisham MB, Meininger C (1989) Superoxide mediates reperfusion-induced leukocyte-endothelial cell interactions. Am J Physiol 257:H1740–1745
95. Gaboury J, Anderson DC, Kuber P (1994) Molecular mechanisms involved in superoxide-induced leukocyte-endothelial cell interactions in vivo. Am J Physiol 266:H637–642
96. Suzuki M, Asako H, Kubes P, Jennings S, Grisham MB, Granger DN (1991) Neutrophil-derived oxidants promote leukocyte adherence in postcapillary venules. Microvasc Res 42:125–138
97. Granger DN, Benoit JM, Suzuki M, Grisham MB (1989) Leukocyte adherence to venular endothelium during ischemia-reperfusion. Am J Physiol 257:G683–688
98. Barroso-Arranda J, Schmid-Schonbein GW, Zweifach BW, Engler RL (1988) Granulocytes and the no-reflow phenomenon in irreversible hemorhagic shock. Circ Res 63:437–447
99. Perry MA, Granger DN (1991) Role of CD11/CD18 in shear rate-dependent leukocyte-endothelial cell interactions in cat mesenteric venules. J Clin Invest 87:1798–1804
100. Jerome SN, Akimitsu T, Korthuis RJ (1994) Leukocyte adhesion, edema, and the development of postischemic capillary no-reflow. Am J Physiol 267:H1329–1336

101. Crinnion JN, Homer-Vanniasinkam S, Hatton R, Parkin SM, Gough MJ (1994) Role of neutrophil depletion and elastase inhibition in modifying skeletal muscle reperfusion injury. Cardiovasc Surg 2:749–753

102. Sisley AC, Desai T, Harig JM, Gewertz BL (1994) Neutrophil depletion attenuates human intestinal reperfusion injury. J Surg Res 57:192–196

103. Shingu M, Nobunaga M (1984) Chemotactic activity generated in human serum from the fifth component of complement by hydrogen peroxide. Am J Pathol 117:201–206

104. de Vries B, Kohl J, Leclercq WK, Wolfs TG, van Bijnen AA, Heeringa P, Buurman WA (2003) Complement factor C5a mediates renal ischemia-reperfusion injury independent from neutrophils. J Immunol 170:3883–3889

105. Haslett C (1992) Resolution of acute inflammation and the role of apoptosis in the tissue fate of granulocytes. Clin Sci (Colch) 83:639–648

106. Cohen GM (1997) Caspases: the executioners of apoptosis. Biochem J 326:1

107. Nicholson DW, Thornberry NA (1997) Caspases: killer proteases. Trends Biochem Sci 2:299–306

108. Hampton MB, Orrenius S (1997) Dual regulation of caspase activity by hydrogen peroxide: implications for apoptosis. FEBS Lett 414:552–556

109. Creagh EM, Carmody RJ, Cotter TG (2000) Heat shock protein 70 inhibits caspase-dependent and –independent apoptosis in Jurkat T cells. Exp Cell Res 257:58–66

110. Kasahara Y, Iwai K, Yachie A, Ohta K, Konno A, Seki H, Miyawaki T, Taniguchi N (1997) Involvement of reactive oxygen intermediates in spontaneous and CD95 (Fas/APO-1)-mediated apoptosis of neutrophils. Blood 89:1748–1753

111. Lundqvist-Gustafsson H, Bengtsson T (1999) Activation of the granule pool of the NADPH oxidase accelerates apoptosis in human neutrophils. J Leukoc Biol 65:196–204

112. Wolfe JT, Ross D, Cohen GM (1994) A role for metals and free radicals in the induction of apoptosis in thymocytes. FEBS Lett 352:58–62

113. Curtin JF, Donovan M, Cotter TG (2002) Regulation and measurement of oxidative stress in apoptosis. J Immunol Methods 265:49–72

114. Suzuki Y, Ono Y, Hirabayashi Y (1998) Rapid and specific reactive oxygen species generation via NADPH oxidase activation during Fas-mediated apoptosis. FEBS Lett 425:209–212

115. Rossi D, Gaidano G (2003) Messengers of cell death: apoptotic signaling in health and disease. Mol Hematol 88:212–218

116. Stridh H, Kimland M, Jones DP, Orrenius S, Hampton MB (1998) Cytochrome c release and caspase activation in hydrogen peroxide- and tributyltin-induced apoptosis. FEBS Lett 429:351–355

117. Saleh A, Srinivasula SM, Acharya S, Fishel R, Alnemri ES (1999) Cytochrome c and dATP-mediated oligomerization of Apaf-1 is a prerequisite for procaspase-9 activation. J Biol Chem 274:17941–17945

118. Higuchi Y (2003) Chromosomal DNA fragmentation in apoptosis and necrosis induced by oxidative stress. Biochem Pharmacol 66:1527–1535

119. Yu S-W, Wang H, Poitras MF, Coombs C, Bowers WJ, Federoff HJ, Poirier GG, Dawson TM, Dawson VL (2002) Mediation of poly(ADP-ribose) polymerase-1-dependent cell death by apoptosis-inducing factor. Science 297:259–263

120. Chiarugi A, Moskowitz MA (2002) PARP-1 – a perpetrator of apoptotic cell death? Science 297:200–201

121. Chandra J, Samali A, Orrenius S (2000) Triggering and modulation of apoptosis by oxidative stress. Free Radic Biol Med 29:323–333

122. Bulotta S, Barsacchi R, Rotiroti D, Borgese N, Clementi E (2001) Activation of the endothelial nitric-oxide synthase by tumor necrosis factor-alpha: a novel feedback mechanism regulating cell death. J Biol Chem 276:6529–6536

123. Stassi G, De Maria R, Trucco G, Rudert W, Testi R, Galluzo A, Giordano C, Trucco M (1997) Nitric oxide primes pancreatic beta cells for Fas-mediated destruction in insulin-dependent diabetes mellitus. J Exp Med 186:1193–1200

124. Lin KT, Xue JY, Nomen M, Spur B, Wong PY (1995) Peroxynitrite-induced apoptosis in HL-60 cells. J Biol Chem 270:16487–16490

125. Almeida A, Bolanos JP (1997) A transient inhibition of mitochondrial ATP synthesis by nitric oxide synthase activation triggered apoptosis in primary cortical neurons. J Neurochem 77:676–690

126. Dobashi K, Pahan K, Chahal A, Singh I (1997) Modulation of endogenous antioxidant enzymes by nitric oxide in rat C6 glial cells. J Neurochem 68:1896–1903

127. Mello Filho AC, Hoffman ME, Meneghini R (1984) Cell killing and DNA damage by hydrogen peroxide are mediated by intracellular iron. Biochem J 218:273–275

128. Jacobson MD (1996) Reactive oxygen species in programmed cell death. Trends Biochem Sci 21:83–86

129. Oda T, Sadakata N, Komatsu N, Muramatsu T (1999) Specific efflux of glutathione from the basolateral membrane domain in polarized MDCK cells during ricin-induced apoptosis. J Biochem (Tokyo) 126:715–721

130. Fernandes RS, Cotter TG (1994) Apoptosis or necrosis: intracellular levels of glutathione influence mode of cell death. Biochem Pharmacol 48:675–681

131. Ghibelli L, Fanelli C, Rotilio G, Lafavia E, Coppola S, Colussi C, Civitareale P, Ciriolo MR (1998) Rescue of cells from apoptosis by inhibition of active GSH extrusion. FASEB J 12:479–486

132. Samali A, Nordgren H, Zhivotovsky B, Peterson E, Orrenius S (1999) A comparative study of apoptosis and necrosis in HepG2 cells: oxidant-induced caspase inactivation leads to necrosis. Biochem Biophys Res Commun 255:6–11

133. Leist M, Single B, Naumann H, Fava E, Simon B, Kuhnle S, Nicotera P (1999) Inhibition of mitochondrial ATP generation by nitric oxide switches apoptosis to necrosis. Exp Cell Res 249:396–403

134. DelaTorre A, Schroeder RA, Kuo PC (1997) Alteration of NF-kappa B p50 DNA binding kinetics by S-nitrosylation. Biochem Biophys Res Commun 238:703–706

135. Tabuchi A, Sano K, Oh E, Tsuchiya T, Tsuda M (1994) Modulation of AP-1 activity by nitric oxide (NO) in vitro: NO-mediated modulation of AP-1. FEBS Lett 351:123–127

136. Chazotte-Aubert L, Pluquet O, Hainaut P, Ohshima H (2001) Nitric oxide prevents gamma-radiation-induced cell cycle arrest by impairing p53 function in MCF-7 cells. Biochem Biophys Res Commun 281:766–771

137. Cassina A, Radi R (1996) Differential inhibitory action of nitric oxide and peroxynitrite on mitochondrial electron transport. Arch Biochem Biophys 328:309–316

138. Brookes PS, Salinas EP, Darley-Usmar K, Eiserich JP, Freeman BA, Darley-Usmar VM, Anderson PG (2000) Concentration-dependent effects of nitric

oxide on mitochondrial permeability transition and cytochrome c release. J Biol Chem 275:20474

139. McCullough KD, Martindale JL, Klotz LO, Aw TY, Holbrook NJ (2001) Gadd153 sensitizes cells to endoplasmic reticulum stress by down-regulating bcl2 and perturbing the cellular redox state. Mol Cell Biol 21:1249–1259

140. Voehringer DW, McConkey DJ, McDonnell TJ, Brisbay S, Meyn RE (1998) Bcl-2 expression causes redistribution of glutathione to the nucleus. Proc Natl Acad Sci USA 95:2956–2960

141. Voehringer DW, Hirschberg DL, Xiao J, Lu Q, Roederer M, Lock CB, Herzenberg LA, Steinman L (2000) Gene microarray identification of redox and mitochondrial elements that control resistance or sensitivity to apoptosis. Proc Natl Acad Sci USA 97:2680–2685

142. Crompton M (2000) Mitochondrial intermembrane junctional complexes and their role in cell death. J Physiol 529:11–21

143. Halestrap AP, Doran E, Gillespie JP, O'Toole A (2000) Mitochondria and cell death. Biochem Soc Trans 28:170–177

144. Crompton M (2003) On the involvement of mitochondrial intermembrane junctional complexes in apoptosis. Curr Med Chem 16:1473–1484

145. Schultz GS, Sibbald RG, Falanga V, Ayello EA, Dowsett C, Harding K, Romanelli M, Stacey MC, Teot L, Vanscheidt W (2003) Wound bed preparation: a systematic approach to wound management. Wound Rep Reg 11 [Suppl 1]:S1–S28

146. Falanga V (2000) Classifications for wound bed preparation and stimulation of chronic wounds. Wound Rep Reg 8:347–352

147. Most D, Efron DT, Shi HP, Tantry US, Barbul A (2001) Differential cytokine expression in skin graft healing in inducible nitric oxide synthase knockout mice. Plast Reconstr Surg 108:1251–1259

148. Wach F, Hein R, Adelmann-Grill BC, Krieg T (1987) Inhibition of fibroblast chemotaxis by superoxide dismutase. Eur J Cell Biol 44:124–127

149. Klyubin IV, Kirpichnikova KM, Gamaley IA (1996) Hydrogen peroxide-induced chemotaxis of mouse peritoneal neutrophils. Eur J Cell Biol 70:347–351

150. Brenneisen P, Briviba K, Wlaschek M, Wenk J, Scharffetter-Kochanek (1997) Hydrogen peroxide (H2O2) increases the steady-state mRNA levels of collagenase/MMP-1 in human dermal fibroblasts. Free Radic Biol Med 22:515–524

151. Sen CK, Khanna S, Gordillo G, Bagchi D, Bagchi M, Roy S (2002) Oxygen, oxidants, and antioxidants in wound healing: an emerging paradigm. Ann N Y Acad Sci 957:239–249

152. Sen CK, Khanna S, Babior BM, Hunt TK, Ellison EC, Roy S (2002) Oxidant-induced vascular endothelial growth factor expression in human keratinocytes and cutaneous wound healing. J Biol Chem 277:33284–33290

153. Sen CK (2003) The general case for redox control of wound repair. Wound Rep Reg 11:431–438

154. Munro JM (1993) Endothelial-leukocyte adhesive interactions in inflammatory diseases. Eur Heart J 14 [Suppl K]:72–77

155. Zweier JL, Broderick R, Kuppusamy P, Thompson-Gorman S, Lutty GAJ (1994) Determination of the mechanism of free radical generation in human aortic endothelial cells exposed to anoxia and reoxygenation. Biol Chem 269:24156–24162

156. Wenk J, Brenneisen P, Wlaschek M, Poswig A, Briviba K, Oberley TD, Scharffetter-Kochanek K (1999) Stable overexpression of manganese superoxide dismutase in mitochondria identifies hydrogen peroxide as a major oxidant in the AP-1-mediated induction of matrix-degrading metalloprotease-1. J Biol Chem 274:25869–25876

157. Galkowska H, Olszewsk WL, Wojewodzka U, Mijal J, Filipiuk E (2003) Expression of apoptosis- and cell cycle-related proteins in epidermis of venous leg and diabetic foot ulcers. Surgery 134:213–220

158. Parks WC (1999) Matrix metalloproteinases in repair. Wound Rep Reg 7:423–432

159. Barrick B, Campbell EJ, Owen CA (1999) Leukocyte proteinases in wound healing: roles in physiologic and pathologic processes. Wound Rep Reg 7:410–422

160. Trengove NJ, Stacey MC, MacAuley S, Bennett N, Gibson J, Burslem F, Murphy G, Schultz G (1999) Analysis of the acute and chronic wound environments: the role of proteases and their inhibitors. Wound Rep Reg 7:442–452

161. Yager DR, Nwomeh BC (1999) The proteolytic environment of chronic wounds. Wound Rep Reg 7:433–441

162. Vaalamo M, Leivo T, Saarialhi-Kere U (1999) Differential expression of tissue inhibitors of metalloproteinases (TIMP-1,-2,-3, and -4) in normal and aberrant wound healing. Hum Pathol 30:795–802

163. Weiss SJ, Peppin G, Ortiz X, Ragsdale C, Test ST (1985) Oxidative autoactivation of latent collagenase by human neutrophils. Science 227:747–749

164. Diegelmann RF (2003) Excessive neutrophils characterize chronic pressure ulcers. Wound Rep Reg 11:490–495

165. Bader DL, Gant CA (1988) Changes in transcutaneous oxygen tension as a result of prolonged pressures at the sacrum. Clin Phys Physiol Meas 9:33–40

166. Polliack A, Taylor R, Bader D (1997) Sweat analysis following pressure ischaemia in a group of debilitated subjects. J Rehabil Res Dev 34:303–308

167. Taylor RP, Polliack AA, Bader DL (1994) The analysis of metabolites in human sweat: analytical methods and potential application to investigation of pressure ischaemia of soft tissues. Ann Clin Biochem 31:18–24

168. Knight SL, Taylor RP, Polliack AA, Bader DL (2001) Establishing predictive indicators for the status of loaded soft tissues. J Appl Physiol 90:2231–2237

169. Hunt TK, Conolly WB, Aronson SB, Goldstein P (1978) Anaerobic metabolism and wound healing: an hypothesis for the initiation and cessation of collagen synthesis in wounds. Am J Surg 135:328–332

170. Ghani QP, Wagner S, Hussain MZ (2003) Role of ADP-ribosylation in wound repair. The contributions of Thomas K Hunt, MD. Wound Rep Reg 11:439–444

171. Trabold O, Wagner S, Wicke C, Scheuenstuhl H, Hussain MZ, Rosen N, Seremetiev A, Becker HD, Hunt TK (2003) Lactate and oxygen constitute a fundamental regulatory mechanism in wound healing. Wound Repair Regen 11:504–509

172. Lingen MW (2001) Role of leukocytes and endothelial cells in the development of angiogenesis in inflammation and wound healing. Arch Pathol Lab Med 125:67–71

173. Petrone WF, English DK, Wong K, McCord JM (1980) Free radicals and inflammation: superoxide-dependent activation of a neutrophil chemotactic factor in plasma. Proc Natl Acad Sci USA 77:1159–1163

174. Steeber DA, Tedder TF (2000) Adhesion molecule cascades direct lymphocyte recirculation and leukocyte migration during inflammation. Immunol Res 22:299–317
175. Salcido R, Donfrio J (1994) Histopathology of pressure ulcers as a result of sequential computer-controlled pressure sessions in a fuzzy rat model. Adv Wound Care 7:23–24
176. Peirce SM, Skalak TC, Rodeheaver GT (2000) Ischemia-reperfusion injury in chronic pressure ulcer formation: A model in the rat. Wound Rep Reg 8:68–76
177. Angel M, Ramasastry SS, Swartz WM, Basford RE, Futrel JW (1987) The causes of skin ulcerations associated with venous insufficiency: a unifying hypothesis. Plast Reconst Surg 79:289–297
178. Goldstein B, Sanders J (1998) Skin response to repetitive mechanical stress: a new experimental model in pig. Arch Phys Med Rehabil 79:265–272
179. Peirce SM Skalak TC, Rieger JM, MacDonald TL, Linden J (2001) Selective A2A adenosine receptor activation reduces skin pressure ulcer formation and inflammation. Am J Physiol Heart Circ Physiol 281:H67–H74
180. Reid RR, Sull AC, Mogford JE, Roy N, Mustoe TA (2004) A novel murine model of cyclical cutaneous ischemia-reperfusion injury. J Surg Res 116: 172–180
181. Chartrain NA, Geller DA, Koty PP, Sitrin NF, Nosster AK, Hottman EP, Billiar TP, Hutchinson NI, Mudgett JS (1994) Molecular cloning, structure and chromosomal localization of human inducible nitric oxide synthase gene. J Biol Chem 269:6765–6772
182. Houwing R, Overgoor M, Kon M, Jansen G, van Asbeck BS, Haalboom JR (2000) Pressure-induced skin lesions in pigs: reperfusion injury and the effects of vitamin E. J Wound Care 9:36–40
183. Sundin BM, Hussein MA, Glasofer S, El-Falaky MH, Abdel-Aleem SM, Sachse RE, Klitzman B (2000) The role of allopurinol and deferoxamine in preventing pressure ulcers in pigs. Plast Reconstr Surg 105:1408–1421
184. Wenk J, Foitzik A, Achterberg V, Sabiwalsky A, Dissemond J, Meewes C, Reitz A, Brenneisen P, Wlaschek M, Meyer-Ingold W, Scharffetter-Kochanek K (2001) Selective pick-up of increased iron by deferoxamine-coupled cellulose abrogates the iron-driven induction of matrix-degrading metalloproteinase 1 and lipid peroxidation in human dermal fibroblasts in vitro: a new dressing concept. J Invest Dermatol 116:833–839

Transport of Fluid and Solutes in Tissues

14

Charles Michel

Introduction

The transport of nutrients and metabolites in tissues involves a series of processes of varying degrees of complexity. Some of these are responsible for the transport of all molecules at a particular stage of the transport pathway. Other mechanisms, particularly those concerned with the transport into and out of cells, are reserved for the transport of solutes of only one or two molecular species. In this chapter we shall consider only processes that apply to all nutrients and metabolites. These are the early steps in the transport pathway of nutrients and the later stages for transport of metabolites where molecules are brought into the tissues or removed from them by the circulating blood. Once nutrient molecules have arrived in the exchange vessels of the microcirculation, they pass through the microvascular walls and then onward through the interstitial fluid.

Transport of solutes through both the walls of small blood vessels and the interstitial spaces is brought about by convection and diffusion. For convective transport to occur there has to be fluid flow, and this flow carries the solutes dissolved in the fluid. Whereas convection involves bulk transport of solutions, diffusion is a mixing process resulting from random thermal movements of molecules within solutions.

We start by considering transport of nutrients and metabolites into and out of tissues by the circulation and their passage through microvascular walls. We then discuss transport through the interstitial spaces and into lymph, noting how the specialised histological features of skin, fat and muscle impose restraints on transport processes.

Transport by the Microcirculation into Tissues

Although recent measurements have suggested that oxygen may be supplied to cells of the epidermis of human skin by diffusion from the atmosphere [1], the velocity of diffusion over distances greater than a few hundred micrometres is too slow to meet the metabolic requirements of nearly all human tissues. The vessels of the microcirculation act as sources from which nutrients can diffuse into the surrounding tissues and as sinks into which metabolites can be cleared. The mean concentrations of solutes within these vessels determine how efficiently their molecules can be transported. These mean concentrations are themselves determined by the rates of consumption or production of the molecules by the metabolising cells and the rate of blood flow through the microcirculation.

The net transport of a solute by the circulation into or out of a tissue is estimated from the conservation of mass. Net solute transport, J_s, is the difference between the total amount of the solute delivered to the tissue by the circulation and the total amount that is leaving. If the blood flow to the tissue is F and the arterial concentration of the solute is equal to C_a, the total amount of solute delivered to the tissue is FC_a. Similarly the total amount of the solute leaving the tissue is FC_v, where C_v is the solute concentration in the venous blood. Thus:

$$J_s = FC_a - FC_v = F(C_a - C_v) \tag{1}$$

A positive value of J_s indicates that a substance is taken up from the blood into the tissue and a negative value indicates a substance is being cleared from the tissue. Although Eq. 1 is no more than a statement of the conservation of mass, it highlights a very important physiological principle. At any given value of J_s, the greater the blood flow the smaller will be the difference in concentration between the arterial and the venous blood. This means that when blood flow is high relative to exchange rate, the concentrations of nutrients in the blood (being delivered to the tissues) is high and the concentration of metabolites (being cleared from the tissues into the blood) is low.

Transport of solutes by the circulation is convective. Convective transport also occurs through the microvascular walls in the stream of fluid that is filtered from microvascular plasma into the tissues but it accounts for only a very small proportion of nutrient transport. Diffusion is the principle mechanism of the transport for most nutrient and metabolite molecules through microvascular walls. Diffusion is essentially a mixing process at a molecular level, the thermal energy constantly displacing molecules relative to one another. Net transport occurs by diffusion when there are initial differences in concentration between different parts of the system through which diffusion is occurring. The mixing process results in net transport of molecules from regions where their concentration is high to regions where it is low. For net transport of molecules to occur from capillary blood to interstitial fluid, therefore, there has to be a concentration difference across the vessel wall. The rate of transport is proportional to this concentration difference. It is also proportional to the permeability of the vessel wall to the diffusing molecule and to the area of vessel wall through which diffusion occurs. If $\hat{C}_c$ is the mean concentration of a nutrient molecule in a capillary and C_i is its mean concentration in the interstitial fluid immediately outside the vessel, then we can write a simple equation, analogous to Eq. 1, describing the net transport of the molecule, J_s, from blood to tissue in terms of the solute permeability, P_d and the surface area of the vessel wall, S, through which transport occurs:

$$J_s = P_d S(\hat{C}_c - C_i) \tag{2}$$

The size, lipid solubility, shape and charge of the solute molecule and the characteristics of the transport pathways through the microvascular wall determine the value of P_d.

The function of the circulation is to maintain the concentrations of nutrients and metabolites immediately outside cells at levels that enable cell metabolism to continue at a rate that is necessary for the organism's survival. Except for highly diffusible molecules such as CO_2 and O_2, the concentration gradients in the interstitial fluid (ISF) are small and C_i approximates to the concentration outside the cells. This means that inspection of equations (1) and (2) reveals how the peripheral circulation is able to maintain levels of nutrients and metabolites in the ISF. For a nutrient, C_i is given by:

$$C_i = \hat{C}_c - \frac{J_s}{P_d S} = \hat{C}_c - \frac{F}{P_d S}(C_a - C_v) \tag{3a}$$

and for a metabolite by:

$$C_i = \hat{C}_c + \frac{J_s}{P_d S} = \hat{C}_c + \frac{F}{P_d S}(C_a - C_v) \tag{3b}$$

The mean concentration of the solute in the exchange vessels, $\hat{C}_c$, must lie between C_a and C_v. Equation 1 indicates that the difference between C_a and C_v is reduced as blood flow is increased, and so the higher the blood flow, the closer is $\hat{C}_c$ to C_a. Thus an increase in blood flow should increase both terms on the right-hand side of Eq. 3a and reduce both terms on the right-hand side of Eq. 3b, and capillary blood becomes a richer source of nutrients and a more effective sink for metabolites.

If the metabolic rate of a tissue increases, a concomitant rise in F can minimise the fall in $\hat{C}_c$. Even if F does increase in proportion to J_s, C_i will fall unless $P_d S$ also increases in proportion to J_s. Thus, if the metabolism of a tissue varies from moment to moment, the nutrients required to sustain metabolism can only be maintained at optimal concentrations for the cells if blood flow and $P_d S$ vary closely with metabolic rate. Metabolism does vary from moment to moment in some tissues (e.g. muscle) and here, blood flow and $P_d S$ also vary closely with metabolic rate. This is called "functional hyperaemia", and apart from heart and skeletal muscle it is seen in association with local variations in metabolic activity in many other tissues (e.g. brain and gastro-intestinal tract). Although the increases in blood flow and $P_d S$ are substantial, they are less than the increases in oxygen consumption. Thus, as the work done by the muscle increases, a point is reached when the O_2 supplied by the circulation can no longer match that required for energy to be supplied by aerobic metabolism. The muscles can continue to work at this rate only by making use of anaerobic metabolism, and the time for which the exercise can continue anaerobically then becomes severely limited.

Even larger variations in blood flow may occur in skin than in muscle; these changes are associated with the regulation of body temperature rather than changes in skin metabolism. Functional hyperaemia probably does occur in the sweat glands during sweating. but this is difficult to detect against the background of high blood flow through the skin, which serves to cool the blood under these conditions. In fat tissue, increases in blood flow do accompany increases in metabolism. Whether this is "true" functional hyperaemia in the sense that the increase in blood flow is secondary to increases in lipolysis has been disputed [2]. The relations between the increments in blood flow and the metabolic rate of fat tissue have not been defined.

Transport of O_2 and CO_2 to the Tissues

Despite its importance in both physiology and pathology, we remain uncertain of many of the details of O_2 transport in tissues. The resistance of microvascular walls to the diffusion of O_2 through them is usually assumed to be the same as that of the tissues surrounding the vessels. This means that O_2 transport in tissues cannot be thought of merely in terms of diffusion through capillary walls without considering the entire process of diffusion through the surrounding tissue.

Diffusion of a solute in one dimension through an area, S, of an aqueous solution is described by Fick's first law of diffusion:

$$J_s = -DS\left(\frac{dC}{dx}\right) \tag{4}$$

where D is the diffusion coefficient of the solute in the medium and (dC/dx) is the concentration gradient across a plane within the solution of area, S. The value of D depends on the size, shape and charge of the diffusing solute molecules. The negative sign is to indicate that the diffusion occurs down the concentration gradient, from high to low concentration.

The diffusion of gases in solution is usually described in terms of gradients of their partial pressure rather than their concentration. This is to distinguish between the concentration of "free" gas molecules in solution from molecules that are in reversible combination with other components. Thus the partial pressure of O_2, PO_2, in a sample of blood is directly proportional to O_2 molecules dissolved in the plasma and red cell water. These dissolved molecules are in equilibrium with O_2 that is reversibly combined with haemoglobin in the red cells. Although the dissolved molecules may be only a tiny fraction of the O_2 that is available in the blood (about 3% of the total O_2 of arterial blood), the PO_2 reflects the activity and potential energy of the O_2, whereas those molecules bound to haemoglobin are a readily available store. One consequence of using gradients of partial pressure rather than concentration as the driving forces of diffusion is that the rate of diffusion becomes dependent on the product of the diffusion coefficient and the solubility of a particular gas rather than upon the diffusion coefficient alone. The importance of the solubility will become apparent when we consider the diffusion of CO_2.

The foundations of our understanding of the oxygen delivery from capillaries to the tissues were laid in a classic series of papers published by the Danish physiologist, August Krogh, in 1919 [3–5]. Krogh was concerned with the delivery of O_2 from the capillaries to the tissues of skeletal muscle at rest and during exercise, when O_2 consumption by the tissues may be increased ten fold or more. Krogh observed the capillaries of muscle are relatively straight and long, running parallel to and between the muscle fibres. He considered that each muscle capillary supplied a cylinder of tissue that surrounded it. From measurements of the O_2 consumption per unit volume of tissue and the diffusion coefficient of O_2 in muscle tissue, he calculated the fall in PO_2 with radial distance. The calculation was based on a mathematical model of oxygen diffusion that had been derived for Krogh by the Danish mathematician, K. Erlang. In this model it was assumed that the O_2 consumption per unit volume of tissue and the diffusion coefficient for O_2 were the same in all parts of the tissue. This led to an expression that showed how PO_2 at a point in the tissue varied with distance from the capillary at the centre of each tissue cylinder. The reasoning is based on Eq. 4 and runs as follows (see Fig. 14.1 a). At a radial distance, x, from the centre of a capillary, O_2 is diffusing outward through a cylindrical surface of area $= 2\pi xL$, where L is the length of the cylindrical surface surrounding the capillary and equal to the length of the capillary. The number of O_2 molecules diffusing through this area should be equal to the number of O_2 molecules that are being consumed by the tissue between x and the outer limit of tissue supplied with O_2 by the capillary at a distance R from the capillary axis. If the O_2 consumption per unit volume of tissue is equal to μ_{O2} (ml min^{-1} ml^{-1} of tissue) the O_2 flux through $2\pi xL$ is $\mu_{O2}(\pi R^2 L - \pi x^2 L) = \mu_{O2}\pi L(R^2 - x^2)$. The gradient of PO_2 across the cylindrical surface is $-dPO_2/dx$ and this can be calculated by re-arrangement of Eq. 4. Substituting for J_S with the flux through the cylindrical surface $2\pi xL$ leads to:

$$-\frac{dPO_2}{dx} = \frac{\mu_{O_2}}{2D_{O2}a_{O_2}}\left(\frac{R^2}{x} - x\right) \tag{5}$$

where D_{O2} and a_{O2} are the diffusion coefficient and solubility of O_2 in the tissue fluids. The equation can be integrated to give values for PO_2 in the tissues between the outside of the capillary wall, where $x = r_c$ and $PO_2 = PO_2(r_c)$, and the outer limit of the tissue cylinder, where $x = R$, i.e.:

$$PO_2(x) = PO_2(r_c) - \frac{\mu_{O_2}}{2D_{o_2}a_{o_2}}\left(R^2 \ln\frac{x}{r_c} - \frac{(x^2 - r_c^2)}{2}\right) \tag{6}$$

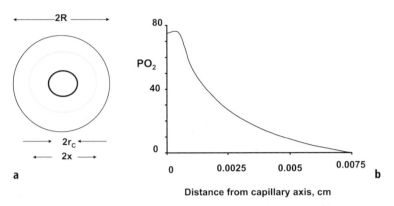

Fig. 14.1 a, b. The Krogh–Erlang model for the supply of oxygen to the tissue surrounding a single capillary. **a** Cross-section through a cylinder of tissue surrounding a capillary where tissue cylinder radius is R and capillary radius is r_c. The model considers the diffusion of O_2 through cylindrical surfaces of tissue (radius$=x$) between r_c and R. **b** Fall in PO_2 (mmHg) at various distances from capillary axis into a tissue cylinder, calculated using Eq. 6 with PO_2 at $r_c=75$ mmHg, $\mu_{O2}=0.01$ ml min^{-1} ml^{-1} tissue, $D_{O2}\,\alpha_{O2}=2.10^{-8}$ ml^{-1} (tissue) mmHg^{-1}cm^{-1}min^{-1}, $R=75$ µm, $r_c=5$ µm

The equation predicts that the PO_2 falls steeply at points immediately outside the capillary but then less and less steeply as the distance from the capillary increases and the area through which the oxygen can diffuse also increases (see Fig. 14.1b). When the tissues are well supplied with O_2, the minimum PO_2 occurs at the boundaries of the tissue cylinders supplied by adjacent capillaries. When blood flow is inadequate, the mean PO_2 in the capillary falls, and the PO_2 in the tissues falls close to zero before the boundary of the cylinder is reached. Unless capillary flow is increased, an outer anoxic part of the tissue cylinder surrounds an inner core of aerobically metabolising tissue. If flow is stopped, the entire tissue becomes anoxic as the store of O_2 in capillaries and the tissues is consumed. Krogh obtained experimental evidence that when a muscle is exercised not only does the velocity of blood flow through the capillaries increase but also new parallel capillaries are opened and perfused. In this way, he argued, the radii of the tissue cylinders is reduced so that a smaller volume of tissue is supplied by each capillary. In this way, O_2 is supplied to the entire tissue by diffusion in spite of a tenfold rise in tissue O_2 consumption.

Krogh's analysis has guided thinking about tissue O_2 transport for over 80 years. Elaboration of the theoretical analysis and measurements of capillary and tissue PO_2 and capillary blood flow have led to a revision of the classical picture, though the principles of the Krogh–Erlang approach have remained intact [6]. Krogh imagined that when blood entered a capillary its PO_2 was equal to that of the arterial blood. We now know that this is not so. Oxygen is lost through the walls of arterioles as blood is brought into a tissue [7–9]. Furthermore, the velocity of blood flow through capillaries in resting muscle may be less than 100 µm s^{-1}. Over distances of 100 µm, the mean diffusion velocity of O_2 is approximately 65 µm s^{-1}, a rate that is comparable with its convective transport by the blood. This means that the diffusion of O_2 along the capillary axis cannot be neglected and can be shown to be important under these conditions. Measurements by Pittman's group [9a] have shown that in resting muscle, O_2 may diffuse from the arterioles feeding the tissue into nearby venules draining it. Thus while the PO_2 in the arteriole is always greater than that in the venule, the PO_2 in the capillaries may be less than that in either the arterioles or the venules. Capillary PO_2 may have no axial gradients, as O_2 can diffuse axially as rapidly as the red cells are flowing through it. There may also be anomalous peaks of PO_2 in regions where an arteriole passes over a network of capillaries, losing some oxygen to them. It has not been possible so far to make similar measurements when a muscle is exercised, but one would predict that this picture would change radically. With much higher flow velocities through the arterioles and capillaries, the fall in PO_2 between the arterioles and capillaries should be minimised and the distribution of PO_2 is expected to approximate more closely to the picture envisaged by Krogh. As techniques for measuring PO_2 continue to be refined there is still much to discover about the distribution and transport of O_2 in tissues.

There have been fewer studies on the transport of CO_2 in tissues than on the transport of O_2. The gradients of CO_2 are much smaller than those for O_2 because the solubility of CO_2 in aqueous solutions is so much greater than the solubility of O_2. Although the diffusion coefficient of CO_2 is slightly less than that for O_2, the product of the diffusion and solubility coefficients of CO_2 is 24 times greater than the magnitude of this product for O_2. Thus if a fall in PO_2 of 48 mmHg is required to achieve a given flux of O_2, the same flux of CO_2 will require a PCO_2 difference of only 2 mmHg.

While the diffusion of CO_2 through tissues occurs relatively rapidly, the storage of CO_2 in the blood occurs more slowly. Most of the CO_2 that can be taken up by blood is stored as bicarbonate ions, HCO_3^-. Both the formation of HCO_3^- and the release of CO_2 from HCO_3^- stores depends on the catalysis of the hydration of CO_2 in the red cells by the enzyme, carbonic anhydrase, and the exchange of HCO_3^- and Cl^- between the red cells and the plasma. The half time for this process is of the order of 0.14 s, five times longer than the half times for the uptake and release of O_2 from haemoglobin in red cell suspensions [10]. About 5% of the CO_2 in blood is in combination with the haemoglobin. Because this can exchange more rapidly than CO_2 in the HCO_3^- store, it is estimated to account for 25–30% of the exchange of CO_2 in the tissues and the lungs. It is possible, however, that CO_2 in the HCO_3^- store of blood can turn over more rapidly in vivo than might be predicted from in vitro measurements of reaction rates. Cytochemical evidence suggests that carbonic anhydrase is present on the luminal surfaces of pulmonary capillary and peripheral microvascular endothelial cells. The potential significance of this has been demonstrated in experiments by Effros and his colleagues [11, 12], who found the fraction of CO_2 that could be released from a bolus of a HCO_3^- solution during a single transit through the lungs or hind limb circulation could be reduced from 30% to 1–2% by pre-treatment with carbonic anhydrase inhibitors.

Carbonic anhydrase is present in muscle, and here its importance may relate to the buffering of the interstitial fluids during anaerobic exercise. Lactic acid released from the muscle cells under these conditions reacts with HCO_3^- to form carbonic acid. This dissociates as a moderately strong acid with a pK of 3.486 [13] and in the absence of carbonic anhydrase would be converted to CO_2 and water relatively slowly (the half time of this reaction at 38 °C is 5.2 s). In the presence of carbonic anhydrase, however, the apparent pK (pK′) is 6.1, with much happier consequences for the tissues.

Transport of Water-Soluble (Lipid-Insoluble) Solutes Across Microvascular Walls

Apart from O_2 and CO_2, the other principal fuels and metabolites of tissues (such as glucose, amino acids, lactic and pyruvic acid), are small water-soluble molecules. Their rates of consumption and production are considerably less than O_2 and CO_2. Consequently their concentration gradients in the tissues are small. For example, if all the O_2 consumed by skeletal muscle were used to burn glucose, then the difference in glucose concentration between the outer surface of the capillary and the most distant point in a Krogh cylinder of tissue would be a few micromoles per litre at rest, rising to 50–100 μmol l^{-1} during severe exercise.

While the gradients of concentration of glucose across the tissues are always small, a large fall in concentration is present across the microvascular walls when glucose uptake is high. This reflects the much greater resistance to diffusion of glucose at capillary walls than through the interstitial space. This is true for all water-soluble molecules. They do not pass through cell membranes rapidly, and their transport between the blood and the tissues is largely confined to narrow spaces between the endothelial cells in vessels where the endothelium is continuous and through the fenestrae in vessels where the endothelium is fenestrated. These different types of endothelium and the pathways through them are illustrated in Fig. 14.2. Fenestrated endothelium is found in capillaries and venules associated with absorptive and secretory epithelia. The exchange vessels of skin, fat, muscle and connective tissue are continuous. The pathway in continuous capillaries can be thought of as a slit, 20 nm wide, between adjacent endothelial cells which, while open at both the luminal and abluminal surfaces of the vessel, is sealed off about 100 nm from the luminal surface over most of its length by tight junctional strands. Small breaks occur in these strands that may account for 1–10% of strand length. In some vessels several tight junctional seals may lie in parallel, forming a set of barriers in series, so the diffusion pathway through the occasional breaks in the barriers may follow a very tortuous course. While the rates at which hydrophilic solutes can exchange are dependent on the area of capillary walls, only a tiny fraction of the total capillary surface area is available for the transport of these solutes.

The permeabilities of microvascular walls to hydrophilic solutes, like their diffusion coefficients, are strongly dependent on molecular size.

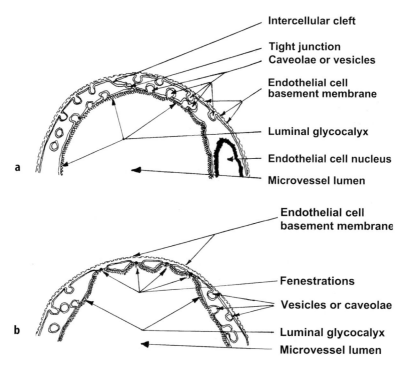

Intercellular cleft

Tight junction
Caveolae or vesicles

Endothelial cell
basement membrane

Luminal glycocalyx

Endothelial cell nucleus

Microvessel lumen

Endothelial cell
basement membrane

Fenestrations

Vesicles or caveolae

Luminal glycocalyx
Microvessel lumen

Fig. 14.2. Diagrams illustrating the ultrastructural features of capillaries with **a** continuous endothelium and **b** fenestrated endothelium

When the permeabilities of these solutes [defined as $J_S/(S\Delta C)$, as in Eq. 2] are plotted against the Stokes–Einstein radii of the molecules, P_d is found to fall considerably as molecular size is increased, becoming 1% or less of the values for P_d of urea or glucose when molecular radius is in the range of 4 nm. This is consistent with diffusion through a molecular filter of water-filled pores with cut-off for molecules with radii in the range 4–5 nm (see Fig. 14.3). While microvascular walls are permeable to macromolecules with larger molecular radii, their transport is confined to a different pathway from that accounting for permeability to small hydrophilic molecules.

At present the strongest evidence for the site of the molecular filter in capillary walls suggests it is a layer of glycoproteins that covers the luminal surface of both continuous and fenestrated capillaries [15]. This is the endothelial surface layer (ESL), and many properties have been ascribed to it, though with little hard evidence. Recent work [16] reveals that it has a quasi-periodic structure consistent with a regular lattice arrangement. The molecular filaments of the lattice have radii of approximately 6 nm and the spacing of these filaments is approximately 20 nm. If the lattice is thought of as a square or cubic arrangement it should severely restrict the passage of molecules greater than 4 nm in radius and be a complete barrier to molecules with radii of 6 nm. One attractive feature of the hypothesis that the ESL acts as the molecular sieve accounts for the fact that the molecular

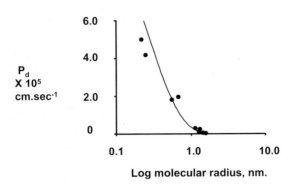

Fig. 14.3. The relations between the permeability of microvessels of mammalian skeletal muscle to hydrophilic solutes and the molecular size assessed as the molecular radius of the solute. Note that the molecular radius has been plotted on a logarithmic scale

sieving properties of both continuous and fenestrated microvascular walls is very similar although the pathways through the endothelium of these two types of vessel are very different.

When permeabilities to solutes with a range of molecular sizes are compared for the exchange vessels of different tissues, it is found that the absolute values of permeability to the smallest molecules may vary by an order of magnitude or more. In contrast, the absolute difference in the permeabilities to macromolecules such as serum albumin show less variation, though considerable differences do exist when the permeabilities are compared to one another.

Permeability of Microvascular Walls to Macromolecules

It has been known for nearly 50 years that, while the permeabilities of microvascular walls to macromolecules are very low, they do not decrease with molecular size in the same way as the permeabilities to small hydrophilic molecules. To account for this, two proposals were made in the 1950s for the mechanism of macromolecular permeability. The debate as to which of these hypotheses is correct continues to this day.

From measurements of the transport of high-molecular-weight dextran polymers from blood to lymph, Grotte [15] proposed that macromolecules were filtered from the plasma into the interstitial fluid through a relatively small number of pores 15 to 20 nm in diameter. Pores of radii 3–4 nm had been proposed a few years earlier by Pappenheimer et al. [16] to account for the permeability of capillary walls to small hydrophilic solutes, and these small pores are now identified with the interstices of the endothelial surface layer. Grotte suggested that there were 32,000 of these small pores for every large pore responsible for the permeability to macromolecules. Figures for the numbers and radii of the large pores have varied over the past 50 years but the idea that something equivalent to large pores is responsible for macromolecular permeability remains one of the two favoured hypotheses. In its present form it is suggested that transport of macromolecules through the large pores occurs almost entirely by convection [17, 18].

The second hypothesis arose from studies on the ultrastructure of microvascular walls. It was found that most endothelial cells contained large numbers of small vesicles (35 nm in diameter). It was shown that electron-opaque macromolecules could be detected inside the vesicles shortly after they had been injected into the circulation. From these observations it was suggested that macromolecules were carried across the endothelial cells by vesicles. The question of which is the more correct of these hypotheses has yet to be resolved. The evidence for the large pore hypothesis is entirely functional, based on the role of convection in the transport of macromolecules from blood to the tissues. It is argued that because the frequency of the large pores is so low, there is no possibility of identifying a large pore in an electron micrograph and being sure that it is not an artefact. Evidence for the vesicle hypothesis was initially based on ultrastructural studies, though more recently it has been buttressed by cell biology [19]. While the existence of vesicles and their labelling by macromolecules is beyond doubt, their active role in the transport of macromolecules across microvascular walls is still questioned [18]. The failure of metabolic inhibitors (including tissue cooling) to inhibit macromolecular transport significantly, while leaving permeability to water and small solutes unchanged, remains

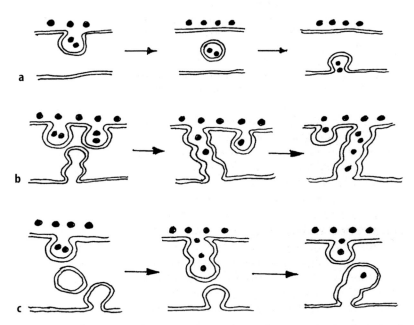

Fig. 14.4 a–c. Various hypotheses to account for the transport of macromolecules through microvascular endothelium by vesicles. a Transcytosis or shuttle or ferry boat of discrete quanta of plasma or ISF containing macromolecules. b Convection through large pores formed by the fusion of endothelial vesicles. c Fission–fusion model: transfer via repeated fusion and separation of adjacent vesicles. Each hypothesis is shown as a sequence of events though in case b stable channels are considered to be a possibility. (Redrawn from Michel CC, Am Rev Respir Dis 1992, 146:S32–S36)

the strongest argument for the large pore hypothesis. Endothelial cell vesicles can form complex structures by fusing with their neighbours, and one possibility is that the vesicles fuse transiently to form large pores. Some of the hypotheses to account for macromolecular permeability of microvascular walls are illustrated in Fig. 14.4.

Fluid Movements Through Microvascular Walls

Net fluid movements between the blood and the tissues occur principally via the pathways available to small hydrophilic solutes, i.e. through intercellular clefts and fenestrations in the endothelia. In addition, approximately 10% of the exchange of water may occur via a route that passes through the cells making use of the water channels (aquaporins) in the endothelial cell membranes [14]. The very low permeability of most microvascular walls to macromolecules means that in most tissues the concentration of plasma proteins is lower in the interstitial fluids than it is in the plasma. This leads to a difference in osmotic pressure of the order of 15–30 cmH$_2$O, which opposes the filtration of fluid down the hydrostatic gradient from the plasma in the microcirculation to tissues. This is the basis of Starling's principle of capillary fluid exchange, which is often written in the form of an equation:

$$J_V = L_p S[(P_C - P_I) - \sigma(\Pi_C - \Pi_I)] \tag{7}$$

where J_V is the rate of fluid filtration from capillaries to tissues, L_p is the hydraulic permeability or hydraulic conductivity of the microvascular wall, P_C is the mean hydrostatic pressure in the microvessel, P_I is the hydrostatic pressure immediately outside the ultra-filter of vessel wall, σ is the mean reflection coefficient to plasma proteins at the vessel wall and Π_C and Π_I are the mean osmotic pressures of the plasma in the vessel and the fluid immediately outside the vessel respectively.

The reflection coefficient of a membrane to a particular solute is an important property. It is both a measure of the ultra-filtration characteristics of the membrane to a solution of that solute and of the fraction of the total osmotic pressure of that solution that can be exerted across the membrane. If a membrane is perfectly semi-permeable to an aqueous solution of glucose, then ultra-filtration of the solution through it results in complete separation of glucose from water, so that pure water emerges from the downstream side of the membrane. Since the membrane "reflects" 100% of the glucose molecules during ultra-filtration it is said to have a reflection coefficient of 1.0. If such a membrane were fitted into a membrane osmometer, the instrument should register the full osmotic pressure of glucose solutions. If during ultra-filtration of the solution, the glucose concentration in the ultra-filtrate were the same as that in the original solution, σ would equal 0 and the glucose solution would be unable to exert an osmotic pressure across such a membrane. If glucose concentration in the ultra-filtrate were 50% of the original solution, σ would equal 0.5 and such a membrane would be able to register up to half of the osmotic pressure set up by differences in glucose concentration in solutions that it separated. The reflection coefficient therefore tells us about convective transport and osmotic pressures. For example, the convective transport of a solute (J_S) carried by ultra-filtration through microvascular walls at a rate J_V (ml s^{-1}) from an initial concentration in the plasma of C_p to the interstitial fluid is:

$$J_s = J_V(1 - \sigma)C_p \tag{8}$$

If ΔC is a difference in concentration of a particular solute across the microvascular wall, this has a total osmotic pressure (Π) of $\phi RT\Delta C$, where RT is the product of the universal gas constant and the absolute temperature (van't Hoff's law) and ϕ, the osmotic coefficient of the solution, is a measure of how well the solution obeys simple molecular theory. The total osmotic pressure will be exerted only if σ for the microvascular wall has a value of 1 for that particular solute. If σ is less than 1.0, a smaller osmotic pressure is exerted. This effective osmotic pressure P_{eff} is defined as:

$$P_{eff} = \sigma\phi RT\Delta C = \sigma\Delta\Pi \tag{9}$$

The reflection coefficient of a molecule at a particular membrane depends upon its size and charge. The larger the molecule, the larger is the value of σ at that membrane. Measurement of the reflection coefficients of neutral hydrophilic molecules at microvascular walls has been used to estimate the dimensions of the pores through which solutions are ultra-filtered.

Because most microvessels are finitely permeable to even the larger of the plasma proteins, the maintenance of the gradients of macromolecular osmotic pressure (or oncotic pressure) is ultimately dependent on continued filtration of fluid from plasma to tissues, albeit at very low rates. This can be understood by considering the consequences if all hydrophilic solutes including macromolecules have initially equal concentrations in the plasma and the interstitial fluid. If the hydrostatic pressure within the exchange vessels of the microcirculation, P_C, is 30–40 cmH$_2$O greater than that in the ISF, it will drive the filtration of fluid from the plasma into the tissues.

Fluid filtration carries solutes from plasma to ISF by convection. The principal hydrophilic solutes, which are small ions such as Na$^+$, Cl$^-$, HCO$_3^-$ and K$^+$, have reflection coefficients of 0.1 or less and relatively high permeabilities. They are carried into the tissues at concentrations only a little less than their values in the plasma. Larger molecules with higher values of σ are present in the ultra-filtrate at concentrations considerably below their plasma values. Thus ultra-filtration gives rise to differences in concentration. In the steady state of ultra-filtration, the concentration of an ultra-filtered solute should equal the ratio of the transport of solute through the wall to the volume flow of fluid (i.e. $C_i = Js/Jv$). If as a first step we assume that convection is only process transporting a solute, its concentration in the ultra-filtrate C_i is:

$$C_I = \frac{J_S}{J_V} = \frac{J_V(1-\sigma)C_p}{J_V} = (1-\sigma)C_p \qquad (10)$$

The concentration difference set up by ultra-filtration across the microvascular wall, $(C_p-C_I)=\Delta C$, is therefore σC_p. Since small molecules have smaller reflection coefficients than macromolecules, one can see immediately that the concentration differences generated for small molecules are small and those for macromolecules with large reflection coefficients will be larger.

So far in this argument, we have neglected diffusion. Net transport by diffusion will occur as soon as the concentration differences, set up by ultra-filtration, develop and it will tend to dissipate them. The extent to which diffusion is effective in doing this depends on the ratio of solute velocity by convection to solute velocity by diffusion. This ratio is known as the Peclet number and is defined as:

$$Pe = \frac{J_V(1-\sigma)}{P_d S} \qquad (11)$$

It can be shown that when diffusion is taken into account the concentration of a solute in the ultra-filtrate, C_I, has a value given by:

$$C_I = \frac{(1-\sigma)C_p}{(1-\sigma e^{-Pe})} \qquad (12)$$

The concentration difference for a particular solute (ΔC) that is ultra-filtered is therefore:

$$\Delta C = (C_P - C_I) = C_p\sigma\frac{(1-e^{-Pe})}{(1-\sigma e^{-Pe})} \qquad (13)$$

The expression on the RHS of Eq. 13 shows that diffusion modifies the concentration difference resulting from ultra-filtration to a degree that depends on the value of the Peclet number. This is exactly what one might expect.

We may use Eq. 13 to give us some idea of the differences in concentration which are likely to develop as a result of ultra-filtration across the capillary walls, assuming that the driving force for ultra-filtration is a pressure difference of 1–10 cmH$_2$O. In most capillaries this would give a small ion such as Na$^+$ a Peclet number of the order of 0.002, and for a macromolecule such as serum albumin the Peclet number would probably be between 0.5 and 1.5. Furthermore, σ to Na$^+$ at the walls of microvessels with continuous endothelia is in the range of 0.1–0.2 and where the endothelium is fenestrated it is in the range of 0.02 to 0.05. The values for σ to albumin at both continuous and fenestrated endothelia are in the range of 0.9–1.0. When these figures are substituted in Eq. 13, it is found that ultra-filtration at these rates should give rise to differences in Na^+ concentration of less than 1% of the plasma concentration, whereas the differences in serum albumin concentration should be of the order of 85–95% of the plasma concentration.

These concentration differences generated by ultra-filtration of fluid through microvascular walls will set up differences in osmotic pressure that oppose fluid filtration (Eq. 5). Since plasma has many solutes, ultra-filtration is opposed by the sum of the osmotic pressures of set up by each solute. Thus Eq. 5 should be written as:

$$J_V = L_P S\left(\Delta P - \sum_i^n \sigma_i \Delta \Pi_i\right). \tag{14}$$

where S is the area of microvascular wall through which filtration is driven by a hydrostatic pressure difference, ΔP, and opposed by the sum of the differences in osmotic pressures of the different solutes $\sum_i^n \sigma_i \Delta \Pi$ (where $i=$ the ith solute). From what has been said about the magnitude of the concentration gradients that arise across microvascular walls with ultra-filtration, it will be immediately appreciated that the osmotic pressure term is dominated by the ultra-filtration of macromolecules and that the contribution of small hydrophilic ions (which are responsible for most of the total osmotic pressure of the body fluids) is negligible.

Equation 14 is a modern statement of Starling's hypothesis of capillary fluid exchange. Net fluid movements between the plasma and the tissues are determined by the differences in hydrostatic and osmotic pressure between the plasma in the exchange vessels and the interstitial fluid surrounding them.

In many textbooks, the statement of Starling's hypothesis is supplemented with the idea that in the tissues around each capillary there is a circulation of fluid. It suggests that at the arterial end the hydrostatic pressure differences exceed the osmotic pressure differences so that here there is net fluid loss from the blood into the tissue, At the venous end of the microvessels, however, ΔP is said to be less than the effective osmotic pressure, so that fluid is continuously absorbed from the tissues into the blood. There are two good reasons to believe that this picture rarely, if ever, represents reality.

The first is that the numbers do not add up [20]. Although the hydrostatic pressure in capillaries at the level of the heart may approximate to osmotic pressure of the plasma proteins, the hydrostatic and osmotic pressures of the surrounding interstitial fluid are not negligible in Eq. 14. When these are taken into account, Eq. 14 predicts that there should always be net fluid filtration from plasma to tissues. There is also the observation that in humans (and any reasonably large animal) most of the exchange vessels are not at heart level and the hydrostatic pressures in the vessels below the heart is very much greater than the total osmotic pressure of the plasma proteins.

The second reason for disbelieving the idea that fluid is continuously re-absorbed from the tissues at the venous end of the exchange vessels follows both from experiments and from the argument outlined above that showed that the concentration differences of macromolecules between the plasma and the ISF arise from ultra-filtration. Because microvascular walls are fi-nitely permeable to macromolecules, the concentration differences of mac-romolecules across them require continuous ultra-filtration to be main-tained and disappear if ultra-filtration ceases. Thus the osmotic pressure gradients that drive uptake of fluid are progressively diminished as absorp-tion continues and the process of fluid absorption can only be short-lived [21]. This prediction has been confirmed in single mesenteric capillaries where the hydrostatic pressures can be controlled [22]. Reabsorption is rapidly curtailed as the concentration of macromolecules surrounding the microvessels rises, diminishing the osmotic pressure difference across the vessel walls.

Continuous absorption of fluid does occur into capillaries of some tis-sues, such as the post-glomerular capillaries of the kidney and the muco-sae of the intestine. In these tissues, however, the local ISF is receiving a continuous input of protein-free fluid from the nearby epithelia and this keeps the concentrations of proteins in the pericapillary fluids low. In tis-sues such as skin, fat and muscle there is no mechanism of this kind. At the venous end of the microcirculation in these tissues, the pressure may sink to levels where fluid reabsorption is transiently possible, but after a few minutes it will attenuate, stop and turn into a low level of filtration. These low levels of filtration are seen as the flow of lymph from the tissue.

In human subjects, the microvascular pressure (P_C) has been measured only in a few types of capillaries, and these measurements have shown that P_C varies greatly with its position relative to the heart. In the skin capillar-ies of the fingers and toes, P_C increases in proportion to the vertical dis-tance, h, between the vessel and the heart. A similar linear relation corre-lates the local arterial and venous pressure, P_V, to h. Whereas the slope of the relation between P_V and h is equal to the product of the density of the blood and the acceleration due to gravity as would expected for a static column of liquid, the slope of P_C against h is considerably less than this [23]. For blood to flow through the circulation from the arteries to the cap-illaries and onward to the veins, P_C must always be less than the arterial pressure and greater than the venous pressure. At heart level, P_C is usually 60–80% of the way from the local arterial to the local venous pressure, but below the heart P_C moves closer to P_V so that in the toes of a man stand-ing still, P_C may only be 1–2 cmH$_2$O above P_V. This is due to a local re-sponse, the veno-arteriolar response, whereby a rise in the local microvas-cular pressures leads to increased constriction of the arterioles. Constric-tion of the arterioles in turn increases the drop in pressure across the arte-rioles, reducing both the rate of perfusion and the pressures within the microcirculation. This is one of possibly several local mechanisms that mini-mise the rate of ultra-filtration into dependent parts of the body under normal circumstances. Not only will the lowered microvascular pressures mean lower filtration rates, but the very slow flow of blood through many of the vessels allows the plasma proteins within to become concentrated to levels where their osmotic pressures again become comparable with the lo-cal microvascular pressure, increasing their effectiveness as brakes on the filtration process.

Increased Permeability

The term "increased vascular permeability" usually refers to an increase in the permeability of microvessels to fluid and macromolecules. It is a char-acteristic change of acute and chronic inflammation. In acute inflammation the increase in permeability to macromolecules is localised to the small ve-nules. It is associated with the appearance of openings in the endothelial lining of these vessels in electron micrographs of the tissue. Until recently it had been assumed that these openings were formed between the endo-thelial cells, but recent reconstructions from serial sections of tissue have shown that in some cases the openings appear to be large pores passing through the peripheral cytoplasm of the endothelial cells close to cell junc-tions [24, 25]. In acute inflammation, mediators such as histamine are re-leased into the ISF from the mast cells and bind to receptors on the venular endothelium. A rise in intracellular Ca^{2+} appears to be the first step in the signalling process, and the activation of guanylate cyclase by nitric oxide occurs as a later step in the process [14]. The cellular mechanics leading the formation of openings in the endothelium remain obscure. For many years it has been believed that the endothelial cells made use of their actin and myosin filaments to contract away from each other, but recent studies cast severe doubts on this.

From a functional point of view, the increased permeability leads to a more rapid filtration of fluid and protein into the tissue. This initially ex-pands the local ISF, which continues to drain into more distant regions of the tissue and into the lymphatics. The rate of drainage by the lymphatics is limited, and if it cannot match the rate of fluid filtration into the tissue, the ISF volume expands progressively and oedema becomes apparent.

Transport Through the Interstitium

While O_2 diffuses through cells as it passes from the capillary blood into the tissues, hydrophilic (lipophobic) molecules have to exchange between the tissues and the blood via the spaces between the cells. These spaces re-present the interstitium and its fine structure varies from tissue to tissue and from point to point in the same tissue.

In skeletal muscle, the interstitium includes both narrow flattened spaces between adjacent muscle cells and the more open spaces surrounding the bundles of muscle cells. Similarly in fat, there are only narrow flattened spaces between the adipocytes within the fat lobules but there are wider spaces between lobules where small arterioles, venules and nerves are found. In narrow intercellular spaces the principal structures are the basement membranes of the adjacent cells. These consist of fine fibrous molecules of type IV collagen that form a two-dimensional lattice with laminin. In the more open regions there are clusters of types I and II collagen fibrils, elastin, hyaluronan and chondroitin. These molecules form the extracellular matrix and the pathways between them are more variable than those in the endothelial glycocalyx with many larger intercommunicating spaces. These spaces form a transport pathway through which fluids and solutes can percolate.

Transport in the interstitium can be thought of as involving two pathways: that between the outside of the exchange vessels and the outside of the cells (which involves solute traffic in both directions) and that between the outside of the exchange vessels and the lymphatics, which is in one direction only. We shall consider the pathway between the microvessels and the terminal lymphatics first.

The Pathway Between the Blood Capillaries and the Lymphatics

The length of this pathway varies considerably from tissue to tissue. In skin, the lymphatic capillaries form a network that underlies the sub-papillary plexuses of arterioles and venules in the superficial dermis. A deeper plexus, separate from the superficial plexus, is found at the lower boundary of the dermis. Blind-ended lymph vessels are present in the papillae and drain into the superficial network. Thus there is a close association between the blood microcirculation and the lymphatics in the most superficial parts of the dermis, implying a short route through the interstitium for newly formed capillary ultra-filtrate to enter the lymph. The same appears to true at the lower border of the dermis, though at intermediate depths within the dermis, the ultra-filtrate may have to flow through tortuous channels for several hundred micrometres before entering terminal lymphatics.

In skeletal muscle, each muscle fibre has several capillaries that run in parallel along its length. Between the capillaries the intercellular space is narrow, but around the capillaries the space is enlarged. The connective tissue is presumably loose around the capillaries, for these vessels become more tortuous as the muscle shortens and straighten as the muscle is stretched. There are nerves but no lymphatics in these spaces. Muscle cells are bound together in bundles or fasciculi by a dense layer of connective tissue called the perimysium. Lymphatic capillaries appear to be confined to the perimysium and to the outermost sheath of connective tissue, the epimysium that encloses the entire muscle. From this picture it appears that fluid filtered from capillaries within a muscle percolates from the centre of a fasciculus to the lymphatics in the perimysium.

The arrangement of the microcirculation and the collecting lymphatics in adipose tissue is somewhat similar to that in skeletal muscle. The fat cells (adipocytes) are packed closely together with little interstitial space between them. These spaces expand only to accommodate narrow capillaries. In transverse sections of human adipose tissue, each adipocyte is surrounded by between two and six capillaries that supply adjacent cells. There are no lymphatics within the fat lobules, but collecting vessels are found in the connective tissue at the boundary of the lobule [26]. As in skeletal muscle, fluid filtered from the capillaries must drain through the narrow intercellular spaces before it enters the lymph at the outer border of the fat lobules.

These histological considerations suggest that the transit of fluid between the microvascular exchange vessels and the lymphatic capillaries might be relatively rapid in skin but greatly delayed in muscle and fat tissue. In muscle, moreover, a wide range of transit times between blood and lymph is to be expected, with much of the ultra-filtrate flowing through a large fraction of the intercellular space to reach the lymphatics. If the muscle bundle is small, highly diffusible molecules may reach the lymphatics before macromolecules. For larger fasciculi where the diffusion distances are great, convection may be the predominant form of transport for both large and small molecules.

In skin, where the lymphatics capillaries appear to be close to most of the exchange vessels, changes in solute concentration in the microvascular ultra-filtrate should be detected fairly rapidly in the lymph. The time taken for the composition of the lymph to represent the altered composition of the ultra-filtrate, however, will be considerably longer. Indeed, the larger molecules might reach their new steady-state concentrations sooner than the smaller molecules, as the volume of ISF with which they can equilibrate may be considerably less than that available for small ions.

Watson and Grodins [27] analysed measurements of the rates of transport of dextrans between blood and lymph in cat hind limbs and found that the mean transit time for the larger molecules was shorter than that for the smaller molecules. They concluded that this reflected the smaller volume of distribution available to the larger molecules in the interstitial space. There is an analogy here with transport through a gel chromatography column. The small molecules appear in the effluent from such a column after the larger molecules as they are distributed in a larger volume within the gel.

Interstitial Fluid and Its Flow Through Tissues

The different volumes of distribution of water-soluble molecules within the extra-cellular spaces influence the distribution of water here. This is most easily understood in terms of a simplified model in which the interstitium is divided into two compartments. The first or free fluid phase represents regions of the ISF where all solutes can enter and move by diffusion and convection. This applies to macromolecules dissolved in the ISF as well as ions and small water-soluble molecules. The second compartment or gel phase represents regions of the interstitial space where the matrix molecules are packed so closely together that they form a barrier to molecules in solution greater than (say) 5 nm in diameter. In this simple model the larger plasma proteins that are present in the free fluid phase are excluded from the gel phase and consequently they exert a small osmotic pressure across the boundary between these two compartments. Another osmotic pressure, developed within the gel, also acts across this boundary in the opposite direction. This pressure, sometimes called the Donnan pressure, is set up by small ions that are associated with the charged groups present on matrix macromolecules. Nearly all the matrix macromolecules have a net negative charge, and for electrical neutrality to be maintained, an excess of positive counter-ions (which are largely Na^+) accumulates around the charged groups in the solution within the gel phase, raising its osmotic pressure. A third factor that plays a part in the distribution of fluid between the free fluid and the gel phases is the strength of the cross-linkages between the matrix molecules, for these oppose expansion of the gel. Thus, at equilibrium, the tendency of fluid to move into the gel under the influence of the Donnan pressure is counterbalanced by the tension on the cross-linkages between the matrix macromolecules and the osmotic pressure of the free fluid phase of the ISF. This description of the distribution of fluid and macromolecules between just two compartments of the interstitium is a considerable simplification. While the concept of a single free fluid phase is reasonable, there are many gel phase compartments that exclude macromolecules of different molecular size and charge.

Because fluid does not flow rapidly within the interstitial spaces of tissues, measurement of its pressure is difficult, and for many years it was uncertain whether the pressure recorded from a fine fluid-filled needle inserted into a tissue was the ISF pressure of that tissue. In the early 1960s, Guyton devised a different approach. He implanted a hollow perforated capsule into the subcutaneous tissues of a dog and allowed it to heal in place. The capsule filled with fluid that Guyton [28] reasonably believed would come to equilibrium with the surrounding ISF reflecting its composition and hydrostatic pressure. When Guyton measured the hydrostatic pressure (by inserting a needle connected to a manometer into the capsular fluid) and reported it was a few millimetres of mercury below atmospheric pressure, this launched a controversy that lasted for nearly 20 years. Guyton and his colleagues implanted capsules at other sites and found that ISF pressure varied considerably from tissue to tissue, being most negative (sub-atmospheric) in lung (–8 to –10 mmHg) and strongly positive in kidney (+4 to +10 mmHg). Scholander [29] devised the wick method, which also recorded negative pressures in many ISFs, and this technique was applied and developed as the wick-in-needle method for use in mammalian tissues by Auckland, Reed and their collaborators [30, 31].

The controversy of the sub-atmospheric values of ISF pressure came to be resolved with more rigorous analyses of the forces acting within gels [32, 33]. Pressure is a measure of the potential energy of a fluid, and the measurement of a sub-atmospheric pressure in the ISF merely signifies that the potential energy of the ISF is slightly less than that of a similar solution contained within an open vessel at atmospheric pressure rather than in the interstices of a gel matrix.

Fluid Flow Through the Interstitium

Fluid flows through the interstitial spaces down gradients of hydrostatic pressure. The resistance to fluid flow is high (hydraulic conductivity low), but the flow velocities are generally very small and consequently so are the pressure gradients.

Levick [34] summarised the data for the hydraulic conductivity of the interstitial space of different tissues that were available from the literature in the mid-1980s. He plotted the values against the concentration of glycosaminoglycans (GAGs) in the tissue (where this was known) and found a strongly inverse relation. A similar relation could be obtained from the rates of sedimentation of synovial hyaluronan in the ultracentrifuge [35]. Levick then examined whether he could account for the correlation between tissue hydraulic conductivity and tissue GAG concentration in terms of the theory of fluid flow through a random network of macromolecular fibres. He found that the variations in hydraulic conductivity could be predicted from the variations of tissue GAG concentration but the absolute values of tissue hydraulic conductivity could only be predicted when the tissue concentrations of collagen and proteoglycans were taken into account.

This important work confirmed what many had already believed about the importance of GAGs to the hydraulic conductivity of a tissue. It also emphasised that contrary to what some had thought, collagen played a significant role. One consequence of the dependence of interstitial hydraulic conductivity upon the concentration of matrix molecules is that hydration of a tissue should lead to a large increase in its hydraulic conductivity. This had been known from the earliest quantitative estimates of tissue conductivity made by Guyton et al. [36].

Although much of the mystery surrounding ISF pressures has now been dispelled, the question of how fluid moves from the interstitium into the terminal lymphatics has been resolved only recently. Simultaneous measurements of the pressure inside the terminal lymphatics and P_{isf} suggested that while the differences were small, lymphatic pressure was greater than P_{isf} for all [37] or most [38] of the time. Hogan [38] worked on lymphatics in the bat wing. where the terminals are contractile, and he was able to make records of the pressures across their walls during repeated cycles of contraction and relaxation. For less than 40% of the time the pressure in the lymphatics was less than P_{isf}. If fluid movement into the lymphatics is driven by this pressure difference, and if the L_P of the lymphatic wall remained constant throughout the cycle, net fluid movement should occur from the lymphatic into the interstitium. Fluid clearly moved in the opposite direction. If the L_P of the terminal lymphatic wall, however, varied during the contractile cycle, so that it was relatively high when P_{ISF} was greater than pressure in the lymphatic and relatively low when the pressure difference was reversed, net fluid movement from interstitium to lymph would occur. This possibility had been suggested by Casley Smith [39] from his observations of electron micrographs of the terminal lymphatic vessels. He noted that when tracers appeared to pass into the lymph there were relatively large gaps between the lymphatic endothelial cells, whereas at other times the junctions between the lymphatic endothelial cells appeared to be closed. He suggested that the peripheral parts of endothelial cells of the terminal lymphatics acted as "flap-valves", opening and closing the fluid-conducting channels between adjacent cells in response to the direction of the pressure gradient across them.

Recent experimental observations by Schmid-Schönbein's group support this idea [40]. When a fluid containing a fluorescent marker is micro-injected into the tissue surrounding a lymphatic capillary, it rapidly enters the vessel. When the same solution is injected directly into the vessel lumen, however, it does not pass out into the tissue. The fluorescent tracer is retained even when the pressure inside the vessel exceeds that outside. At the present time it is not known whether the simple flap valve suggested by Casley Smith [39] is the mechanism of the rectification of flow through the lymphatic endothelium. It is hoped that the approach used by Schmid-Schonbein and his colleagues [40] can be used to investigate and to extend our understanding here.

Mathematical models of fluid circulation through the tissues, from blood capillaries via interstitium to lymphatics and back to blood again, have been used for many years to help clarify our understanding of fluid balance and the regulation of blood volume [41]. Considerations of the structure of the interstitium were introduced around 1970 [42, 43], and these models have become more sophisticated and detailed with time [44, 45]. Of considerable interest is the combined theoretical and experimental approach to ISF drainage into the lymphatics of the rat tail by Swartz and her colleagues [46]. This tissue has a superficial, regular network of lymphatic capillaries that can be visualised by fluorescent tracers. When fluid is infused into the tissues near the tip of the tail, it flows centrally through the interstitium, from where it is cleared into the lymphatic network. Close to the infusion site, the fluid flow through the interstitium may exceed flow through the lymphatic network, but more of the infused fluid is carried by the lymphatics as one moves nearer to the base of the tail, until at some point lymphatic clearance exceeds interstitial flow. Swartz et al. [46] developed a mathematical model to describe these phenomena that assumed the specific hydraulic conductivity of the tissue remained constant at different infusion rates and the fluid entered the lymphatics down a pressure gradient with a constant conductivity of the walls of the lymphatic vessels. In the laboratory, they infused a physiological saline solution containing 0.1% FITC dextran (MW 2000 kDa) into the tips of rat tails and observed that the tissues filled with fluorescent tracer for a well-demarcated distance towards the base before the lymphatic network became clearly visible and the tissue fluorescence faded. The length of the region filled with fluorescent tracer was directly related to the pressure applied to the infusion system, and this was consistent with the theoretical model, which assumed linear relations between infusion pressure and the infusion rate. The model could then be used to extract information about the hydraulic conductivity of the interstitium and of the lymphatic system. One problem with this study is its limited applicability to other situations. The rat tail is enclosed in a tough sleeve so that overall volume changes in the vicinity of the infusion site could be assumed to be negligible. This property also enables the assumption to be made that the hydraulic conductivity of the tissue is independent of the rate of fluid flow through it. Neither of these assumptions may be made for normal skin or subcutaneous tissue. As demonstrated by Guyton et al. [36] and subsequently others, infusion of fluid into subcutaneous tissue leads to a large increase in hydraulic conductivity of the interstitium.

The resistance to fluid flow through the interstitium is not just important for flow between the capillaries of the cardiovascular and lymphatic systems. It governs fluid flow into and out of specialised body cavities, e.g. joint cavities, pleural and peritoneal spaces and the anterior chambers of the eye. In all tissues, it stabilises the ISF, preventing its rapid flow under gravity with changes in the position of the tissues with respect to the heart. It also contributes to the stiffness of the tissues, determining the rate of flow of fluid out of compressed regions.

A simple calculation reveals that even the highest estimates for the hydraulic conductivity of subcutaneous tissues are low enough to protect tissue from rapid changes in ISF volume with changes in posture. When a human subject moves from a lying to a standing position, there will be a tendency for the ISF to drain from the upper parts of the body to the feet. The vertical pressure gradient is 1 cmH_2O per centimetre of vertical height. Taking the highest value for the specific hydraulic conductivity of subcutaneous tissue as 10^{-6} cm s^{-1} cmH_2O^{-1}, the flow per unit area of interstitial tissue is 10^{-6} cm s^{-1}. If the cross-sectional area of the lower part of the leg just above the ankle is approximately 8 cm^2, ISF flows down each leg into the feet of standing subjects at a rate of just less than 0.03 ml per hour or less than 0.5 ml per 16-hour day. This figure contrasts with estimates on the order of 30 ml per hour for microvascular filtration of fluid into the feet of sitting and standing subjects.

In articular cartilage, the hydraulic resistance of the interstitium protects the cells when the tissue is compressed. Here, the specialised matrix occupies the greater part of the tissue volume and acts as a highly efficient hydraulic buffer. In tissues such as skin and muscle, however, ISF is unlikely to protect the cells from compression, as its volume is normally less than

20% of the tissue volume. We have already noted that when the ISF volume is expanded in oedema, the hydraulic resistance of the interstitium falls dramatically. This is seen in the clinical demonstration of pitting oedema. The clinician applies pressure with his thumb over an area of oedematous tissue for a few tens of seconds, displacing excess ISF from this area and leaving an indentation or pit in the tissue that slowly refills.

Summary and Speculations

In this review of transport of fluid and solutes through tissues, we have seen that fluid flows through tissues down gradients of hydrostatic pressure. Even osmotic flows are the result of gradients of hydrostatic pressure within the pores of the membrane through which the flow occurs. The volume of fluid flowing down a given pressure gradient, either within microvascular walls or in the interstitium, is determined by the ultrastructure of the fluid-conducting pathways in these tissues. Considerable progress has been made over the past 25 years in developing a clear understanding of this aspect of structure and function. Solutes are transported through tissues by convection and diffusion. Diffusion is effective for transport of small molecules over microscopic distances. For transport over greater distances, only convection would appear to be adequate. Once again the ultrastructure of the pathways is an important determinant of the actual flux of solute, whether it is by convection or diffusion. Because the pathways have dimensions similar to those of the larger molecules that are being transported, the size, charge and lipid solubility of a molecule all influence its rate of transport. This is most obvious when we consider transport through microvascular walls, where the molecular sieving effects give rise to concentration differences between the plasma and the interstitial fluids. In the interstitium it is responsible for regions that only the smallest molecules can penetrate. While molecular sieving has the effect of favouring transport of small molecules over large molecules through microvascular walls, it may also favour the more rapid passage of macromolecules than smaller solutes through the interstitial space between the microvessels and the lymph.

What relevance does this information about healthy tissues have for the investigation of the pathophysiology and management of pressure ulcers? As a starting pointing let us consider the needs of tissues such as skin, fat and muscle over relatively short periods such as an hour or two. We might then speculate on how far these can be met if external pressure compresses a local region of tissue to an extent that blood flow here is halted. We will also consider whether any new transport problems might arise as a consequence.

We know that under normal conditions skin, muscle and fat require a constant supply of oxygen and the constant clearance of CO_2, and these are dependent on convective transport by the circulation into and out of the microvessels plus diffusion between the microvessels and the mitochondria in cells that surround them. It might also be thought that glucose, fatty acids and amino acids need to be supplied by the circulation. While this would be true of certain tissues (e.g. brain requires a constant supply of glucose), in muscle and fat this is less important as there are sufficient stores of carbohydrate and fat within the cells to meet the metabolic needs of resting tissue for an hour or two. A continuous flux of glucose from the microcirculation to the cells does occur in resting muscle, but this is to maintain the levels of glycogen in the cellular stores.

If the tissues lie between bone and the external surface, pressure applied to a small circular area on the surface could compress a cylinder of tissue between the surface and the bone to an extent that the circulation within this tissue cylinder is stopped (see Fig. 14.5 a). Any transport to or from the cells within the compressed tissue must occur across the boundary of the cylinder and the surrounding tissue. If the circulation within the compressed region is arrested, transport can only occur by diffusion. Convection of interstitial fluid would be brought to a halt shortly after the circulation was arrested for it depends on pressure gradients across microvascular walls, within the interstitium and between the interstitial fluid and the terminal lymphatics. Even if interstitial fluid continued to flow within the compressed tissue, its rate of flow could not exceed its flow in normal tissues when it is a fraction of 1% of that in the microcirculation. It would therefore be incapable of delivering nutrients to the cells at the rates they require.

To estimate how much of the compressed tissue can be supplied with oxygen by diffusion from its surroundings, we can use the same sort of argument that Krogh and Erlang developed to determine how much tissue could be supplied with O_2 by diffusion from a single capillary. It is useful to start by making the following assumptions: (a) that diffusion can just supply all the compressed tissue within the cylinder; (b) that the O_2 consumption of the tissue and the O_2 diffusion coefficient and solubility are uniform throughout the tissue; and (c) that O_2 consumption of the tissue is independent of the local PO_2 providing the latter is greater than 1 or 2 mmHg.

In Fig. 14.5 b, R is the radius of the cylinder of locally compressed tissue and x is a point along the radius measured from its boundary with the surrounding tissue. The rate at which O_2 diffuses past x, $Jo_2(x)$, is related to the oxygen consumption of the tissue of the inner cylinder that has a radius of $(R-x)$ and an outer surface of $2\pi(R-x)$. If a is the solubility of oxygen in tissue fluid expressed in terms of ml O_2 ml^{-1} $mmHg^{-1}$, and μO_2 is the O_2 consumption per unit volume of tissue, we can use Eq. 4 to derive an expression for PO_2 at different distances along from the boundary towards the centre of the cylinder of compressed tissues. This is analogous to Eq. 6, i.e.

$$PO_2(x) = PO_2(surface) - \frac{\mu O_2}{2Da}\left(Rx - \frac{x^2}{2}\right).$$ (15)

Equation 15 can be evaluated since Krogh [3] determined values for μO_2 and Da in muscle that have been confirmed by more recent work and values also exist for these parameters in skin tissue. Krogh expressed Da as a

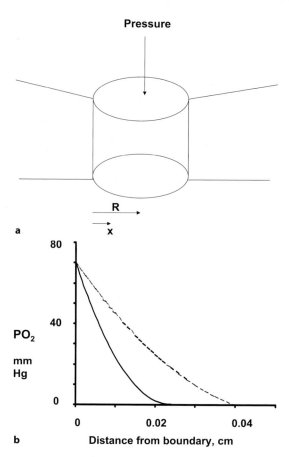

Fig. 14.5 a, b. Simple theoretical model to investigate diffusion into a locally compressed region of tissue. **a** Cylinder of tissue compressed from above where R is the radius of the cylinder measured from its circumference and x is any distance along R. **b** Fall in PO_2 from perimeter of cylinder to centre calculated using Eq. 15 for skin tissue (*upper curve*) and muscle (*lower curve*)

single constant that is now generally referred to as the Krogh constant and has a value of 2×10^{-8} ml of O_2 per ml of muscle per mmHg per cm per minute. Estimates of μO_2 for resting muscle lie in the range of 0.005 to 0.01 ml O_2 ml^{-1} tissue min^{-1} and for skin in the range of 0.0018–0.002 ml·ml^{-1} min^{-1}. Substituting these values in Eq. 15 suggests that a cylinder of compressed skin tissue with a diameter of 0.8 mm could continue to consume O_2 at its normal rate when O_2 was transported from its boundary entirely by diffusion, providing that the PO_2 in the surrounding tissue had a mean value of 70 mmHg. Diffusion from surrounding tissues could meet the resting O_2 requirements of compressed resting muscle only if the cylinder of compressed tissue were less than 0.5 mm in diameter.

Although the distances to which O_2 can penetrate are small, Fig. 14.5 b does indicate that they are different for muscle and skin, reflecting their different basal metabolic rates. It seems possible that this might also reflect differing degrees of damage to skin and muscle during a prolonged period of compression involving both tissues.

When compressed tissues are deprived of O_2, anaerobic metabolism is activated with the formation of lactic acid and its release into the interstitial space. In the absence of blood flow, the lactic acid has to diffuse out of the compressed tissue, and this raises several interesting problems. While it is generally assumed that acid is buffered by HCO_3^- ions, it has been pointed out that this would be efficient only if carbonic anhydrase were readily available in the interstitial fluid to convert the large quantities of carbonic acid into dissolved CO_2. While it seems possible that the muscle carbonic anhydrase serves this purpose, and an alternative source of carbonic anhydrase might be that of the red cells trapped in the tissues, if insufficient carbonic anhydrase were available the pH of the tissues might fall to lethal values, depending on the rate of lactate release.

A second problem concerns the level to which lactate might rise in a compressed region of tissue if its only means of clearance were by diffusion into surrounding tissues. One may use analogous expressions to Eq. 15 to estimate the concentration of lactate as it diffuses out of a compressed cylinder of tissue. When one attempts to evaluate these expressions one finds the fundamental data are even more uncertain than they are for oxygen. Although reasonable estimates may be made for the rates of lactate production in skeletal muscle during anaerobic exercise, the values for rates of lactate formation per unit volume of ischaemic muscle or skin can only be guessed. If anaerobic metabolism in resting ischaemic muscle were to yield the same turnover of ATP molecules as aerobic metabolism, then the formation of lactate would be of the order of 2–3 μmol ml^{-1} tissue min^{-1}. Clearance of lactate by diffusion from the cylinder of compressed tissue 1 cm in diameter could match these levels only if the concentration at the centre was 10–20 molar! Clearly anaerobic metabolism could not continue under these conditions, but what the calculations reveal is how much more needs to be discovered to understand what actually happens.

While the calculations and discussion in the last few paragraphs are highly speculative, they are included because they do draw attention to areas of uncertainty. If the principles of tissue transport that have been clarified in healthy tissues are applied to guide investigations of tissue ischaemia, it is hoped that they may not only raise questions but also assist in the formulation of rational answers.

References

1. Stücker M, Struk A, Altmeyer P, Herde M, Baumgärtl H, Lubbers DW (2002) The cutaneous uptake of atmospheric oxygen contributes significantly to the oxygen supply of the human dermis and epidermis. J Physiol 538:985–994

2. Rosell S (1984) Microcirculation and transport in adipose tissue. In: Handbook of physiology. The cardiovascular system. Microcirculation, sec 2, vol IV, pt 2.
   American Physiological Society, Bethesda, MD, pp 949–967
3. Krogh A (1919) The rate of diffusion of gases through animal tissues with some remarks on the coefficient of invasion. J Physiol 52, 391–408
4. Krogh A (1919) The number and distribution of capillaries in muscles with calculations of the oxygen pressure head necessary for supplying the tissue. J Physiol 52:409–415
5. Krogh A (1919) The supply of oxygen to the tissues and the regulation of the capillary circulation. J Physiol 52:457–474
6. Kruezer F (1982) Oxygen supply to tissues: the Krogh model and its assumptions. Experientia 38:1415–1426
7. Duling BR, Berne RM (1970) Longitudinal gradients in peri-arteriolar oxygen tension: a possible mechanism for the participation of oxygen in the local regulation of blood flow. Circ Res 27:669–678
8. Kuo L, Pittman RN (1990) Effect of systemic hemodilution on arteriolar oxygen transport in hamster striated muscle. Am J Physiol 259:H1694–H1702
9. Filho IPT, Kerger H, Intaglietta M (1996) PO2 measurements in arteriolar networks. Microvasc Res 51:202–212
9a. Ellsworth M, Ellis CG, Popel AS, Pittman RN (1994) Role of microvessels in oxygen supply to tissues. News in Physiol Sci 9:119–123
10. Michel CC (1974) The transport of oxygen and carbon dioxide by the blood. In; MTP International Reviews of Sciences. Physiology Series 1 vol 2. Respiratory physiology. Butterworths, London, pp 67–104
11. Effros RM, Weissman ML (1979) Carbonic anhydrase activity of the cat hind leg. J Applied Physiol 47:1090–1098
12. Effros RM, Shapiro L, Silverman P (1980) Carbonic anhydrase activity of rabbit lungs. J Appl Physiol 49:589–600
13. Roughton FJW (1964) Transport of oxygen and carbon dioxide. In: Handbook of physiology, sec 3, vol 1. American Physiological Society, Bethesda, MD, pp 767–825
14. Michel CC, Curry FE (1999) Microvascular permeability. Physiol Rev 79:703–761
15. Grotte G (1956) Passage of dextran molecules across blood-lymph barrier. Acta Chir Scand Suppl 211:1–84
16. Pappenheimer JR, Renkin EM, Borrero LM (1951) Filtration, diffusion and molecular sieving through peripheral capillary membranes. A contribution to the pore theory of capillary permeability. Am J Physiol 167:13–46
17. Rippe B, Haraldsson B (1994) Transport of macromolecules across microvascular walls: the two pore theory. Physiol Rev 74:163–219
18. Rippe B, Rosengren B-I, Carlsson O, Venturoli D (2002) Transendothelial transport: the vesicle controversy. J Vasc Res 39:375–390
19. Schnizter JE, Allard J, Oh P (1995) NEM inhibits transcytosis, endocytosis and capillary permeability; implication of caveolae fusion in endothelia. Am J Physiol 268:H48–H55
20. Levick JR (1991a) Capillary filtration- absorption balance reconsidered in the light of dynamic extravascular factors. Exp Physiol 76:825–857
21. Michel CC (1984) Fluid movements through capillary walls. In: Handbook of physiology. The cardiovascular system. Microcirculation, sec 2, vol IV, pt 1, chap. 9. American Physiological Society, Bethesda, MD, pp 375–409

22. Michel CC, Phillips ME (1987) Steady state fluid filtration at different capillary pressures in perfused frog capillaries. J Physiol 388:421–435
23. Levick JR, Michel CC (1978) The effects of position and skin temperature on the capillary pressures in the fingers and toes. J Physiol 274:97–109
24. Neal CR, Michel CC (1995) Transcellular gaps in microvascular walls of frog and rat when permeability is increased with the ionophore A23187. J Physiol 488:427–437
25. Feng DJ, Nagy J, Hipp K, Pyne K, Dvorak HF, Dvorak AM (1997) Re-interpretation of endothelial gasp induced by vasoactive mediators in guinea pig, mouse and rat: many are transcellular pores. J Physiol 504:747–761
26. Ryan TJ (1995) Lymphatics and adipose tissue. Clin Dermatol 13:493–498
27. Watson P, Grodins F (1978) An analysis of the effects of the interstitial matrix on plasma-lymph transport. Microvasc Res 16:19–41
28. Guyton AC (1963) A concept of negative interstitial pressure based on pressures in implanted perforated capsules. Circ Res 12:399–414
29. Scholander P, Hargens AR, Miller SL (1968) Negative pressure in the interstitial fluid of animals. Science 161:321–328
30. Auckland K, Nicolaysen G (1981) Interstitial fluid volume: local regulatory mechanisms. Physiol Rev 61:556–643
31. Auckland K, Reed RK (1993) Interstitial lymphatic mechanisms in the control of extracellular fluid volume. Physiol Rev 73:1–78
32. Silberberg A (1981) The significance of hydrostatic pressure in the fluid phase of a structured tissue space. In: Hargens AR (ed) Tissue fluid pressure and composition. Williams & Wilkins, Baltimore, pp 71–73
33. Granger DN, Mortillaro NA, Kvietys PR, Taylor AE (1981) Regulation of interstitial fluid volume in the small bowel. In: Hargens AR (ed) Tissue fluid pressure and composition. Williams & Wilkins, Baltimore, pp 173–183
34. Levick JR (1987) Flow through interstitium and other fibrous matrices. Q J Exp Physiol 72:409–437
35. Preston BN, Davies M, Ogston AG (1965) The composition and physicochemical properties of hyaluronic acids prepared from ox synovial fluid and from a case of mesothelioma. Biochem J 96:449–474
36. Guyton AC, Scheel K, Murphee D (1966) Interstitial fluid pressure. III. Its effects on resistance to tissue fluid mobility. Circ Res 19:412–419
37. Clough GF, Smaje LH (1978) Simultaneous measurement of the pressure in the interstitium and the terminal lymphatics of the cat mesentery. J Physiol 283:457–468
38. Hogan RD (1981) The initial lymphatics and interstitial fluid pressure. In: Hargens AR (ed) Tissue fluid pressure and composition. Williams & Wilkins, Baltimore, pp 155–163
39. Casley Smith JR (1972) The role of the endothelial intercellular junctions in the function of the initial lymphatics. Angiologica 9:106–131
40. Trzewik J, Mallipattu SK, Artmann GM, Delano FA, Schmid-Schönbein GW (2001) Evidence for a second valve system in lymphatics: endothelial microvalves. FASEB J 15:1711–1717
41. Guyton AC, Granger H, Taylor AE (1975) Circulatory physiology II. Dynamics and control of the body fluids. Saunders Philadelphia
42. Wiederhielm CA (1972) The interstitial space. In: Fung YC, Perrone N, Anliker M (eds) Biomechanics: its foundations and its objectives. Prentice Hall, Englewood Cliffs, NJ, pp 273–286

43. Zweifach BW, Silberberg A (1979) The interstitial–lymphatic flow system. In: Guyton AC, Young DB (eds) Int Rev Physiol Cardiovascular Physiol III, vol 1. University Park Press, Baltimore, pp 215–260
44. Bert JL, Martinez M (1995) Interstitial fluid transport. In: Reed RK, McHale NG, Bert JL, Winlove CP, Laine GA (eds) Interstitium, connective tissue and lymphatics. Portland Press Proceedings, pp 101–117
45. Taylor DG (1995) Systems analysis and mathematical modelling of interstitial transport and microvascular exchange. In: Reed RK, McHale NG, Bert JL, Winlove CP, Laine GA (eds) Interstitium, connective tissue and lymphatics. Portland Press Proceedings, pp 119-135
46. Swartz M, Kaipainen A, Netti PA, Brekken C, Boucher Y, Grodzinsky AJ, Jain RK (1999) Mechanics of interstitial-lymphatic fluid transport: theoretical foundation and experimental validation. J Biomech 32:1297–1307

Skin Model Studies

15

Yak-Nam Wang, Joan Sanders

Introduction

The skin is the largest single organ of the body, forming 15–20% of the weight. Several roles of the skin have been identified and are of critical importance, including transmission of stimuli, protection and temperature regulation.

The skin is a fibrous composite material composed of collagen and elastin fibres within an amorphous matrix of mucopolysaccharides traditionally known as the ground substance. It is a very complex structure also containing nerve fibres, sweat glands, small blood vessels and lymph vessels [1–3]. The skin can be divided into two main layers: the epidermis and the dermis (Fig. 15.1).

The epidermis is an avascular superficial layer of ectodermal origin, which lies adjacent to the dermis. Its thickness depends on which part of the body it covers, varying between 60 μm and 100 μm over most areas, and reaching 600 μm in the plantar and palmar regions [1]. The epidermis consists of five layers of stratified squamous epithelial cells, namely the stratum basale, stratum spinosum, stratum granulosum, stratum lucidum (not present in thin skin) and stratum corneum at the top surface.

The basal layer of the epidermis, the stratum basale, interdigitates with the underlying dermis by projections from both the epidermis and dermis, known as epidermal pegs and dermal papillae, respectively. This is known as the dermal–epidermal junction. The keratinocytes in the basal layer are living and actively proliferate. However, as they migrate through the progressive layers towards the surface, these cells become more keratinized, forming at the top surface the stratum corneum consisting of dead keratinized cells. Although this layer is relatively flexible, strong and inextensible, it contains a plane of weakness where it can rupture under shear due to the low strength of the bonding between the cell layers.

The dermis accounts for the greatest proportion of the skin thickness. It can be divided into two main layers: the papillary layer (pars papillaris) and the reticular layer (pars reticularis). The former is the thinner of the two and interdigitates with the epidermis. The reticular layer lies beneath the papillary layer and gives the skin its toughness and strength, as a direct result of the dense mass of interweaving connective tissue fibres [5].

The dermis is much thicker than the epidermis, ranging between 1 mm and 4 mm [1]. It is a vascularized fibrous layer supplied with nerves,

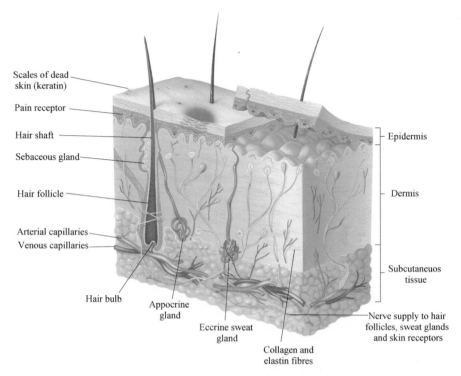

Scales of dead skin (keratin)

Pain receptor

Hair shaft

Sebaceous gland

Hair follicle

Arterial capillaries
Venous capillaries

Hair bulb

Appocrine gland

Eccrine sweat gland

Collagen and elastin fibres

Epidermis

Dermis

Subcutaneuos tissue

Nerve supply to hair follicles, sweat glands and skin receptors

Fig. 15.1. Section through healthy skin. Adapted from Weston [4]

lymph vessels, hair follicles, sweat glands, sebaceous glands and smooth muscle. The vasculature within the dermis has three principle functions, namely nutrition, oxygenation and thermoregulation. In a survey of older individuals (60–80 years), regional differences in blood capillary density of the human papillary dermis were found to be greater in the head and neck region than in lower parts of the body [6].

It is well accepted that there is a high incidence of ulcer formation in aged patients. The changes that occur in the structure of skin with age may be partially responsible for this high incidence. Chronologically aged skin is dry, wrinkled, lax, and both the dermis and epidermis are thinner [7]. Banwell et al. [8] observed effacement and blunting of the epidermal ridges and dermal papillae causing flattening of the dermal–epidermal junction in a patient population. This would result in a smaller area of contact and decreased adhesion between the epidermis and dermis. This weakening of the dermal–epidermal junction can lead to blistering or rupture at lower shear forces and friction. It has also been observed that with increased age, there is a loss of capillary loops in the dermal papillae and a decreased vascularity in the reticular dermis. Other aspects of chronologically aged skin are thinning of blood vessel walls, reduction and thickening of collagen, increases in collagen cross-links leading to brittle mechanical characteristics and fragmentation of elastin, resulting in compromised viscoelastic properties of the skin.

Skin Model Studies

Although the cause of pressure ulcers is multifactorial, it is widely accepted that pressure ischaemia and the following reperfusion play a critical role. It is well documented that skin is less susceptible to pressure-induced ischaemia than fat and muscle [9, 10] because it has a lower metabolic demand than muscle or fat [11]. Animal studies have shown that pressure ulcers can occur from muscle upwards or from the upper dermis downwards [12, 13]. However, animal models also indicate that skin is more susceptible to breakdown than deep tissue under certain loading conditions (i.e. forces that include shear). Models looking at ulcer formation only in the skin (Table 15.1) are particularly relevant to patient groups where there is a lack of significant underlying muscle and where the skin is relatively thin (e.g. the elderly). Although sacral ulcers have the highest incidence, heel ulcers are considered to be more serious because they frequently lead to foot or leg amputation due to complications and infection.

Due to the multiple variables found in the human environment, the aetiology of pressure ulcers has been difficult to study in a clinical setting. Unlike the tissue-engineered muscle models described in Chap. 16, currently there are no cell models or tissue-engineered models that have been developed specifically for pressure ulcer research. Most of the research on pressure ulcers has been carried out using animal models, and only a handful of these investigations have focused on the skin. The closest to tissue-engineered models is the use of skin organ cultures [14–20]. Although the animal models and other lab models lack the mechanical history and elements present in the human environment, certain hypothesis can be researched to gain more fundamental understanding of pressure ulcer formation in order to explain the complex processes involved.

Animal Studies

In 1942 Groth [21] observed that pressure ulcers similar to those in humans can be produced in animals, and there have since been many animal studies dedicated to pressure ulcer research. The rat model has been one of the most common animal models used in skin pressure ulcer research. The use of this model not only offers advantages in terms of cost and size of animals, but more is known about the effects of pharmacological intervention on pharmacokinetics in rats than any other species. However, rats, along with rabbits and dogs, have heavy, thick hair and loose skin with minimal subcutaneous tissue so the pressure distribution within the skin may or may not be similar to that found in humans [22]. This problem has, to some extent, been minimized by the use of hypotrichotic fuzzy rats which also means that there is no need for depilation [23–25].

There are limitations in the interpretation of results obtained from animal studies as the structure of animal skin, aside from swine, cannot be

Table 15.1. Overview of skin models

Reference	Model	Type of stress	Method of stress application	Applied stress in mmHg (kPa)	Time in hours	Site	Comments
Kosiak [28]	Dogs	Normal	Hypodermic syringe	100–550 (13–73)	1–12	Trochanter, ischial tuberosity	Microscopic pathologic changes observed in tissue after 1 h of stress at 60 mmHg
Dinsdale [29]	Swine	Normal with and without friction	Indenter	160–1100 (21–147) with and without friction	3	Iliac spine	Presence of friction in paraplegic pigs significantly increased formation of pressure sores
Nola and Vistnes [30]	Rats	Normal	Hypodermic syringe	100–110 (13–14.5)	6 (over 4 days)	Skin over muscle, skin over tibia	Pressures that caused 100% damage in skin over bone did not necessarily cause damage in skin over muscle
Herman et al. [25]	Rat	Normal	Indenter	92 (12.3)	5	Greater trochanter (pre-stressed and unstressed)	Baseline perfusion levels were elevated in pre-stressed skin
Salcido [23, 24]	Rat	Normal	Indenter	145.3 (19.4)	6 (over 5 days)	Greater trochanter	Skin ulceration seen under indenter. Damage may be due to neutrophil-mediated activation

Table 15.1 (continued)

Reference	Model	Type of stress	Method of stress application	Applied stress in mmHg (kPa)	Time in hours	Site	Comments
Goldstein and Sanders [17]	Swine	Normal and shear; cyclic at 1 Hz	Indenter	0.1–21 (0.2–2.9) normal ±0.1–8 (0.2–10.7) shear 4–8 (0.5–1) normal ±0.1–2.7 (0.2–0.4) shear	10–40 min 40 min/day (up to 3 weeks)	Greater trochanter	Skin breakdown occurred earlier as shear was increased. Adaptation observed in long-term experiments
Peirce et al. [39]	Rat	Compression	Magnet and steel plate	50 (6.5) (pressure with recovery)	2+R 1+R (5 cycles over 1–5 days)	Dorsal skin	Tissue damage increased with duration of ischaemia and increase in total I-R cycle
Houwing et al. [44]	Swine	Normal	Indenter	47.8 (63.7)	2 (skin collected. 0–336 h after loading)	Greater trochanter	Onset of damage was only seen in tissue collected 1–2 h into the reperfusion period

easily compared to human tissue. It is suggested that the porcine model is the most suitable animal model in which to research the aetiology of human pressure ulcers. This is because porcine skin provides the best match in terms of skin properties, histology, connective tissue morphology, cell kinetics, immunoreactivity and physiological structure and function. Furthermore, pigs and humans are similarly susceptible to conditions such as diabetes and paraplegia [26, 27]. In addition, the use of miniature pigs allows pressure ulcer research to be carried out on mature animals without the size of the animal causing technical difficulties. The use of hairless pigs eliminates the need for depilation [27].

Like deep tissue breakdown studies, skin ulcers studies have concentrated on one or a combination of factors known to promote ulceration. Kosiak [28] was one of the first to focus on the effect of pressure on ulcer formation in the epidermis. In this study, one ischaemic period (1–2 h) was induced by static pressures ranging from 60 mmHg to 550 mmHg. The lowest pressure and duration (60 mmHg for 1 hr) investigated was reported to be enough to induce significant histological changes within the skin. Damage observed included inflammatory cell infiltration, extravasation and hyaline degeneration. Kosiak concluded from this investigation that low pressure for long durations was the primary cause of pressure ulcers although damage to tissue would occur at high pressures for short durations.

Dinsdale [29] investigated the effects of different types of loading on normal and paralysed swine. Pressures ranging from 160 to 1020 mmHg were applied to the iliac supine, with and without friction, for 3 h. Damage ensued in the dermis after 24 h of loading, and ulcer formation was significantly increased in the presence of friction.

Studies have also investigated the application pressures on multiple days. Nola and Vistnes [30] compared the effects of 6 h of pressure (100–110 mmHg) per day, over 4 days, on skin over bone and skin over muscle over bone. It was found that a pressure regimen that caused 100% skin ulceration over bone did not necessarily cause skin ulceration when muscle was present, suggesting that the mechanisms behind skin breakdown and deep tissue breakdown are distinctly different.

The effects of pressure on tissue vasculature are accepted as playing an integral role in susceptibility to ulceration, and thus many studies have investigated perfusion and blood flow. In a study of capillary pressure, using micro-injection, Landis [31] found an average pressure of 32 mmHg in the arteriolar limb, 22 mmHg in the mid-capillary bed and 12 mmHg on the venous side. From these data it has been widely recognized that pressure at the surface of the skin, or interface pressure, in excess of 32 mmHg will lead to occlusion of the capillary bed and consequent tissue ischaemia. However, the relationship between pressure and perfusion is rather dubious. Herrman et al. [25] applied pressures to the hip over the greater trochanter of fuzzy rats until perfusion reached an apparent minimum, measured by laser Doppler flowmetry. Skin perfusion was observed to increase with low levels of surface pressure and then decrease with further increases in pressure until a minimum was reached. It is probable that the tissue was able to withstand the initial increases of surface pressure while maintaining good perfusion because of: (1) the stiffness of the connective tissue; (2) the increased tissue internal pressure due to loss of water causing an increased proteoglycan concentration; and (3) vasodilation and recruitment of vessels. However, as pressure increases, the ability of this system to compensate is overcome. When an additional ischaemic period was applied to the same region for 5 h followed by a 3-h reperfusion period the response of stressed and unstressed skin was significantly different. In comparison with the unstressed rats, the pre-stressed rats had elevated control perfusion levels (63% greater than controls); loss of the initial increase in perfusion with low levels of increasing pressure; a depression (45% lower than controls) in the hyperaemic response with delayed recovery time; and a decreased (54% lower than controls) amplitude of low-frequency rhythms in skin perfusion. This would suggest the tissue needs sufficient time for recovery before normal tissue behaviour is returned.

Salcido et al. [23, 24] used hypotrichotic fuzzy rats to investigate the relationship between pressure duration and blood perfusion. Pressure was applied to the trochanter region of the rat for 6 h per day over 5 consecutive days. After 5 days of loading, ulceration was observed in the skin directly under the area covered by the indenter. Tissue damage was characterized by the presence of white cells and evidence of oedema. The blood flow measurements revealed an exponential relationship between pressure and blood flow, similar to the widely accepted relationship between pressure and time, as describe in previous chapters. At 80 mmHg blood flow was completely cut off. The authors suggested that some of the damage may be due to neutrophil-mediated activation and infiltration followed by the generation of oxygen-derived free radicals and subsequent cell necrosis. Salcido and colleagues [23] suggested that infarction was the precursor to pressure ulcer formation resulting in the formation of oxygen free radicals.

Most of the research into the aetiology of pressure ulcers has focused on damage caused by ischaemia and neglected the fundamental role of the ischaemia–reperfusion (I-R) mechanism in ulcer formation. I-R injury has been defined as the injury, at a cellular level, resulting from the reperfusion of blood to a previous ischaemic tissue [32]. Much of the research on I-R injury has previously been focused on the heart, liver, brain and kidneys. It has been shown from such research that I-R injury is distinctly different from injury caused by ischaemia alone [33–36]. It was not until the past two decades that I-R injury was documented as an important factor in the formation of skin wounds such as pressure ulcers [23, 37–40]. There is therefore inadequate knowledge of the role of I-R injury in ulcer formation. Of the few models that investigate I-R injury in pressure sore formation, many only look at a limited number of I-R cycles and use high pressures to induce ulceration. Such loading regimens are not particularly relevant to the clinical situation.

At a cellular level, tissue metabolism may be reduced after significant ischaemic periods to preserve function. However, this inherent protective mechanism can steer the tissue towards a cascade of detrimental effects as the blood supply is restored [37, 38]. The sudden decrease in oxygen tension within the extracellular matrix and the cells themselves results in the activation of control mechanisms to maintain steady state. This leads to the slowing down or ceasing of ATP generation. A major consequence of a decrease in ATP concentration is the down-regulation of various energy-requiring processes such as protein synthesis and ion pumps. Such effects have been reported to occur as early as 5 min after ischaemia [41]. With the restoration of the blood supply during reperfusion, oxygen-derived free radicals are formed in amounts that exceed the capacity of natural free-radical scavenging mechanisms. Under oxidative stress, free-radical scavengers are decreased and this attenuates the problem. Neutrophils that have migrated into damaged areas are also a source of oxygen-derived free radicals. Sundin et al. [22] therefore proposed three concepts for the underlying mechanism of pressure ulcer formation: ischaemic, neurotrophic and metabolic. When present in excess, oxygen-derived free radicals can damage the endothelium of blood vessels, resulting in an accumulation of platelets and granulocytes. Decreasing blood flow and the resulting thrombosis can lead to tissue necrosis.

There have been only a handful of studies investigating the effects of I-R injury on skin ulceration. The most clinically relevant study was carried out by Peirce et al. [39]. The authors developed and characterized an animal model for a reproducible investigation of I-R injury. Clinically relevant pressures (50 mmHg), equivalent to those found at the trochanter–mattress interface [43, 44] were applied cyclically following loading and unloading patterns measured in hospitals as a result of scheduled turning regimens. During the procedure, the animal was not anaesthetized so as to further mimic the clinical setting. Pressure was applied using an implanted steel plate and an externally applied magnet (see Fig. 12.1 e).

Tissue damage was quantified by skin thickness, leucocyte extravasation, skin blood flow, $TcPO_2$ and area of necrotic tissue. From these studies it was found that the degree of tissue damage increased with the total number of I-R cycles (maximum of 10). Similarly, tissue damage was significantly increased when the duration of ischaemia was increased from 1 h 2 h or the total frequency was increased from one I-R cycle on 1 day to 10 I-R cycles per day for 5 days. It was clear that the effects of ischaemia and reperfusion were more damaging than those of ischaemia alone. The application of five I-R cycles over 10 h resulted in 13% necrotic tissue, compared to 8% of necrotic tissue resulting from 10 h of ischaemia alone. Total tissue damage was clearly related to the number of cycles, the duration of ischaemia and the I-R cycle frequency. This data sheds new light on fundamental pressure-relieving protocols such as scheduled turning regimens and self-pressure relief by lifting oneself out of a wheel chair. Indeed, it appears that such practices may potentially subject the individual to premature ulcer formation through I-R injury.

In a study by Houwing et al. [44] pressures were applied to an area above the greater trochanter in a porcine model for 2 h and biopsies taken immediately on unloading and at 2 h to 2 weeks after unloading (during reperfusion). Tissue sections were evaluated histologically and damage was assessed by neutrophil infiltration and biochemical analysis for indicators of oxidative stress. No visible skin damage was observed after pressure application except for non-blanching erythema which lasted a few days. At a microscopic level, specimens taken immediately after removal of pressure showed no histopathological signs of damage. However, an increase in infiltration of the tissue with neutrophils was observed 1–2 h after removal of pressure and this increased with time up to 2 weeks. Oedema was present after 2 h but had diminished after 1 week. Notwithstanding, after 2 days of extended reperfusion, histological examination revealed damage to muscle, sweat glands and fat. At the end of the designated reperfusion phase (2 weeks) some repair to the tissue was observed with the presence of new connective tissue. At this point damage was observed in the skin directly under the pressure applicator. Damage was also evident distal to the pressure applicator, suggesting that the resulting damage was due to reperfusion rather than the pressure itself. Indeed, even after 10 h of pressure application, damage was only seen 1–2 h after pressure removal. The increase of hydrogen peroxide and decrease of antioxidants in the reperfused tissue suggests that the tissue undergoes a state of oxidative stress. This conclusion was supported by the fact that tissue damage was significantly reduced by presence of vitamin E, an antioxidant. Other animal studies have shown that the administration of free-radical scavengers improves survival and function of skin [22, 45].

Temperature is one of the least explored factors of pressure ulcer formation. There is an increase of about 10% in the metabolic rate and oxygen consumption of tissues for every 1 °C increase in temperature [46]. It has been shown by Kokate et al. [47] that a greater amount of tissue damage occurs at higher temperatures. Static pressures and temperatures (ranging from 25° to 45 °C) were applied along prone swine's backs using pressure–temperature applicators. The pressures applied (100 mmHg) stimulated pressures that can be experienced by bedridden patients. It was found that epidermal and dermal damage, determined histologically, occurred at higher temperatures (above 40°C) but no skin damage was observed at lower temperatures despite the possible presence of deep tissue damage. These results suggest a relationship between temperature and pressure in pressure ulcer formation similar to that found between pressure and time.

The only study that looked extensively at the effects of pressure combined with shear was developed by Goldstein and Sanders [17]. In this investigation the greater trochanters of swine were subjected to cyclic stresses (normal ± shear at a frequency of 1 Hz) in two studies to look at the short-term effects (10–40 min) and long-term adaptation (40 min/day over 3 weeks) using a custom-designed load applicator (indenter dimensions 10.2×7.8 mm) [48]. In the short-term study, normal forces of 1–16 N were applied with shear forces of 1–6 N in different combinations. A relationship between normal force, shear force and breakdown was obtained (Fig. 15.2).

Figure 15.2 shows the force combinations that resulted in tissue breakdown or slippage of the load applicator. It was found that at higher shear

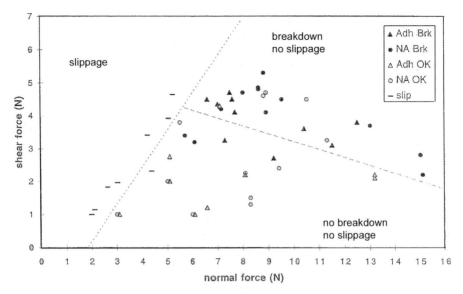

Fig. 15.2. Force combinations of shear and normal force resulting in breakdown or slippage. *Adh*, Adherent; *Brk*, breakdown; *NA*, non-adherent. Adapted from Goldstein and Sanders [17]

stresses breakdown occurred at shorter loading durations. In the long-term adaptation studies, below threshold forces (3–6 N normal ± 1–2 N shear) were applied every day for 40 min for up to 3 weeks to the greater trochanter. It was found that after this time the skin adapted without skin breakdown [17, 18].

Human Studies

All of the human pressure ulcer studies conducted to date have looked at the effects of 'safe' pressures on tissues of healthy and/or debilitated people or have examined damaged areas of patients. However, the morphological picture of human skin ulceration has not been well documented. Most histological studies have been in animal models [11, 13, 28]. Most human studies have focused on physiological changes such as blood flow and temperature measurements. Only a few studies have looked at human pressure ulcer formation using histological techniques [12, 49, 50].

Arao et al. [50] investigated the morphology of dermal papillae in skin associated with sacral ulceration post mortem. The dermal papillae provide oxygen and nutrition to the epidermis. These structures are of great importance in maintaining the integrity of the skin and protecting the body from external forces. Despite the role of the papillary dermis, there has been little research into papillary morphological changes and how the connective tissue changes during the course of ulcer formation. The studies by Arao and colleagues revealed distinct morphological differences between healthy, boundary (between healthy tissue and ulcer), and damaged areas. In healthy areas, a finger-like configuration of the dermal papillae was observed at high density and regular arrangement. In contrast, at the boundary, irregular shape and arrangement of the papillae was observed, and in the damaged area there were no papillae and collagen fibrils were destroyed. In healthy tissue the reticular fibres anchored down the epidermis to the underlying dermis. This interface is paramount in the provision of oxygen and nutrients to the epidermis. Therefore, the rupture of this layer will result in necrosis.

The most wide ranging and clinically relevant histological study was carried out by Witkowski and Parish [12]. Fifty-nine ulcers from a wide range of patient groups, with different ulcerations at varying stages of damage, were investigated in order to gain better insight into the histological changes that occur during different phases of ulceration in human tissue. It was found that early stages of ulceration were observed to occur in the upper dermis with dilation of capillaries, swelling and separation of the endothelial cells. This was followed by oedema and infiltration of the papillary dermis. Along with the vascular changes, in the early ulcer necrosis of the sweat glands and fat was evident. Epidermal necrosis was documented to occur late in the course of ulcer formation and was characterized into four types depending on the cause.

Skin water comprises 70% of the cutaneous mass [51] but varies, especially in the upper dermis, during the course of the day and in response to manipulations such as those observed in the socket of amputees [52]. It is easily exchangeable and plays an important role in fluid homeostasis in the body. It is well accepted that the resilience, elasticity and protective function of the skin is affected by water content, which in turn can be affected by age, disease and nutrition (i.e. during ageing of the skin water is generally lost in the lower dermis; diseases such as chronic venous insufficiency lead to skin oedema). Ryan [53, 54] hypothesizes that pressure at the surface of the skin could be harmful if it were to remove fluid and increase the rigidity of the epidermis.

Organ Culture Models

Only a limited number of studies have used organ cultures to investigate concepts relating to skin ulceration, and these studies have only begun within the past few years. However, such models are important when investigating the effects of mechanical stimulation without the effects of the circulation.

It has been shown by Edsberg and co-workers [14–16] using skin organ cultures that pressure has a direct effect on the mechanical properties of the skin. Foreskin tissue collected from newborn circumcisions was placed in culture and subsequently tested in a loading system designed to apply static or cyclic pressures simulating the loading situation at the human heel. Foreskin was chosen as the epidermal thickness is comparable to that of the heel and both tissues are from regions with little fat present. Changes in mechanical properties of the skin were observed with successive loading. Stress softening (Mullins effect) was observed, where a smaller load is required in the second loading compared to the first loading to produce the same amount of elongation of the skin [14]. Static loads were found to be more damaging to the skin than dynamic loading. It was suggested that the changes in the skin's mechanical properties can have serious implications with regard to the tissue's ability to sustain potentially damaging loads, especially in tissues normally associated with greater stiffness, such as skin over bone [55]. Changes in the mechanical properties may therefore contribute to the formation of ulceration. However, the same effect has not been investigated in aged or damaged skin.

The precursor to ulcer formation may be changes in the microstructure of the skin in response to the loading conditions. Testing of skin taken from ulcerations revealed a significantly lower strain at peak stress in tension than in healthy tissue [15, 16]. At a microscopic level, the changes in the ulcer tissue were found to be so severe that tensile testing did not further alter the damaged tissue microstructure. In normal healthy tissue, microscopic changes may lead to tissue adaptation; in aged or impaired tissue, however, changes may result in ulceration. Indeed, changes in the skin structure in response to pressure and shear have also been shown in other studies [14–19] depending on the type and duration of load. With the application of 170 mmHg static and 110–170 mmHg dynamic pressures, Edsberg and colleagues observed early changes in the skin microstructure 4 h after loading. The statically loaded tissue showed parallel alignment of the collagen and elastin fibrils to the loaded surface and the surface undulations were flattened out in the skin subjected to 110–170 mmHg dynamic pressure displayed an elongated capillary component that showed parallel alignment with the collagen and elastin fibrils to the loaded surface.

The lack of blood supply in Edsberg's model eliminates the artefacts associated with perfusion. Instead, the changes are solely a result of the loading conditions. The function of the skin microstructure in the development of the pressure ulcer has largely been overlooked. The elastic fibres of the dermis play an important role in facilitating tissue recovery from deformation. It has been suggested by Hagisawa et al. [56] that if blood capillaries and elastic fibres are not densely distributed in a loaded area, tissue recovery from ischaemia will be delayed, leading to increasing tissue insult. This was partially supported by morphological examination of capillary and elastin density in at-risk bony sites (sacrum and ischial tuberosity) and a non-bony site (gluteus maximus). Collagen fibres act to buffer external pressures. It was suggested by Bridel [57] that since the collagen content of the dermis decreases with age, and alters with disease and malnutrition, the figure of 32 mmHg capillary closing pressure, determined by Landis [31], will vary with age. Indeed, Crenshaw and Vistnes [58] observed that skin necrosis originates in the dermis where the collagen is located.

Sanders and Daly [59] used organ cultures to examine the adaptive response of skin to mechanical stimulus. Full-thickness skin from the pig hind limb was removed from an anaesthetized animal and immediately placed in culture. These full-thickness skin explants were then subjected to normal and shear stresses using a custom-designed closed-loop biaxial force controller [48] following a waveform found at the stump/socket interface. It was found that the skin adapted to the mechanical stress by increases in collagen fibril diameter and decrease in collagen fibril density. Although a mechanism behind this adaptation has been hypothesized [60] the actual mechanism has not been shown. Further studies are currently under way to investigate this adaptive mechanism in more detail.

Pressure and Shear

As emphasized in this book, the application of pressure is instrumental in ulcer formation. In 1841, Hunter [61] stated that 'pressure external to the body stimulates and gives signs of increased strength with increases in thickening of the skin. However, if the pressure exceeds the stimulus of thickening, then the pressure becomes an irritation'. Indeed, it is well established that there is a pressure and time threshold above which ulceration is more likely, and at levels below threshold skin adaptation has been observed using animal [18] and skin organ culture models [19]. It is generally accepted that a combination of the loading conditions results in an increase in the occurrence of ulceration [58]. Tangential shear forces act in a direction parallel to the supporting interface and occur when adjacent anatomical structures internal to the body slide across one another. These forces are coupled with normal pressures which act perpendicular to the tissue surface.

There have been several theories proposed concerning the effects of the shear on weight-bearing soft tissues. Shear forces, such as stretching and pulling on the skin, damage the perforating vessels to the skin causing thrombosis of the vessels [61, 62]. Shear forces are one of the most dangerous problems affecting semi-recumbent patients or those in chairs, or whenever tissue is being slid along the surface of a bed such as when patients are being lifted up or when the head of the bed is lifted (Fowler's position) [63, 64]. Shear forces are inevitable in the presence of normal pressures. However, it has been claimed that it is practically impossible to confidently measure the forces involved in pressure ulcer formation. It is especially difficult to measure shearing of the skin [65]. Although the role of shear in the formation of pressure ulcers is still unclear, its importance cannot be underestimated. One theory is that shear stress causes a decrease in fibrinolytic activity, which is believed to be associated with tissue necrosis [58, 66].

Bader et al. [66] investigated the effects of shear force on healthy skin of the volar aspect of the forearm. Skin was stretched between two points, and tissue vasculature and blood flow was monitored. It was found that there was an increase in the number of vertical and horizontal blood vessels in the skin that collapsed with increase in shear applied to the skin. Similarly, Bennett and colleagues [67, 68] and Dinsdale [29, 70] showed

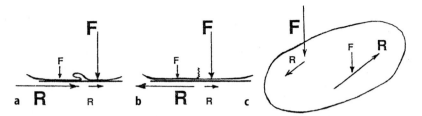

Fig. 15.3. Possible skin loading conditions corresponding to **a** the wrinkled carpet effect; **b** stretching of the skin; **c** shearing or twisting of skin. *F*, Vertical force; *R*, tangential force. Reprinted with permission from Davis [71]

that at a sufficiently high level of shear, the pressure necessary to occlude vessels was almost half that when little shear was present.

Further, Davis [71] hypothesized that particular combinations of pressure and shear are more damaging than others. Davis suggests that there are three possibilities of loading (Fig. 15.3) (1) 'wrinkled carpet effect', where one region of the skin slips towards another that is stationary; (2) 'stretching effect' where one region of the skin slips away from another; and (3) 'torsion effect' where one region of skin slips parallel to another region (Fig. 15.3). A number of studies [72–75] have shown that elevated plantar pressures play a major role in the aetiology of skin ulcerations. However, Pollard et al. [76] showed that diabetic neurotrophic ulceration occurred at sites of maximum stress under the foot. Studies focused on the effects of shear stresses on the foot [77–79] have been limited by the difficulties in the measurement of shear. These instrumental limitations often result in underestimation of maximum shear stress, since the maximum shear stress is a vector addition of medial–lateral and anterior–posterior components and instruments are limited to detecting shear forces in one of the directions only. Sanders and co-workers [52, 59, 80] have measured the interface pressures and shear stresses at the residual limb/prosthetic socket interface using custom-designed interface stress transducers.

Frictional forces can be classified as a subset of tangential shear forces as they are shear forces limited to the skin and superficial fascia. Friction normally occurs between the skin and the support surface when the skin moves against the support surface. Friction results in stripping of the epidermis leading to the formation of a superficial ulcer. Dinsdale, Waterlow and Dealey [29, 64, 81] demonstrated that the application of pressure and friction increased the susceptibility of the skin to ulceration.

With the multifactorial aetiology of pressure ulcer formation, it is clear that single interface pressure measurements may not provide a sufficient description of the consequences of these factors in human tissue. Also, due to the difficulties in measuring shear and friction in clinical situations it is difficult to use these to monitor a patient's susceptibility to skin breakdown. Although the infiltration of inflammatory cells has been widely used to determine the extent of damage, this is not possible in the clinical situation. Other tissue markers must therefore be used.

Tissue Markers

Although several different factors are well accepted as being important in the development of skin ulceration, their measurements are not trivial. This leads to problems in detecting the onset of ulceration despite the need for early detection.

Aside from pressure and shear measurements, an alternative method to assess conditions within the skin involves the non-invasive monitoring of blood flow in the skin subjected to I-R. A wide range of techniques have been proposed and examined, including thermography [82–84], laser Doppler [85, 86], radioisotope clearance [87, 88], reflectance spectroscopy [89] and the measurement of partial pressure of tissue oxygen tension (TcPO$_2$) [90–92]. The effectiveness of these measurements is variable; however, TcPO$_2$ measurement has shown great potential and has proved an accurate and repeatable indicator of the metabolic status of the tissue. It has been suggested by Trott [93] that tissue oxygen measurements may be a useful technique for predicting the likely success of healing venous ulcers.

Bader et al. [94] investigated cyclic loading of sacral tissue of normal and debilitated subjects using TcPO$_2$ measurements. It was found that the TcPO$_2$ levels in all of the healthy subjects and some of the debilitated subjects showed complete recovery from the load within a short period of time. However, a significant proportion of the debilitated subjects demonstrated a delayed recovery to the cyclic loading (Fig. 15.4).

This would suggest that there are certain groups of people that are at high risk of ulceration that can be detected by measuring TcPO$_2$. Schubert et al. [95] compared tissue oxygen tension, skin blood flow and tissue perfusion in normal individuals and a patient group. It was found that occlusion of skin blood flow occurred at significantly lower external skin pressure in at-risk patient groups than in young and healthy controls.

It has been demonstrated using animal models and organ cultures that pathological changes occur in skin as a result of pressure. Even during the

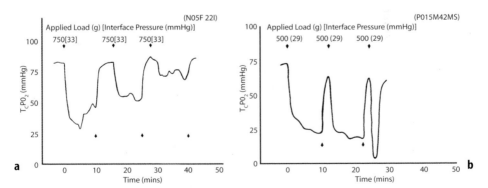

Fig. 15.4. Tissue response to repeated loading at the sacrum showing **a** normal response; **b** impaired response. Adapted from Bader [94]

early stages of ulceration, there will be significant changes in the biochemistry of the skin. These biochemical changes have been detected both invasively and non-invasively, as detailed in Chap. 8. Measurement of metabolites obtained from sweat samples is the most promising technique as it is non-invasive, sensitive, easy to use and of low cost.

Barnett and Ablarde [96] described the temperature response of healthy skin during and after short durations of sitting using video thermography. Thermography has also been used to characterize the response of damaged tissue in order to predict the occurrence of ulceration [82–84]. Damaged tissue does not exhibit the characteristic temperature increase observed in healthy skin during reperfusion. It has, therefore, been suggested that lack of temperature increase may be use to identify damaged tissue [46]. However, thermography may only be a slight improvement to visual inspection by monitoring skin colour. Sprigle et al. [97] evaluated temperature differences between areas of erythema and surrounding healthy tissue in a number of outpatients and inpatients of a hospital using perfusion monitors. It was found that 62% of erythematous sites had increased temperature; 23% had decreased temperatures and 15% were no different to surrounding healthy tissue. The increase in temperature found in the majority of damaged tissue supported the theory that erythema is caused by increased perfusion or an inflammatory response. It was suggested that sites with decreased temperatures resulted from stagnation of the blood flow and thus can indicate microcirculatory damage.

Meijer et al. [98] found that susceptible patients had substantially prolonged recovery times in terms of blood flow. This has also been observed in other studies [94]. In a study by Sanders [99], the thermal recovery time (TRT) was measured in skin after pressure with shear was applied to the skin of three healthy subjects for up to 10 min. The TRT was defined as being the time interval between cessation of the load and the attainment of either a maximum or a stabilization in the temperature. An infrared sensor was used to monitor the temperature changes. It was found that increased shear pressure and higher stress levels resulted in longer TRTs. However, the clinical relevance of this response is still to be determined. Sanada et al. [100] measured blood flow in a patient group using laser Doppler flowmetry in the skin over the iliac and sacral bony prominences. The results suggested that there may be a correlation between the degree to which blood flow is decreased and the severity of tissue damage. It has been suggested by van Marum et al. [101] that impairment of the local blood flow response may be the result of endothelial damage. Gidlof et al. [102] observed that the degree of endothelial damage was inversely related to the degree of vasodilation and reactive hyperaemia.

It has been reported by Spector et al. [103] that darkly pigmented individuals are more likely to enter long-term-care facilities with pressure ulcers and there is a disproportionate incidence of stage IV pressure ulcers in this patient group [104]. This may be the result of poor early detection. Matas et al. [105] developed a spectroscopic blanch test that was able to detect the blanch response in light and darkly pigmented skin through the measurement of total haemoglobin. This study showed that this technology may be a clinically useful tool to detect blanch response.

Wound Healing

Pressure ulcers are known to have a notoriously poor healing tendency. There is a high mortality rate associated with pressure ulcers. Despite this, the reason for the protracted healing is not well researched and thus not well understood. However, factors such as infection, impaired microcirculation, poor tissue oxygenation and decreased fibrinolytic activity are important. In order for tissue to be replaced by itself, cells must be able to proliferate and migrate. Seiler et al. [20] observed that epidermal cells at the ulcer edge exhibited a delayed start in growth, decreased growth rate and decreased area of outgrown cells. This would suggest that the cells have decreased mitotic and/or migration potentials. However, due to in vivo evidence of epidermal hyperplasia, it was hypothesized that the decreased growth observed in culture was due to a decrease in migration potential. The cause for the impairment of migration is still unknown. However, it was suggested by Seiler and colleagues [20] that the impaired vascularization in the area will result in insufficient supply of growth factors and cells needed in migration. In addition, motility-related proteins such as tubulin may have been damaged.

Factors such as malnutrition will affect the skin's mitogenic capacity. Healing of pressure ulcers has been shown to be suppressed in malnourished animals. This was due to reduction in fibroblast proliferation, capillary formation, macrophage infiltration and low level of general cell proliferation. Both Bullough and Elisa [106, 107] and Takeda et al. [108] have shown that there is a deep depression in the mitogenic activity in the dermis of the malnourished. This may be due to a shortage of carbohydrates in the epidermal cells. A decrease in glucose that was noted in malnourished subjects could also account for the decrease in epidermal mitotic rate.

Langerhans cells play an important role in the immune defence of the skin. It was observed by Kohn et al. [109] that there was a lower percentage of Langerhans cells in the epidermis of patients with pressure ulcers than in a control population. It was found that there was an absence of dendrites in 30–50% of Langerhans cells in patients with ulceration, in both the damaged area and in healthy tissue. In healthy individuals (young and old), only 13% of the cells were without dendrites. In addition, the percentage of Langerhans cells present in individuals with ulcerations was found to be significantly lower in both the damaged area and in healthy tissue than in tissue taken from healthy individuals. The results suggest a depressed immunity in the epidermis which, in addition to other factors, may contribute to difficulties in healing pressure ulcers.

Future Perspectives

Due to the multifactorial nature of the aetiology of skin ulcers it is important to be able to isolate the effects of different factors from complications that are found in the clinical setting. Cell-culture models and tissue-engineered models allow for this. Muscle models have already been developed and used, as detailed in Chap. 14, to determine the direct effects of pressure on myoblasts. However, this has not yet been done for skin. The development of tissue-engineered skin would be useful to study the effects of pressure on the skin alone or in conjunction with muscle models.

References

1. Rushmer RF, Buettner KJ, Short JM, Odland GF (1966) The skin. Science 154(747):343–348
2. Kenedi RM, Gibson T, Evans JH, Barbenel JC (1975) Tissue mechanics. Phys Med Biol 20(3):699–717
3. Lanir Y (1981) The fibrous structure of the skin and its relation to the mechanical behaviour. In: Marks R, Payne PA (eds) Bioengineering and the skin. MTP Press, Lancaster
4. Weston T(1990) Atlas of anatomy. Marshall Cavendish
5. Odland GF (1991) Structure of the skin. In: Goldsmith LA (ed) Physiology, biochemistry, and molecular biology of the skin. Oxford University Press, New York
6. Pasyk KA, Thomas SV, Hassett CA, Cherry GW, Faller R (1989) Regional differences in capillary density of the normal human dermis. Plast Reconstr Surg 83(6):939–945; discussion 946–947
7. Witkowski JA, Parish LC (2000) The decubitus ulcer: skin failure and destructive behavior. Int J Dermatol 39(12):894–896
8. Banwell P, Withey S, Holten I (1998) The use of negative pressure to promote healing. Br J Plast Surg 51(1):79
9. Goode PS, Allman RM (1989) The prevention and management of pressure ulcers. Med Clin North Am 73(6):1511–1524
10. Lowthian PT (1995) An investigation of the uncurling forces of indwelling catheters. Br J Nurs 4(6):328, 330–334
11. Willms-Kretschmer K, Majno G (1969) Ischemia of the skin. Electron microscopic study of vascular injury. Am J Pathol 54(3):327–353
12. Witkowski JA, Parish LC (1982) Histopathology of the decubitus ulcer. J Am Acad Dermatol 6(6):1014–1021
13. Daniel RK, Priest DL, Wheatley DC (1981) Etiologic factors in pressure sores: an experimental model. Arch Phys Med Rehabil 62(10):492–498
14. Edsberg LE, Mates RE, Baier RE, Lauren M (1999) Mechanical characteristics of human skin subjected to static versus cyclic normal pressures. J Rehabil Res Dev 36(2):133–141
15. Edsberg LE, Cutway R, Anain S, Natiella JR (2000) Microstructural and mechanical characterization of human tissue at and adjacent to pressure ulcers. J Rehabil Res Dev 37(4):463–471

16. Edsberg LE, Natiella JR, Baier RE, Earle J (2001) Microstructural characteristics of human skin subjected to static versus cyclic pressures. J Rehabil Res Dev 38(5):477–486
17. Goldstein B, Sanders J (1998) Skin response to repetitive mechanical stress: a new experimental model in pig. Arch Phys Med Rehabil 79(3):265–272
18. Sanders JE, Goldstein BS (2001) Collagen fibril diameters increase and fibril densities decrease in skin subjected to repetitive compressive and and shear stresses. J Biomech 34(12):1581–1587
19. Sanders JE, Mitchell SB, Wang YN, Wu K (2002) An explant model for the investigation of skin adaptation to mechanical stress. IEEE Trans Biomed Eng 49(12 Pt 2):1626–1631
20. Seiler WO, Stahelin HB, Zolliker R, Kallenberger A, Luscher NJ (1989) Impaired migration of epidermal cells from decubitus ulcers in cell cultures. A cause of protracted wound healing? Am J Clin Pathol 92(4):430–434
21. Groth KE (1942) Clinical observations and experimental studies of the pathogenesis of decubitus ulcers. Acta Chir Scand Suppl 76:1–209
22. Sundin BM, Hussein MA, Glasofer S, El-Falaky MH, Abdel-Aleem SM, Sachse RE, Klitzman B (2000) The role of allopurinol and deferoxamine in preventing pressure ulcers in pigs. Plast Reconstr Surg 105(4):1408–1421
23. Salcido R, Donofrio JC, Fisher SB, LeGrand EK, Dickey K, Carney JM, Schosser R, Liang R (1994) Histopathology of pressure ulcers as a result of sequential computer-controlled pressure sessions in a fuzzy rat model. Adv Wound Care 7(5):23–24, 26, 28 passim
24. Salcido R, Fisher SB, Donofrio JC, Bieschke M, Knapp C, Liang R, LeGrand EK, Carney JM (1995) An animal model and computer-controlled surface pressure delivery system for the production of pressure ulcers. J Rehabil Res Dev 32(2):149–161
25. Herrman EC, Knapp CF, Donofrio JC, Salcido R (1999) Skin perfusion responses to surface pressure-induced ischemia: implication for the developing pressure ulcer. J Rehabil Res Dev 36(2):109–120
26. Meyer W, Schwarz R, Neurand K (1978) The skin of domestic mammals as a model for the human skin, with special reference to the domestic pig. Curr Probl Dermatol 7:39–52
27. Lavker RM, Dong G, Zheng PS, Murphy GF (1991) Hairless micropig skin. A novel model for studies of cutaneous biology. Am J Pathol 138(3):687–697
28. Kosiak M (1959) Etiology and pathology of ischemic ulcers. Arch Phys Med Rehabil 40:62–69
29. Dinsdale SM (1974) Decubitus ulcers: role of pressure and friction in causation. Arch Phys Med Rehabil 55(4):147–152
30. Nola GT, Vistnes LM (1980) Differential response of skin and muscle in the experimental production of pressure sores. Plast Reconstr Surg 66(5):728–733
31. Landis EM (1930) Microinjection studies of capillary blood pressure in human skin. Heart 15:209–228
32. Pretto EA Jr (1991) Reperfusion injury of the liver. Transplant Proc 23(3):1912–1914
33. Wolfson RG, Millar CG, Neild GH (1994) Ischemia and reperfusion injury in the kidney: current status and future direction. Nephrol Dial Transplant 9:1529–1533
34. Kurokawa T, Nonami T, Harada A, Nakao A, Takagi H (1996) Mechanism and prevention of ischemia-reperfusion injury of the liver. Semin Surg Oncol 12(3):179–182

35. Harris AG, Skalak TC (1996) Effects of leukocyte capillary plugging in skeletal muscle ischemia-reperfusion injury. Am J Physiol 271(6 Pt 2):H2653–H2660

36. Quinones-Baldrich WJ, Caswell D (1991) Reperfusion injury. Crit Care Nurs Clin North Am 3(3):525–534

37. McCord JM (1985) Oxygen-derived free radicals in postischemic tissue injury. N Engl J Med 312(3):159–163

38. McCord JM (1987) Oxygen-derived radicals: a link between reperfusion injury and inflammation. Fed Proc 46(7):2402–2406

39. Peirce SM, Skalak TC, Rodeheaver GT (2000) Ischemia-reperfusion injury in chronic pressure ulcer formation: a skin model in the rat. Wound Repair Regen 8(1):68–76

40. Angel MF, Ramasastry SS, Swartz WM, Basford RE, Futrell JW (1987) The causes of skin ulcerations associated with venous insufficiency: a unifying hypothesis. Plast Reconstr Surg 79(2):289–297

41. Osorino AR, Berezesky IK, Mergner MJ, Trump BF (1980) Mitochondrial membrane fusions in experimental myocardial infarction. Fed Proc Fed Am Soc Exp Biol 39:634–642

42. Ratliff C, Donovan A, Schuch J (1998) Hospital replacement mattresses: do they stand the test of time? 30th Annual Wound Ostomy and Continence Conference, Salt Lake City, Utah

43. Whittemore R (1998) Pressure-reduction support surfaces: a review of the literature. J Wound Ostomy Continence Nurs 25(1):6–25

44. Houwing R, Overgoor M, Kon M, Jansen G, van Asbeck BS, Haalboom JR (2000) Pressure-induced skin lesions in pigs: reperfusion injury and the effects of vitamin E. J Wound Care 9(1):36–40

45. Cetinkale O, Bilgic L, Bolayirli M, Sengul R, Ayan F, Burcak G (1998) Involvement of neutrophils in ischemia-reperfusion injury of inguinal island skin flaps in rats. Plast Reconstr Surg 102(1):153–160

46. Mahanty SD, Roemer RB (1979) Thermal response of skin to application of localized pressure. Arch Phys Med Rehabil 60(12):584–590

47. Kokate JY, Leland KJ, Held AM, Hansen GL, Kveen GL, Johnson BA, Wilke MS, Sparrow EM, Iaizzo PA (1995) Temperature-modulated pressure ulcers: a porcine model. Arch Phys Med Rehabil 76(7):666–673

48. Sanders JE, Garbini JL, Leschen JM, Allen MS, Jorgensen JE (1997) A bidirectional load applicator for the investigation of skin response to mechanical stress. IEEE Trans Biomed Eng 44(4):290–296

49. Barnett SE (1987) Histology of the human pressure sore. CARE Science, Practice 5:13–18

50. Arao H, Obata M, Shimada T, Hagisawa S (1998) Morphological characteristics of the dermal papillae in the development of pressure sores. J Tissue Viability 8(3):17–23

51. Gniadecka M (2000) Studies on cutaneous water distribution and structure. Forum for Nordic Dermato-Venereology 5(2a Suppl 1):1–24

52. Sanders JE, Zachariah SG, Baker AB, Greve JM, Clinton C (2000) Effects of changes in cadence, prosthetic componentry, and time on interface pressures and shear stresses of three trans-tibial amputees. Clin Biomech (Bristol, Avon) 15(9):684–694

53. Hu D, Phan TT, Cherry GW, Ryan TJ (1998) Dermal oedema assessed by high frequency ultrasound in venous leg ulcers. Br J Dermatol 138(5):815–820

54. Ryan TJ, Thoolen M, Yang YH (2001) The effect of mechanical forces (vibration or external compression) on the dermal water content of the upper dermis and epidermis, assessed by high frequency ultrasound. J Tissue Viability 11(3):97–101

55. Sangeorzan BJ, Harrington RM, Wyss CR, Czerniecki JM, Matsen FA, 3rd (1989) Circulatory and mechanical response of skin to loading. J Orthop Res 7(3):425–431

56. Hagisawa S, Shimada T, Arao H, Asada Y (2001) Morphological architecture and distribution of blood capillaries and elastic fibres in the human skin. J Tissue Viability 11(2):59–63

57. Bridel J (1993) The aetiology of pressure sores. J Wound Care 2(4):230–238

58. Crenshaw RP, Vistnes LM (1989) A decade of pressure sore research: 1977–1987. J Rehabil Res Dev 26(1):63–74

59. Sanders JE, Daly CH (1993) Normal and shear stresses on a residual limb in a prosthetic socket during ambulation: comparison of finite element results with experimental measurements. J Rehabil Res Dev 30(2):191–204

60. Wang YN, Sanders JE (2003) How does skin adapt to repetitive stress to become load tolerant? Med Hypothesis 61(1):29–35

61. Hunter JA, McVittie E, Comaish JS (1974) Light and electron microscopic studies of physical injury to the skin. II. Friction. Br J Dermatol 90(5):491–499

62. Reichel SM (1958) Shearing force as a factor in decubitus ulcers in paraplegics. JAMA 166:762–768

63. Versluysen M (1986) How elderly with femoral fractures develop pressure sores in hospital. Br Med J 292:1311–1313

64. Waterlow J (1988) Tissue viability. Prevention is cheaper than cure. Nurs Times 84(25):69–70

65. Lowthian P (1997) Notes on the pathogenesis of serious pressure sores. Br J Nurs 6(16):907–912

66. Bader DL, Barnhill RL, Ryan TJ (1986) Effect of externally applied skin surface forces on tissue vasculature. Arch Phys Med Rehabil 67(11):807–811

67. Bennett L, Kavner D, Lee BK, Trainor FA (1979) Shear vs pressure as causative factors in skin blood flow occlusion. Arch Phys Med Rehabil 60(7):309–314

68. Bennett L, Lee BY (1988) Vertical shear existence in animal pressure threshold experiments. Decubitus 1(1):18–24

69. Hunter J (1941) The blood, inflammation and gunshot wounds. In: The complete works of John Hunter (ed JF Palmer). Haswell Barrington and Haswell, Philadelphia

70. Dinsdale SM (1973) Decubitus ulcers in swine: light and electron microscopy study of pathogenesis. Arch Phys Med Rehabil 54(2):51–56 passim

71. Davis BL (1993) Foot ulceration: hypotheses concerning shear and vertical forces acting on adjacent regions of skin. Med Hypotheses 40(1):44–47

72. Cavanagh PR, Ulbrecht JS (1991) Biomechanics of the diabetic foot: a quantitative approach to the assessment of neuropathy, deformity and plantar pressure. In: Jahss MH Disorders of the foot and ankle. Saunders, Philadelphia

73. Ctercteko GC, Dhanendran M, Hutton WC, Le Quesne LP (1981) Vertical forces acting on the feet of diabetic patients with neuropathic ulceration. Br J Surg 68(9):608–614

74. Sims DS, Jr., Cavanagh PR, Ulbrecht JS (1988) Risk factors in the diabetic foot. Recognition and management. Phys Ther 68(12):1887–1902

75. Stokes IA, Faris IB, Hutton WC (1975) The neuropathic ulcer and loads on the foot in diabetic patients. Acta Orthop Scand 46(5):839–847
76. Pollard JP, Le Quesne LP, Tappin JW (1983) Forces under the foot. J Biomed Eng 5(1):37–40
77. Pollard JP, Le Quesne LP (1983) Method of healing diabetic forefoot ulcers. Br Med J (Clin Res Ed) 286(6363):436–437
78. Tappin JW, Pollard JP, Becket EA (1980) Method of measuring shearing forces in the sole of the foot. Clin Physics Physiol Meas 1(1):83–85
79. Tappin JW, Robertson KP (1991) Study of the relative timing of shear forces on the sole of the forefoot during walking. J Biomed Eng 13(1):39–42
80. Sanders JE, Lam D, Dralle AJ, Okumura R (1997) Interface pressures and shear stresses at thirteen socket sites on two persons with transtibial amputation. J Rehabil Res Dev 34(1):19–43
81. Dealey C (1997) Managing pressure sore prevention. Mark Allen, Salisbury
82. Bergtholdt HT, Brand PW (1975) Thermography: an aid in the management of insensitive feet and stumps. Arch Phys Med Rehabil 56(5):205–209
83. Newman P, Davis NH (1981) Thermography as a predictor of sacral pressure sores. Age Ageing 10(1):14–18
84. Benbow SJ, Chan AW, Bowsher DR, Williams G, Macfarlane IA (1994) The prediction of diabetic neuropathic plantar foot ulceration by liquid-crystal contact thermography. Diabetes Care 17(8):835–839
85. Cobb J, Claremont D (2001) An in-shoe laser Doppler sensor for assessing plantar blood flow in the diabetic foot. Med Eng Phys 23(6):417–425
86. Mayrovitz HN, Sims N, Taylor MC (2002) Sacral skin blood perfusion: a factor in pressure ulcers? Ostomy Wound Manage. 48(6):34–42
87. Bennett L, Kavner D, Lee BY, Trainor FS, Lewis JM (1984) Skin stress and blood flow in sitting paraplegic patients. Arch Phys Med Rehabil 65(4):186–190
88. Sorensen JL, Hauge EN, Wroblewski H, Biering-Sorensen F (1994) Cutaneous and subcutaneous blood flow rates in paraplegic humans investigated by 133xenon wash-out. Methodological considerations. Clin Physiol 14(3):281–289
89. Hagisawa S, Ferguson-Pell M, Cardi M, Miller SD (1994) Assessment of skin blood content and oxygenation in spinal cord injured subjects during reactive hyperemia. J Rehabil Res Dev 31(1):1–14
90. Newson TP, Rolfe P (1982) Skin surface PO2 and blood flow measurements over the ischial tuberosity. Arch Phys Med Rehabil 63(11):553–556
91. Bader DL, Gant CA (1988) Changes in transcutaneous oxygen tension as a result of prolonged pressures at the sacrum. Clin Phys Physiol Meas 9(1):33–40
92. Knight SL, Taylor RP, Polliack AA, Bader DL (2001) Establishing predictive indicators for the status of loaded soft tissues. J Appl Physiol 90(6):2231–2237
93. Trott A (1992) Chronic skin ulcers. Emerg Med Clin North Am 10(4):823–845
94. Bader DL (1990) The recovery characteristics of soft tissues following repeated loading. J Rehabil Res Dev 27(2):141–150
95. Schubert V (2000) The influence of local heating on skin microcirculation in pressure ulcers, monitored by a combined laser Doppler and transcutaneous oxygen tension probe. Clin Physiol 20(6):413–421
96. Barnett RI, Ablarde JA (1995) Skin vascular reaction to short durations of normal seating. Arch Phys Med Rehabil 76(6):533–540

97. Sprigle S, Linden M, McKenna D, Davis K, Riordan B (2001) Clinical skin temperature measurement to predict incipient pressure ulcers. Adv Skin Wound Care 14(3):133–137

98. Meijer JH, Germs PH, Schneider H, Ribbe MW (1994) Susceptibility to decubitus ulcer formation. Arch Phys Med Rehabil 75(3):318–323

99. Sanders JE (2000) Thermal response of skin to cyclic pressure and pressure with shear: a technical note. J Rehabil Res Dev 37(5):511–515

100. Sanada H, Nagakawa T, Yamamoto M, Higashidani K, Tsuru H, Sugama J (1997) The role of skin blood flow in pressure ulcer development during surgery. Adv Wound Care 10(6):29–34

101. van Marum RJ, Meijer JH, Ribbe MW (2002) The relationship between pressure ulcers and skin blood flow response after a local cold provocation. Arch Phys Med Rehabil 83(1):40–43

102. Gidlof A, Lewis DH, Hammersen F (1988) The effect of prolonged total ischemia on the ultrastructure of human skeletal muscle capillaries. A morphometric analysis. Int J Microcirc Clin Exp 7(1):67–86

103. Spector WD, Kapp MC, Tucker RJ, Sternberg J (1988) Factors associated with presence of decubitus ulcers at admission to nursing homes. Gerontologist 28(6):830–834

104. Meehan M (1994) National pressure ulcer prevalence survey. Adv Wound Care 7(3):27–30, 34, 36–38

105. Matas A, Sowa MG, Taylor V, Taylor G, Schattka BJ, Mantsch HH (2001) Eliminating the issue of skin color in assessment of the blanch response. Adv Skin Wound Care 14(4):180–188

106. Bullough WS (1949) The relation between the epidermal mitotic activity and the blood-sugar level in the adult male mouse. J Exp Biol 26:83–99

107. Bullough WS, Elisa EA (1950) The effects of graded series of restricted diets on epidermal mitotic activity in the mouse. Br J Cancer 4:321–328

108. Takeda T, Koyama T, Izawa Y, Makita T, Nakamura N (1992) Effects of malnutrition on development of experimental pressure sores. J Dermatol 19(10):602–609

109. Kohn D, Kohn S (1993) Langerhans' cells of elderly patients with decubital ulcers. J Dermatol 20(7):413–417

In Vitro Muscle Model Studies

16

Debby Gawlitta, Carlijn Bouten

Introduction

Studies of soft tissues under mechanical loading have shown that skeletal muscle tissue is highly susceptible to sustained compression, eventually leading to tissue breakdown in the form of deep pressure ulcers [1, 2]. This breakdown starts at the cellular level with disintegration of contractile proteins and damage to the cell membrane and nucleus, followed by inflammatory reactions.

Although it is clear that both the duration and magnitude of compression affect muscle cell damage, the aetiological pathways whereby tissue compression leads to cell damage are not completely understood. To date, theories have mainly focussed on the impairment of metabolite and oxygen transport through the tissue [2–4], whereas the direct damaging effects of cell deformation due to compressive straining have only recently been identified as a cause of deep pressure ulcer development [5]. Most probably the aetiology is multifactorial in nature and both processes play a role. Tissue compression may (partially) occlude blood vessels and the smaller capillaries, which then no longer provide enough oxygen to the tissue, resulting in local ischaemia. Due to the impaired tissue perfusion, transport of nutrients and waste products to and from the metabolically active muscle cells is affected, while closure of the lymphatic system may result in additional transport problems, as waste products, excess fluids and proteins are no longer properly removed from the tissue. The restoration of transport during tissue *re*perfusion can be extremely harmful because of reactive oxygen species accumulating in the tissue upon load removal. Cell deformation, on the other hand, triggers a variety of effects such as altered membrane stresses, volume changes and cytoskeletal reorganisation, which may be involved in early cell damage. It has been shown that the response of muscle cells to deformation during tensile or shear straining is crucial to cellular degeneration or adaptation [6, 7], and a comparable response might be expected for compressive straining.

As it is impossible to study the effects of reduced transport and cell deformation independently of each other and other predisposing factors in human studies, these aspects should be studied using model systems. Ideally, a hierarchy of model systems ranging from single-cell in-vitro models to animal models (Chap. 12) and human studies should provide information about the relative contribution of, for example, cell deformation, local ischaemia, and reperfusion in the aetiology of pressure ulcers.

This chapter reviews the use of in-vitro models of muscle cells and muscle tissue to study the aetiology of deep pressure ulcers. In general, in-vitro models offer better experimental control and fewer ethical considerations than in-vivo (animal) studies. Literally, 'in vitro' means 'in glass' and these model systems are defined as cells or tissues cultured in the laboratory under artificial conditions, outside the human body. One of the benefits of in-vitro cell culture is the fact that the same cell clone or cell line can be used in different studies and in different laboratories to improve reproducibility of results. Moreover, the same cell line can be used when creating muscle models using the concept of tissue engineering.

Skeletal Muscle Cell and Tissue Culture

Skeletal muscle tissue is a highly differentiated, well-organised, anisotropic tissue that produces force by contraction. During myogenesis muscle precursor cells, or myoblasts, fuse into parallel aligned arrays of multinucleated myotubes [8, 9]. The mechanisms responsible for producing this orderly structure are poorly understood but require myoblasts to come together, orient and align prior to fusion. After fusion, the myotubes assemble their contractile proteins and become mature contractile myofibres, which eventually become organised in parallel bundles. This organisation is essential for effective muscle contraction and force transmission.

Thus, like many cell types, skeletal muscle cells cannot be conceived as isolated structures. They are well organised and surrounded by extracellular matrix, to form a functional tissue. Therefore, it is likely that compression-induced muscle cell damage is influenced by cell–cell interactions, cell–matrix interactions, and three-dimensional (3D) tissue configuration. To study the relationship between muscle (cell) compression and cell damage a series of complementary in-vitro model systems is adopted, ranging from single cells to monolayers and three-dimensional tissue-engineered muscle analogues under compressive strain. This chapter describes model systems all employing the C2C12 mouse skeletal muscle cell line. Single-cell studies are used to quantify cell deformation and resulting cell damage, whereas 3D (engineered) constructs are used to introduce more complexity and reality to the model. Although it is currently not possible to create a functional capillary network in tissue-engineered models, the presented model systems offer the potential to study the influence of conditions such as ischaemia by strictly controlling the culture conditions (e.g. oxygen supply and diffusion).

Single-Cell Studies

Comprehensive studies on the compression of individual C2C12 myoblasts were performed by Peeters et al [10–13]. Although such a single-cell model is very distinct from a patient at risk of developing pressure ulcers, it can provide fundamental understanding of the response of the smallest units in the human body to compressive loading. Through a hierarchical approach, the cellular response may assist in explaining the tissue response to compressive loading [14].

The single-cell studies were performed using a specially designed loading device that enabled monitoring of the morphological and biomechanical response of the cells to compression [10]. The device (Fig. 16.1) consisted of an incubation chamber (37°C and 5% CO_2) for the cells and a set of micromanipulators and piezo-actuators for very precise compression of individual cells with a glass indenter. This indenter, with a diameter of 60 μm, was built-in and connected to a force transducer, capable of measuring forces with 10 nN resolution. The C2C12 cells were grown on a cover glass at the bottom of the incubation chamber. The complete device was then mounted onto the stage of an inverted confocal microscope for real-time monitoring of cell morphology and viability. Viability monitoring was facilitated by the use of a fluorescent dye (propidium iodide, see below) to indicate cell death with high spatio-temporal resolution. The cells were seeded at a low density and could therefore be individually loaded in unconfined compression until bursting. Experiments with this device showed that stepwise compression (0.5 μm per step) resulted in structural membrane changes, starting at 50% axial compression or strain, while cell deformation perpendicular to the axis of compression was anisotropic and mainly determined by the organisation of the actin cytoskeleton within the cell [11]. When studied in more detail [12], the cells clearly started to form membrane bulges at about 60%

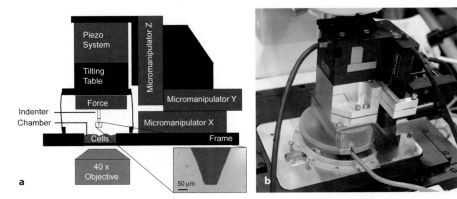

Fig. 16.1. a Schematic representation showing the individual components of the single-cell loading device; the inset shows the glass indenter. b Photograph of the complete device on the stage of a confocal microscope. Adapted from Peeters et al. [10]

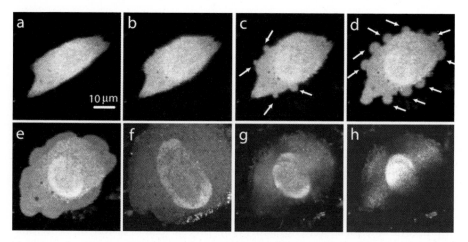

Fig. 16.2 a–h. Membrane bulging (*arrows*) during compressive straining (up to ~90%) of C2C12 mouse skeletal myoblasts. a–f The same cell during downward compression; g, h the indenter moves up again. Adapted from Peeters et al. [11]

compression (see Fig. 16.2). This bulging continued until the cell membrane burst at ±72% compressive strain, as evidenced by a dip in the force measurement and a subsequent influx of propidium iodide into the cell plasma. In a subsequent experiment C2C12 cells were cyclically loaded until cell death was observed [13]. In these dynamic experiments, a predefined strain magnitude was imposed on the cells for 10 cycles with a frequency of 10^{-1}, $10^{-0.5}$, 10^{0}, $10^{0.5}$, and 10^{1} Hz before repeating the experiment with an increased strain magnitude until the cell burst. Again, membrane bulging was observed, but now at strains exceeding 40%. Initially, bulging seemed reversible and tended to disappear within seconds after removing the load. However, with increased strain magnitude, bulging was irreversible and the size of the bulges increased until cell death was indicated by a marked entry of propidium iodide into the cell (at ~54%). With respect to the frequency of loading, cell membranes tended to rupture at high frequencies rather than at lower frequencies.

Muscle Tissue Constructs

The single-cell studies by Peeters et al. yield considerable information on the response of individual myoblasts to compression. In a tissue, however, these cells are surrounded by other cells and extracellular matrix. In this configuration, compressive tissue loads are transferred to the individual cells in a different way, resulting in altered relationships between compressive straining and cell damage or death. In addition, in muscle tissue the myoblasts have fused to form multinucleated myotubes, which may react differently to compressive straining.

Bouten et al. [5] studied compression of C2C12 cells fused into myoblasts and seeded in a 3% low gelling temperature agarose gel. For this purpose myoblasts were allowed to grow for 4 days in agarose constructs supplemented with growth medium (as compared to an attachment and migration period of 16 h) and subsequently shifted to differentiation medium for another 8 days. The resulting cell population in the agarose gel then consisted of three subpopulations: 50% spherical myoblasts, 35% spherical myotubes, and 15% elongated rod-shaped myotubes. Only deformations of the first two subpopulations were considered when studying the effects of construct compression on cell damage. Using a specially designed compression rig mounted to the stage of a confocal microscope, the agarose constructs were loaded in unconfined compression up to 40% compressive strain. Cell deformation was monitored in time using the viable fluorescent cytoplasm probe Calcein-AM and the change in cell diameters parallel to the axis of compression. Overall, the cells changed from their spherical appearance to a more "UFO-shaped" morphology during compression. Cell strains in the direction of compression were similar to the applied construct strain. On a smaller scale, the myoblast subpopulation showed membrane buckling at 30–40% strain, while myotubes already showed signs of buckling at 20% strain. In a second experiment the influence of prolonged compressive straining (0–24 h, at 0, 10, and 20% strain) was studied. Cell/agarose constructs were compressed in a specially designed cell straining device inside a testing machine (Dartec, UK), capable of simultaneous compression of up to 24 constructs at different strains (Fig. 16.3). Cell damage was quantified from histology to identify membrane damage and/or nuclear condensation and fragmentation. At 10% strain a significant increase in cell damage was observed after 2 h of compression, whereas cell damage remained fairly constant after 4 h of compression. At 20% strain the percentage cell damage increased from about 40% at 1 h to almost 100% at 24 h compression (see Fig. 16.4). In the control gel the percentage of damaged cells remained constant throughout the entire loading period. It should be noted that the level of 20% construct strain corresponds to a compressive load of about 32 mmHg or 4.3 kPa. This level of compression has long been considered as a causal factor for pressure ulcers, since it is traditionally quoted as the capillary closing pressure. Pressures exceeding this value were assumed to result in ischaemia-induced pressure ulcers. The described experiments, however, prove that in the absence of capillaries and blood perfusion, the mere deformation of cells alone can cause considerable damage with time.

Clinically relevant compression studies using the same muscle model of cell/agarose constructs were performed by Wang et al. [16]. Again, using the Dartec loading device gross static strains of 10 and 20% were applied (for 0–12 h), corresponding to pressures of 18 and 32 mmHg, respectively, but now apoptotic (DNA nick translation) and necrotic (haematoxylin & eosin staining) cellular breakdown were discriminated. The total amount of non-viable cells at 10% compressive straining increased significantly after 4 h of straining and a maximum percentage of 54% non-viable cells was found at 12 h of straining. The DNA nick translation revealed that the major-

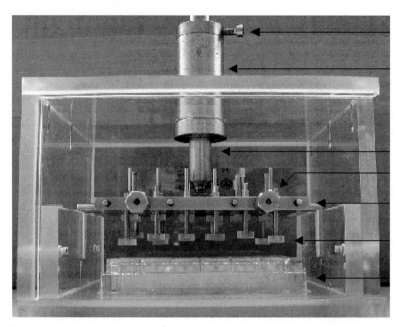

Fig. 16.3. Compressive training device used for simultaneous compression (static or dynamic) of up to 24 tissue analogues

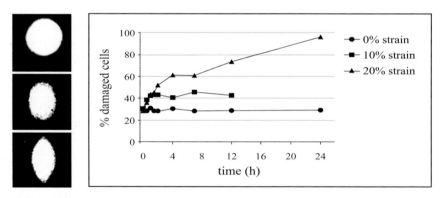

Fig. 16.4. Percentage cell damage with time at 0, 10 and 20% compressive strain. The images at *left* show gross cell deformation at 0% (*top*), 10% (*middle*), and 20% (*bottom*) strain

ity (70%) of the non-viable cells were undergoing apoptosis after 8 h and 12 h of compression.

A significantly different tendency was found for the 20% strained constructs. Here the percentage non-viable cells was already significantly higher than in unstrained controls after 0.5 h and reached a maximum value of 76% at 12 h (control 30%). Again, about 70% of these cells were undergoing apoptosis. The subpopulation of elongated myotubes seemed to be especially sensitive to compression, as all of these cells had died within 1.5 h.

Tissue-Engineered Muscle Equivalents

The work of Wang et al. and Bouten et al. was based on a parsimonious in-vitro model of C2C12 cells in agarose gel. The proportion of cells actually fusing into elongated myotubes was rather small in these constructs (15%). Furthermore, most cells remained spherical due to the lack of anchorage points in the gel. In actual skeletal muscle tissue the predominant cell population consists of elongated multinucleated myotubes.

Therefore, Breuls et al. [17] made an attempt to direct the cell morphology towards a more natural one, using a modification of the cell–gel suspension protocol proposed by Vandenburgh et al. [18]. C2C12 myoblasts were suspended in a collagen/matrigel mixture and kept in growth medium

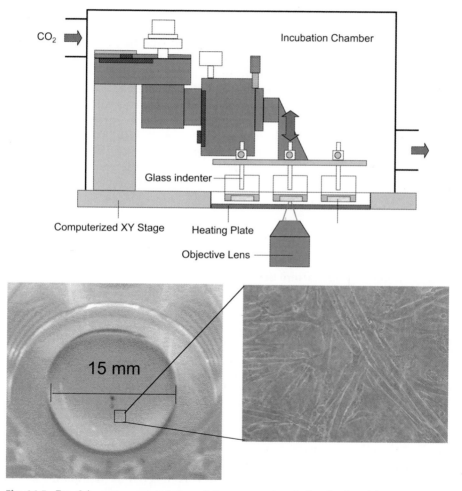

Fig. 16.5. *Top:* Schematic representation of the compression device developed by Breuls et al. [17]. *Bottom:* Engineered skeletal muscle tissue with myotubes showing in the inset

for 3 days to allow the cells to proliferate. After another 7 days in differentiation medium (2% horse serum) the constructs were used in compression experiments. These constructs were disc-shaped with a diameter of approximately 10 mm (Fig. 16.5, bottom). For the compression experiments a device was designed, containing an incubation chamber and glass indenters with a diameter of 5 mm (Fig. 16.5, top). This device was mounted onto the stage of a confocal microscope to compress the constructs, while visualising cell morphologies and damage. Four levels of strain were applied: 0, 0+, 30, or 50%, where the 0% strain group represents unstrained samples and the 0+% group represents constructs that were loaded with the tare strain of the resting indenter on the construct, but without compression. This group served to study the effect of a non-porous indenter on diffusion of oxygen and nutrients into the construct. During the compression experiments, cells inside the constructs were monitored in real time with viable fluorescent probes [19] to quantify cell viability after 0, 1, 2, 4, 6, and 8 h.

The mere application of strain alone invoked significant initial cell damage immediately after load application: ±8% in the 30% strain group and ±14% in the 50% group. At 30% strain a further increase in the percentage of cell death was observed between 2 h and 6 h, whereas at 50% strain additional cell death was found between 1 h and 4 h. After these periods the percentage of dead cells remained constant. This is in agreement with the inverse relation between amplitude and duration of tissue compression and observed tissue damage in animal studies (see reference [20] in Chap. 12). The plateau values for the percentage of damaged cells reached maximum values of just over 50% (at 30% strain) and above 80% (at 50% strain).

Clinical Implications of In-Vitro Studies

The combined results from the above studies can provide better insight into thresholds for muscle damage development in terms of magnitude and duration of applied strains. The most important observations are summarised in Table 16.1.

From the work performed by Breuls et al. it can be concluded that in compressed muscle tissue damage may start to develop immediately after load application (up to 14% at 50% strain) and continues to develop within the following hours. Considering these results traditional clinical practices, such as 2-h patient-turning regimens, need to be carefully evaluated. Nowadays patients are turned for pressure relief, but this may be very harmful for the newly loaded body side if damage occurs immediately after load application. Also, in many cases muscle tissue is loaded continuously for hours when turning is impossible, such as during operations or in intensive care patients, who may be intubated or connected to monitors.

Figure 16.6 shows the percentage of viable cells from all compression experiments described in this chapter as a function of magnitude and time

Table 16.2. Summary of the major findings of the 'in vitro' studies presented in this chapter. After [5, 10, 16, 17]

Authors	Model	Time scale compression	Main results
Peeters et al. [10]	Single myoblasts	Seconds	Stepwise strain >50% causes structural cell damage Strain >60% causes membrane bulging 72% strain: cells start to burst Dynamic straining: bulging at 40%, bursting at 54% Cells more sensitive to high frequency than low frequency
Bouten et al. [5]	Myoblasts and myotubes in agarose	1–24 h	Strain >20%: buckling of myotubes Strain >30–40%: buckling of myoblasts Increase in damage in cell after 1 h of straining
Wang et al. [16]	Myoblasts and myotubes in agarose	0.5–12 h	At 10% strain: increase in damage after 4 h compression At 20% strain: increase in damage after 0.5 h compression 60–70% of cell death due to apoptosis Myotubes more sensitive to straining than myoblasts
Breuls et al. [17]	Myoblasts and myotubes in collagen/matrigel mixture	1–8 h	At 30 and 50% strain: immediate cell damage At 30% strain: 50% damaged at 8 h At 50% strain: 80% damaged at 8 h

of compression. Clearly, the proportions of viable cells decreased with increasing strain magnitude. Furthermore, at constant strain magnitude, cell viability decreased with time of compression. It should be noted that these inverse relationships between magnitude and time of compression were related to cell deformation alone, rather than to impaired transport due to ischaemia, lymphatic occlusion, or reperfusion, which were not incorporated in the in-vitro models. The relative contribution of impaired oxygen transport to the observed cell damage, however, remains to be elucidated. So far, the effect of compression on the permeability of the tissue constructs for oxygen has not been quantified. Also, the effect of construct compression on the washout of waste products is not known. For example, in the work by Breuls et al., constructs were compressed under a 5-mm-diameter indenter and up to 50% strain, which could have limited transport

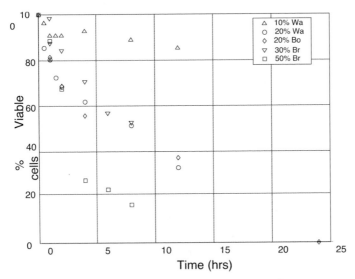

Fig. 16.6. Combined percentages of viable cells in time from Bouten et al., (*Bo* [5]) Wang et al. (*Wa* [16]), and Breuls et al. (*Br* [17]). Percentages are normalised for the percentage cell death in unstrained controls

processes. If this effect is added to the possible squeezing out of oxygen upon load application, 'ischaemia' could have influenced the observed cell damage. Nevertheless, the distribution of cell death under the indenter was homogeneous and not dependent on the distance of the cells to the edge of the indenter, as one might have expected to occur in oxygen diffusion-related damage evolution.

In patient and animal studies the observed tissue damage is generally related to the pressure measured at the skin surface (or interface pressure). This pressure, however, is not representative of the local stresses and strains inside the tissue, which are relevant for tissue breakdown [21–24]. Local strains can differ considerably from externally applied loads and global tissue deformation at the body surface, as they are dependent on tissue geometry, tissue mechanical properties and local inhomogeneities, such as bony prominences. Likewise, the (damaging) strains applied in the current in-vitro models cannot be directly translated to clinically relevant interface pressures. For this purpose computational models that link stresses and strains at the cellular level to those at the tissue (surface) level are required [25].

Several authors have made attempts to estimate the strains arising near bony prominences in skeletal muscle tissue, using computational models (see Chap. 10). In a buttock model described by Oomens et al. [21], incorporating all tissue layers covering the ischial tuberosities, the overall strain throughout the muscle layer was determined to be about 15% during sitting (80-kg male). Considering the presented in-vitro results, this strain magnitude is damaging when applied for several hours. In another study, by Linder-Ganz and Gefen [26], the pelvic region of a lying subject (60-kg male) was modelled in more detail. Here tissue strains of up to 6% were found to occur in the longissimus muscle. These strains increased to 10% when bodyweight increased to 80 kg. Reger et al. [27] monitored deep tissue deformations in the pelvic region using MR imaging. Here, tissue deformation during compression was compared between paraplegic and normal female subjects. A clear difference in total tissue deformation between the two groups illustrates the importance of the physical condition of the patient. The tissue thicknesses from bone to skin at the trochanter and ischial tuberosities, were reduced by application of surface loads up to 60 mmHg. As a result, the compressive strains in the paraplegic group were in the range of 42–67%, whereas the normal group exhibited strains between 20 and 35%. The majority of the deformation was observed in the muscle tissue. Again considering the results summarised in Fig. 16.6, these strains can cause substantial damage with time. That is, taking into account that this figure is based on measurements in a murine cell line and not on human tissue.

Obviously, apart from the duration and magnitude of tissue strains and possibly resulting transport impairments, other predisposing factors play a role in the onset of deep pressure ulcers. These may include factors such as immobility, age, malnutrition, medication, and dehydration, which affect the load-bearing capacities of the tissues, and factors like temperature and incontinence which influence the loads on the tissue. In-vitro models can contribute to the understanding of the fundamental processes underlying pressure ulcer development. The ability to control most predisposing factors independently of each other in these models can facilitate the quantification of the relative contribution of these factors to the aetiology of pressure ulcers.

Future Perspectives and Experiments

The most important advantage of studying damage development in 'in vitro' models of skeletal muscle is that the model can be very reproducible and easily controlled and manipulated. Cells can be genetically modified [18, 28], or stained to visualise the whole cell or a cellular protein of interest. For tissue engineering purposes also the ratio of tissue components (cells vs matrix) can be varied, and culture conditions can be monitored. The latter is especially relevant when studying the effects of external/risk factors on tissue damage. Hence, with respect to deep pressure ulcers, a tissue-engineered muscle model can be loaded with stress factors, such as anoxia or altered nutrient supply, via the surrounding medium and other culture conditions to simulate the influence of external risk factors on tissue viability.

In order to study the influence of such predisposing factors on the development of deep pressure ulcers, an extended model system was designed in our lab. This system consists of three key components:

1. A tissue-engineered skeletal muscle
2. A device that controls normal culture conditions, such as temperature and humidity, but that can also impose risk factors, such as compression and anoxia
3. A probe for real-time damage assessment, by monitoring expression of fluorescent markers and damage molecules that can be quantified in the culture media.

With this model system, information can be obtained on the effect of several degrees of clinically relevant compressive strains (0, 20, 40%) with or without the effects of anoxia (0% O_2) or normoxia (20% O_2) on tissue viability. For both factors, compression and anoxia, damage development in time can be monitored and quantified, from viable (fluorescent) stainings and the release of cellular proteins in the culture medium. Muscle cell-specific proteins, such as myoglobin and creatine kinase, have the potential to serve as a future marker for pressure ulcer development in patients and hence are relevant candidate markers. In addition, specific fluorescent probes can provide information about the pathways of cell death (e.g. apoptosis vs necrosis).

Extensions of this model can be employed to study the relative and combined contribution of compression, ischaemia, nutritional conditions, presence of reactive oxygen species, etc., on tissue breakdown with time and to discriminate between major and minor risk factors. This would result in stress–damage relationships as indicated in Fig. 16.7, which provides thresholds for irreversible tissue damage and hence guidelines for pressure ulcer prevention.

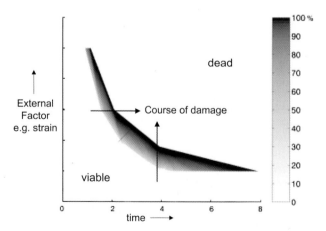

Fig. 16.7. Graph indicating the suggested response (from reversible damage to cell death) of muscle tissue to a predisposing factor for pressure ulcer development, such as strain, decreased oxygen tension or accumulation of metabolic waste products

Summary

Currently feasible in-vitro models of skeletal muscle cells and tissue assist in understanding the fundamental processes that underlie the development of pressure ulcers in muscle. In this chapter, several predisposing factors for deep pressure ulcer development are reviewed in combination with available in-vitro models. In particular, the influence of sustained cell deformation on the onset of tissue breakdown is described. The results of a series of deformation studies are summarised and demonstrate that cell deformation due to tissue compression plays a prominent role in the onset of tissue breakdown, where tissue breakdown is related to the time and magnitude of compression. The well-controllable in-vitro models have considerable potential for establishing damage thresholds in response to mechanical loading (tissue compression) with or without additional risk factors of pressure ulcer development.

References

1. Nola GT, Vistnes LM (1980) Differential response of skin and muscle in the experimental production of pressure sores. J Plast Reconstruct Surg 66:728–733
2. Daniel RK, Priest DL, Wheatley DC (1981) Etiologic factors in pressure sores: an experimental model. Arch Phys Med Rehabil 62:492–498
3. Kosiak M (1959) Etiology and pathology of ischemic ulcers. Arch Phys Med Rehabil 40:62–69
4. Peirce SM, Skalak TC, Rodeheaver GT (2000) Ischemia-reperfusion injury in chronic pressure ulcer formation: a skin model in the rat. Wound Repair Regen 8:68–76
5. Bouten CV, Knight MM, Lee DA, Bader DL (2001) Compressive deformation and damage of muscle cell subpopulations in a model system. Ann Biomed Eng 29:153–163
6. Cheng W, Li B, Kajstura J, Li P, Wolin MS, Sonnenblick EH, Hintze TH, Olivetti G, Anversa P (1995) Stretch-induced programmed myocyte cell death. J Clin Invest 96:2247–2259
7. Vandenburgh HH, Hatfaludy S, Karlisch P, Shansky J (1991) Mechanically induced alterations in cultured skeletal muscle growth. J Biomech 24 Suppl 1:91–99
8. Emerson CP Jr (1993) Embryonic signals for skeletal myogenesis: arriving at the beginning. Curr Opin Cell Biol 5:1057–1064
9. Wigmore PM, Dunglison GF (1998) The generation of fiber diversity during myogenesis. Int J Devel Biol 42:117–125
10. Peeters EA, Bouten CV, Oomens CW, Baaijens FP (2003) Monitoring the biomechanical response of individual cells under compression: a new compression device. Med Biol Eng Comput 41:498–503
11. Peeters EA, Bouten CV, Oomens CW, Bader DL, Snoeckx L, Baaijens FP (2004) Anisotropic, three-dimensional deformation of single attached cells under compression. Ann Biomed Eng 32(10):1443–1452

12. Peeters EA, Oomens CW, Bouten CV, Bader DL, Baaijens FP (2005) Load-bearing properties of single attached cells under compression. J Biomech (in press)
13. Peeters EA, Oomens CW, Bouten CV, Bader DL, Baaijens FP (2005) Viscoelastic properties of single attached C2C12 myoblasts. J Biomech Eng (IN PRess)
14. Bouten CV, Oomens CW, Baaijens FP, Bader DL (2003) The etiology of pressure ulcers: skin deep or muscle bound? Arch Phys Med Rehabil 84:616–619
15. Bouten CV, Breuls RG, Peeters EA, Oomens CW, Baaijens FP (2003) In vitro models to study compressive strain-induced muscle cell damage. Biorheology 40:383–388
16. Wang YN, Bouten CV, Lee DA, Bader DL (2004) Compression induced damage in a muscle cell model 'in vitro'. Eng Med 219 part H:1–12
17. Breuls RG, Bouten CV, Oomens CW, Baaijens FP (2003) Compression induced cell damage in engineered skeletal muscle tissue: an in-vitro model to study pressure ulcer aetiology. Ann Biomed Eng 31:1357–1364
18. Vandenburgh HH (1998) Attenuation of skeletal muscle wasting with recombinant human growth hormone secreted from a tissue-engineered bioartificial muscle. Hum Gene Ther 9:2555–2564
19. Breuls RG, Mol A, Petterson R, Oomens CW, Baaijens FP, Bouten CV (2003) Monitoring local cell viability in engineered tissues: a fast, quantitative and non-destructive approach. Tissue Eng 9:269–281
20. Reswick J, Rogers J (1976) Experiences at Rancho Los Amigos Hospital with devices and techniques to prevent pressure sores. In: Kennedy RM, Cowden JM, Scales JJ (eds) Bed sore mechanics. Macmillan, London, pp 301–310
21. Oomens CW, Bressers OF, Bosboom EM, Bouten CV, Bader DL (2003) Can loaded interface characteristics influence strain distributions in muscle adjacent to bony prominences. Comput Methods Biomech Biomed Eng 6:171–180
22. Chow C, Odell E (1978) Deformations and stresses in soft body tissues of a sitting person. J Biomech Eng 100:79–86
23. Dabnichki P, Crocombe A, Hughes S (1994) Deformation and stress analysis of supported buttock contact. Proc IME part H: J Eng Med 208:9–17
24. Todd B, Thacker J (1994) Three-dimensional computer model of the human buttocks, in vivo. J. Rehab Res Dev 31(2):111–119
25. Breuls RG, Oomens CW, Bouten CV, Bader DL, Baaijens FP (2003) A theoretical analysis of damage evolution in skeletal muscle tissue with reference to pressure ulcer development. J Biomech Eng 125:902–909
26. Linder-Ganz E, Gefen A (2004) Mechanical compression-induced pressure sores in rat hindlimb: muscle stiffness, histology, and computational models. J Appl Physiol 96:2034–2049
27. Reger SI, McGovern TF, Chung KC (1990) Biomechanics of tissue distortion and stiffness by magnetic resonance imaging. In Bader DL (ed) Pressure sores: clinical practice and scientific approach. Macmillan, London, pp 177–190
28. Vandenburgh H, Del Tatto M, Shansky J, Lemaire J, Chang A, Payumo F, Lee P, Goodyear A, Raven L (1996) Tissue-engineered skeletal muscle organoids for reversible gene therapy. Hum Gene Ther 7:2195–2200

Imaging Tissues for Pressure Ulcer Prevention

17

MARTIN FERGUSON-PELL

Introduction

Every day, clinicians determine tissue status by visual and physical assessment. These practices, although technologically simple, belie the complex range of physiological responses of the tissues that may be detected by clinical assessment. Observations made by clinicians are used to assess the integrity of tissues and their response to the mechanical, physical and chemical environment. Clinical observation, however, is limited in a number of important ways. Qualitative clinical assessment is difficult to record accurately, particularly when observations require recording of subtly different levels in tissue status or response. Different observers also often record qualitative observations differently. This often results in difficulties when working in teams or shifts, or when information is assessed over time.

Imaging often requires qualitative interpretation of the information recorded, but the image at least captures information in a way that allows multiple assessors to view the same primary dataset. However, the nature of imaging systems in healthcare settings usually requires them to be operated by clinical and technical specialists working in a dedicated setting. They are usually used for diagnosis and screening in order to detect early evidence of pathologies, or to assist in the provision of interventions, such as surgery or radiotherapy.

The potential for using imaging systems for the prevention and management of pressure ulcers is an altogether different proposition. With the prevalence of pressure ulcers in district general hospitals reported to be between 15 and 20% [1], use of specialist imaging facilities to assess wound status, or to identify particularly vulnerable patients, would create an overwhelming demand for scarce resources. Practical imaging systems to assist in pressure ulcer management must therefore be simple enough to use at the bedside. It may also be desirable for these systems to make measurements of parameters associated with the interaction of the patient with the bed or seating system, as it is here that problems with tissue integrity first occur.

The cost of managing and preventing pressure ulcers certainly could justify the use of quantitative methods for tissue risk assessment and for monitoring the healing of ulcers. At present, however, confidence in the value of these technologies is modulated by their complexity, their cost and the lack of evidence of their efficacy.

From the technology developers' perspective most of the technical requirements for instruments to provide reliable measurements of physiological or mechanical parameters can be fulfilled. However, a significant barrier to their development is the lack of sound physiological and aetiological understanding of pressure ulcer pathology, as highlighted in Chap. 1. Without a direct link to validated aetiological models, the design of effective clinical tools cannot be accomplished with confidence. For this reason many of the tools in use clinically have their origins as research instruments to measure specific physiological or mechanical parameters. They are most effectively used by clinicians, who use the information provided by these instruments to supplement their clinical skills and intuition.

Much can, however, be learnt from work to date, from technologies developed for related application areas and from the use of instruments by researchers seeking to develop an improved understanding of the pressure ulcer problem. This chapter reviews many of these technologies and the insight they can provide into pressure ulcer aetiology.

Wound Assessment

X-rays have in the past been used to assess the extent of necrotic undermining by injecting contrast media into the wound. The disadvantages of needing to use dedicated imaging services are obvious.

A very simple way to record pressure ulcer dimensions is to use photography. With the advent of digital photography and the introduction of digital patient records it is much more practical for clinicians to record the progress of wound healing and to make simple measurements of changes in wound dimensions. Of course, a major limitation is that simple photography only yields information in two dimensions and therefore measurements of wound depth are not reliable from simple photographs. The Vision Engineering Research Group (VERG; Winnipeg, Canada) has produced a simple-to-use wound measurement system (VeV MD) using digital photography that provides reliable three-dimensional information. To achieve this, the VeV MD software uses target plates placed in the field of the image to determine the camera position and orientation in relation to the wound and corrects for the distortion caused by the curvature of the lens. With these correction techniques it is possible to record the area, length, width, perimeter, depth and volume, along with the hue of different regions of the wound. Easy-to-use software enables the clinician to track changes in all the parameters over time so that the progression of the wound healing process can be monitored. Figure 17.1 shows the target plate in position along with the margins of the wound that are detected automatically by the software. Of course, in cases where the tissues are undermined this system would fail to detect the full extent of tissue damage. Ultrasound imaging offers a more comprehensive means of wound assessment in these cases.

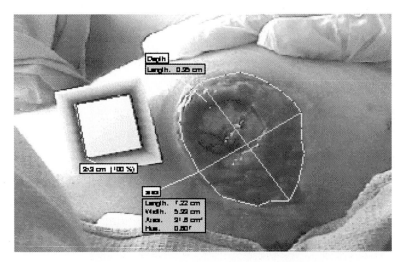

Fig. 17.1. The VeV MD system in use, showing the target plate used to calculated wound dimensions and the margins of the wound detected by the software

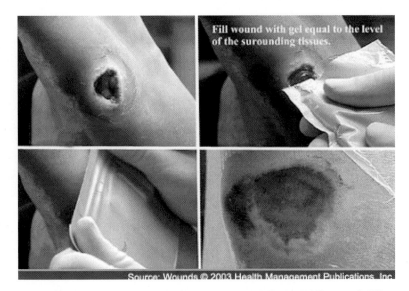

Fig. 17.2. Use of B-mode ultrasonography for wound assessment (after Wendelken et al. [2])

The use of B-mode ultrasonography to provide a non-invasive record of the extent of wound undermining has been described in detail by Wendelken et al. [2]. This approach allows accurate monitoring of wound dimensions by filling the wound with a sterile wound-mapping gel and film dressing (Hudson Diagnostic Imaging). The wound is scanned by slowly moving the probe across the wound and a series of images captured digitally. (Fig. 17.2). Measurements of the wound can then be made using the digital

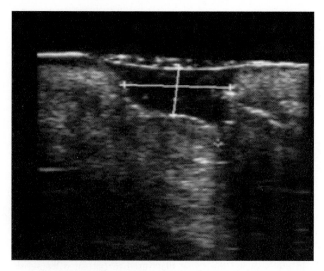

Fig. 17.3. Ultrasound image of stage IV pressure ulcer being measured using digital callipers (after Wendelken et al. [2])

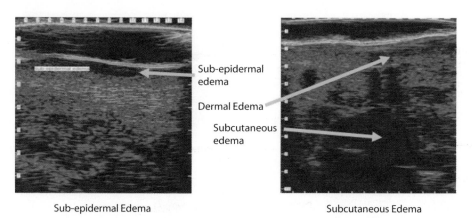

Sub-epidermal edema

Dermal Edema

Subcutaneous edema

Sub-epidermal Edema   Subcutaneous Edema

Fig. 17.4. Use of high-frequency ultrasonography to detect early pressure ulcer development (after Lyder [3])

callipers provided with the instrument's software package, as indicated in Fig. 17.3.

Lyder [3] has used higher-frequency ultrasonography (Longport Inc., Swarthmore, PA, USA) to detect more subtle changes in tissues associated with a developing pressure ulcer. Lyder claims that experienced users of the system can differentiate phases of development, including pockets of oedema, inflammatory changes and frank breakdown (Fig. 17.4). Assessment of these images is a skilful process and open to differences in interpretation.

Elastography is a non-invasive method for imaging tissues based on differences in the tissue stress–strain modulus associated with different tissue constituents and structures. Srinivasan et al. [4] have developed a technique using ultrasound that measures tissue strain and a nano-indenter which measures tissue modulus. By comparing the results from these two techniques on tissue phantoms they have demonstrated that there is an intrinsic relationship between tissue modulus and tissue strain. This offers a promising technique for future imaging of tissues where modulus changes are associated with pathology, for example the oedema associated with early pressure ulcer onset. A further development of elastographic technologies has been demonstrated by Sinkus et al. [5]. In this case, magnetic resonance imaging (MRI) is coupled with mechanical wave propagation. The tissue modulus can be inferred from the MRI data by taking a sequence of synchronised measurements at the maximum and minimum induced strains in the tissues during the application of the vibration. Further discussion of MRI applications is provided in Chaps. 12 and 18.

Although these more advanced techniques do not at present offer practical everyday tools for patient assessment they are of real value in developing a more detailed understanding of pressure ulcer aetiology. With an improved understanding of the problem, more practical imaging techniques may well be evolved.

Pressure Measurement

Numerous devices have been produced for single-point measurements, of which most successful for routine clinical measurements was the Talley-Scimedics Pressure Evaluator developed by Reswick and Rogers [6] for assessment of wheelchair cushion pressures. It comprised a thin elliptically shaped air bladder, approximately 100×80 mm, with a copper foil grid laminated to opposing surfaces of the inside of the bladder forming a switch. When the bladder was inflated the grid switches were 'open', and when sufficient pressure was applied externally to the bladder it collapsed, causing the switch to 'close'. This device had a number of technical limitations, not least its fragility and tendency to under-read when pressure was concentrated within its sensing area. However, it had the distinct advantages of low cost and ease of use, becoming widely adopted by clinicians needing a tool to measure interface pressures when assessing patients for wheelchair cushions and seating. A smaller sensor was later produced, based on similar principles, for making more localised single-point measurements; this device was thin enough to be considered suitable for measuring pressure beneath pressure garments and bandages. Its size and flexibility made it only practical to place directly on the skin prior to making interface measurements, whereas the Talley-Scimedics sensor could be positioned beneath the fully-clothed patient.

The introduction of these interface pressure measurement systems into the clinical setting raised important issues about interpretation of the data and their validity. These concerns continue to be debated by clinicians, researchers and manufacturers of support surfaces who use pressure measurement to promote their products. Ferguson-Pell [7] proposed specifications for interface pressure sensors, pointing out that the sensors can introduce errors by locally perturbing the measurement region in which it is placed. The author proposed minimum specifications for the aspect ratio (ratio of thickness to diameter) of pressure sensors for different applications. Later, Ferguson-Pell and Cardi [8[demonstrated the limitations of pressure-mapping systems in terms of their potential to hammock across the measurement region, in addition to measurement errors introduced by creep and hysteresis in the sensors. These studies and others have contributed to the widely established view that pressure-measurement systems are of clinical value when making comparisons between different support surfaces for an individual, where essentially qualitative information is required. The imaging of pressure between the body and a support surface is not a new technology. The earliest images were produced by Aronovitz et al. [9] and Reswick et al. [10] using a multicellular inflatable mat with 1886 independent reading of pressure made in rapid succession. A similar device was developed by Garber et al. [11], who produced the first commercial pressure-mapping system (TIPE System), which provided a spatial resolution of 144 sensors on a pad measuring 400×400 mm. This system was later modified by Jaros et al. [12] to enable the data to be displayed on a computer. Bader and Hawken [13] introduced the Oxford Pressure Monitor (OPM; Talley, UK), which used a novel pneumatic sensor to monitor 12 sensors placed at approximately 25 mm centres. In the early 1990s a number of pressure-mapping systems were introduced, filling the void left by the removal of the TIPE from the market due to man-

Table 17.1. Summary of four commercially produced pressure-mapping systems

System	Novel Pliance	Tekscan	Xsensor	FSA
Manufacturer	Novel GmbH, Munich, Germany	Tekscan Inc., Boston, USA	Xsensor Technology Corp., Calgary, Canada	Vista Medical, Winnipeg, Canada
	There are five models for wheelchairs			
Sensor type	Capacitive	Conductive ink	Capacitive	Conductive rubber
Single sensor area	600 mm^2– 196 mm^2	103 mm^2	135 mm^2	298 mm^2
Sensor pitch	25 mm– 14 mm	10 mm	13 mm	25 mm
Number of sensors	256–1344	1558	1296	225

ufacturing difficulties. Talley Medical Devices produced a 96-sensor array (Mk III, Talley Pressure Monitor). In Canada the QAPad was introduced, providing an electropneumatic system similar to the TIPE with 256 sensors placed on a 400×400 mm sensing area. Further developments were introduced using capacitive arrays of sensors by Novel (Munich, Germany) and by Xsensor (Calgary, Canada). Simultaneously, Vista Medical introduced the Force Sensing Array and Tekscan the SEAT System using semiconductor materials that decrease in resistance with increasing applied axial stress. Sample images are shown and the characteristics of these four systems are outlined in Table 17.1.

As can been seen in Fig. 17.5, dramatic differences in pressure distribution are noted when a buttock phantom is loaded on a wide range of wheelchair cushions. The loading conditions are identical in each case, but the pressure distribution is significantly different due to the properties of the cushion.

With the advent of the ability to measure interface pressure distributions came questions about how to interpret them (also discussed in Chap. 5). A number of proposals have been made for "peak acceptable pressures", many of them linked to physiological studies to determine capillary closure pressure. However Kosiak [14] and later Reswick and Rogers [6], emphasised the multi-factorial nature of pressure ulcer aetiology, not least that there is a nominal inverse relationship between applied pressure and the duration of its application to initiate a pressure ulcer. This inverse relationship is thought to be substantially modulated by other clinical risk factors and the loading history of the tissues. Bader [15], using tissue partial pres-

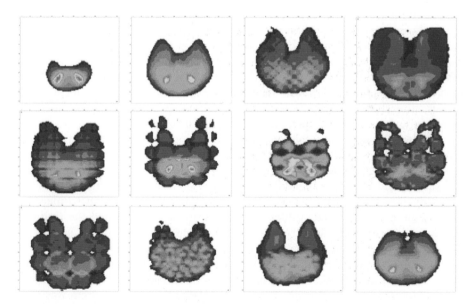

Fig. 17.5. Pressure maps generated by a gel-covered cushion loading indenter for a range of commercial cushions. The pressure map at *top left* is for a rigid surface for reference purposes

sure of oxygen measurements, demonstrated how, under repetitive loading conditions, there were changes in tissue response with increasing number of loading cycles.

Of course, pressure mapping images draw attention to differences in the way pressure is distributed spatially and thereby introducing third and fourth dimensions (pressure: amplitude, two spatial dimensions and time) to the measurements obtained from simpler instruments that are relevant to pressure ulcer aetiology. Drummond et al. [16] undertook an important study by measuring the distribution of pressure in wheelchairs beneath children with spina bifida. They defined an index by taking the ratio of the sum of the pressure readings in the sacral–ischial region to the sum of all readings on the cushion. Those children whose index was high, indicating that a greater proportion of the body weight was transferred to the cushions through their sacral–ischial tissues, were found to develop significantly more pressure ulcers. This study, coupled with that of Ferguson-Pell et al. [17], was the first to show in human subjects a link between pressure measurement parameters and actual pressure ulcer incidence. Subsequently Geyer et al. [18] undertook a comprehensive randomised prospective study which showed that peak pressure and average pressure were correlated with increased pressure ulcer incidence in a group of frail elderly people in a nursing home setting.

Discussion of pressure measurement is not complete without addressing reasonable concerns for the biomechanical validity of these measurements. Interface pressure measurement strictly measures localised axial stresses that occur between two loading surfaces. These stresses are often referred to as contact stresses. Off-axis, or shear, stresses are known to occur and are thought to be of considerable clinical significance. Transducers to measure shear stresses have, however, presented significant technological challenges, although a number have been produced for research purposes. The level of shear stress is influenced by the direction of load transfer between the body and the support surface and the frictional properties of the interface. Interposing sensors will result in substantial changes in local shear unless the shear sensor matches the frictional properties of the interface materials. A satisfactory technological solution is still elusive.

However, recognising that it is the physiological response of tissues to local mechanical stresses that determines their viability, many have suggested that measures of tissue deformation would yield measures more closely linked to the influence of a support surface on pressure ulcer risk. Cheung [19] and Sprigle et al. [20] employed instrumentation to measure the shape of the buttocks under loaded conditions and related the findings back to interface pressure readings. They found in a group of spinal injured participants that there were distinctive differences in loaded buttock shape linked to level of injury. They suggested that custom contoured seating could be used to accommodate these differences and thereby minimise tissue deformation during sitting. A buttock shape-sensing system was produced (Fig. 17.6) which enabled a record to be taken and input to a numerically controlled milling machine. Although the cushions did not match

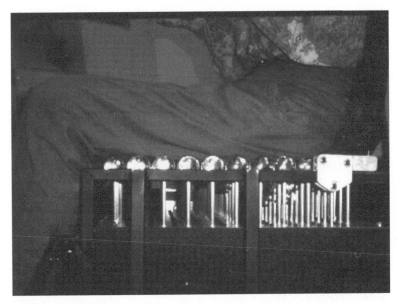

Fig. 17.6. Spring-loaded displacement sensors used to measure loaded buttock contour

the undeformed buttock shape, because the measurements were made with the tissues loaded on spring-loaded displacement sensors, this approach was thought to reduce tissue deformation compared with a planar cushion. There are concerns, however, that cushions formed to create an intimate fit might restrict opportunities to produce pressure redistribution through changes in posture. Nonetheless buttock shape-capturing technologies are being widely used for patients needing sophisticated postural management and where the risk of pressure ulcer development is relatively low.

Monitoring Tissue Response to Load

Given the many limitations of pressure mapping, interest has been directed towards the use of physiological monitoring where the body's response to a support system is used to indicate its suitability.

A number of discrete sensing systems have been used for this purpose, including transcutaneous measurements of the partial pressure of oxygen in the tissues [15], tissue reflectance spectroscopy (TRS) [21–23] and laser Doppler flowmetry (LDF) [24]. In all cases these instruments measure physiological changes in tissues associated with either the application of load generating ischaemia, or the reperfusion response (reactive hyperaemia) when the load is removed.

Figure 17.7 illustrates TRS and LDF responses for a heel placed on an alternating pressure mattress during an inflation and deflation cycle. The cyclic variations in the LDF signal are associated with vasomotion.

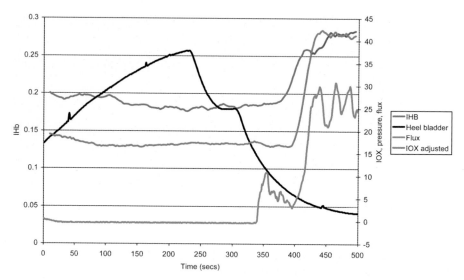

Fig. 17.7. Tissue response for a heel of a healthy subject placed on an alternating pressure mattress. The internal bladder pressure in one of the cells of an alternating pressure mattress is represented in *black*. The indices for skin blood content and oxygenation are indicated in *blue* and *red*, respectively, and the laser Doppler flux is represented in *green*

Laser Doppler Flowmetry

Laser Doppler flowmetry imaging uses a stable monochromatic laser light source directed through a fibre optic to illuminate the tissue. Backscattered light is collected using a second fibre optic placed closed to the source (approximately 1.5 mm centres). The backscattered light will be slightly frequency shifted if the scattering medium, namely blood, is moving either towards (blue shift) or away from (red shift) the point of measurement. The net effect is for the bandwidth of the frequency spectrum of the backscattered light to be broadened by an amount proportional to the average velocity of the scattering medium. The tissue thickness sampled is typically 1 mm, the capillary diameters 10 μm and the velocity spectrum measurement 0.01–10 mm/s.

Most LDF systems make single-point measurements providing an index of the blood flow rate. However, one scanning system (LDF Imager; Moor Instruments, Devon, UK) produces images of the blood flow in tissues by using a mirror to move the laser beam across the region of measurement in a raster pattern. This system can measure regions of tissue from 50×50 mm up to 500×500 mm, taking approximately 5 min to complete the scan. The maximum resolution of the system is 100 μm. A typical image of a healing burn is shown in Fig. 17.8.

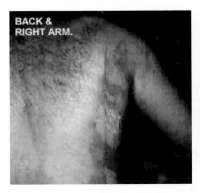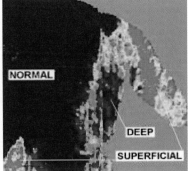

Fig. 17.8. Laser Doppler flowmetry image of healing burn with corresponding photograph (after Moor Instruments)

Transcutaneous Oxygen Measurement

TcPO$_2$ sensors employ a polarographic Clark electrode which comprises a platinum cathode held at 0.7–0.9 V relative to an anode usually made from silver. An oxygen-permeable membrane isolates the electrode from the skin. In order to measure the partial pressure of oxygen in the tissue the electrode is heated to 42–44 °C. This induces maximal vasodilation, so that the oxygen diffusing through the skin is equilibrated closely with arterial oxygen tension. Only discrete measurements are possible at present using TcPO$_2$ sensors; however, a four-sensor system is available commercially for multi-point measurements (Perimed, Järfälla, Sweden). These sensors have been used extensively by Bader [15]. Their repeatability for clinical applications is discussed by Coleman et al. [25].

Tissue Reflectance Spectroscopy

Oxy- and deoxyhaemoglobin have distinctly different absorption spectra, particularly in the green and red regions of the spectrum as well as in the near infra-red (NIR) region of between 700 and 850 nm.

A number of approaches have been adopted to use the absorption spectrum of light in the visible region to characterise the blood content and oxygenation of the superficial vasculature of the skin. Dawson et al. [26] employed the points on the absorption spectra for oxy- and deoxyhaemoglobin, known as the isobestic points (Fig. 17.9). The level of oxygenation does not influence the absorption of light at these wavelengths. These wavelengths are influenced by the concentration of blood in the sample volume and other factors, such as melanin. By taking ratios of neighbouring isobestic points (absorption = L_{xxx} at wavelength xxx), it is possible to derive indices for the blood concentration (H) in the sample volume, and its level of oxygenation (O_x). The indices proposed by Feather et al. [26] were:

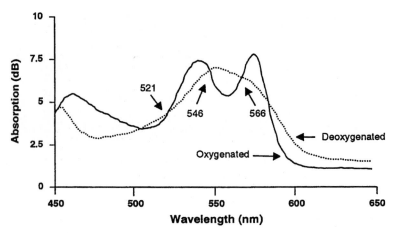

Fig. 17.9. The absorption spectrum of blood indicating the isobestic wavelengths

$$H = \left[\frac{(L_{544} - L_{527})}{16.5} - \frac{(L_{573} - L_{544})}{29} \right] \cdot 100 \qquad (17.1)$$

$$O_x = 100 \cdot [(L_{573} - L_{558}) - (L_{558} - L_{544})]/(14.5H) \qquad (17.2)$$

As the blood concentration tends to zero, then O_x becomes indeterminate (one cannot measure haemoglobin oxygenation if there is no blood!) and in practice for low blood concentrations the signal-to-noise ratio becomes very low.

Subsequently Ferguson-Pell and Hagisawa [22] proposed a slightly modified form of these equations for spectrometers with improved resolution. The isobestic wavelengths are shown in Fig. 17.9.

Scattering is the dominant photon–tissue interaction in skin in the NIR wavelengths, whereas in the visible region light is strongly absorbed and therefore only penetrates the most superficial layers of the skin. Hebden and Delpy [27] and Hebden et al. [28] have demonstrated, using arrays of TRS optodes, that in the NIR it is possible to create images showing regions of differing blood oxygenation of the neonate brain. In Fig. 17.10 this technique is demonstrated for the forearm.

It is also interesting to note that in the NIR an important terminal enzyme in the cellular respiratory chain (cytochrome oxidase, CtOx) produces in its oxidised state a broad peak around 830 nm [29]. This is not present for the enzyme in its reduced state. Thus it may prove possible to monitor and image the degree of oxygenation in tissues at a cellular level. However, due to the relatively strong absorption at these wavelengths this technique presents practical difficulties when decoupling the simultaneous contributions to the absorption spectrum of haemoglobin and CtOx.

Ferguson-Pell and colleagues made discrete sensors to measure tissue reflectance spectra at interfaces between the body and support surfaces, and

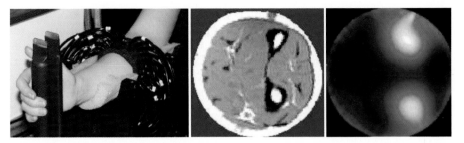

Fig. 17.10. NIR imaging of arm (*left*: optode array around circumference of arm; *centre*: X-ray image; *right*: NIR image) (after Elwell and Hebden [29])

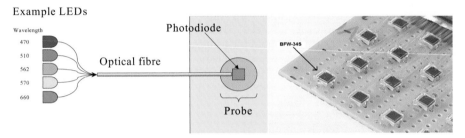

Fig. 17.11. Schematic representation of a prototype array of sensors that use high-intensity LED illumination at centre wavelengths consistent with the isobestic points used by tissue reflectance spectroscopy to estimate levels of blood content and oxygenation

sample data are presented in Fig. 17.11. The dimensions of these sensors (10 mm diameter, 2.5 mm thickness) is approaching the aspect ratio requirement for pressure sensors at body–support interfaces [7]. They have also produced an array of sensors that offer the potential to image these parameters, using high-intensity light-emitting diodes with emission wavelengths close to the isobestic points used in the equations above (Fig. 17.9).

Summary

Imaging techniques are available both to measure the interaction of the body with support surfaces and to assess tissue status. Ultrasound provides an effective method for assessing wound status, particularly in determining the extent of undermining of the wound. Photogrammetry techniques permit accurate measurement of wound dimensions using simple digital photography.

Mechanical interaction with a support surface can be visualised using pressure mapping. There are, however, concerns regarding the accuracy of these devices and their influence on the supporting characteristics of some cushions and mattresses.

The physiological response of tissues to ischaemia can be determined with a range of different techniques that provide information about blood flow, tissue oxygenation, and blood content and oxygenation. Imaging physiological parameters is challenging, especially if information is required while the tissue is under load. However, recent advances in electro-optics are reducing both the size and cost of sensors, suggesting a promising future for using the tissues as a direct indicator of their status, rather than drawing inferences from simple observation or pressure measurements alone.

References

1. Clark M, Bours G, de Flour T (2002) Summary report on the prevalence of pressure ulcers. Report European Pressure Ulcer Advisory Panel
2. Wendelken ME Markowitz L Patel M Alvarez OM (2003) Objective, non-invasive wound assessment using B-Mode ultrasonography. Wounds 15(11) 351–360
3. Lyder CHB (2004) Battling pressure ulcers: consistency means success. Nursing Homes Long Term Care Management 53(1):72–73
4. Srinivasan S, Krouskop T, Ophir J (2004) A quantitative comparison of modulus images obtained using nanoindentation with strain elastograms. Ultasound Med Biol 30(7):899–918
5. Sinkus R, Lorenzen J Schrader D, Lorenzen M, Dargatz M, Holz D (2000) High-resolution tensor MR elastography for breast tumour detection. Phys Med Biol 45:1649–1664
6. Reswick J, Rogers J (1976) Experience at Rancho Los Amigos Hospital with devices and techniques to prevent pressure sores. In: Kenedi RM, Cowden JM, Scales JT (eds) Bed sore biomechanics. MacMillan, London, pp 301–310
7. Ferguson-Pell MW (1980) Design criteria for the measurement of pressure at body/support interfaces. Eng Med 9:209–214
8. Ferguson-Pell MW, Cardi MD (1993) Prototype development and comparative evaluation of a wheelchair pressure mapping system. Assistive Technol 5:78–91
9. Aronovitz R, Geenway R, Lindan O, Reswick J, Scanlan J (1963) A pneumatic cell matrix to measure the distribution of contact pressure over the human body. Proc 16th Ann Conf Eng Med Biol, Baltimore 5:62–63
10. Reswick JB, Lindan O, Lippay A (1964) A device to measure pressure distribution between the human body and various supporting surfaces. Report No. EDC 4-6407, Medical Engineering Group, Case Institute of Technology and Highland View Hospital, Cleveland, Ohio
11. Garber SL, Krouskop TA, Carter RE (1978) A system for clinically evaluating wheelchair pressure-relief cushions. Am J Occup Ther 32:565–570
12. Jaros LA, Levine SP, Kett RL, Koester DJ (1988) The spiral pressure monitor. Proceedings of 3rd International Conference on Rehabilitation Technology, RESNA 308–309
13. Bader DL, Hawken MB (1986) Pressure distribution under the ischium of normal subjects. J Biomed Eng 8:353–357
14. Kosiak M (1961) Etiology of decubitus ulcers. Arch Phys Med Rehab 42:19–29
15. Bader DL (1990) The recovery characteristics of soft tissues following repeated loading. J Rehabil Res Dev 27:141–150
16. Drummond D, Breed AL, Narechania R (1985) Relationship of spine deformity and pelvic obliquity on sitting pressure distributions and decubitus ulceration. J Pediatr Orthop 5:396–402

17. Ferguson-Pell MW, Wilkie IC, Reswick JB, Barbenel JC (1980) Pressure sore prevention for the wheelchair-bound spinal injury patient. Paraplegia 18:42–51
18. Geyer MJ, Brienza DM, Karg P, Trefler E, Kelsey S (2001) A randomized control trial to evaluate pressure-reducing seat cushions for elderly wheelchair users. Adv Skin Wound Care 14:120–129
19. Cheung KC (1987) Tissue contour and pressure distribution on wheelchair cushions. PhD Thesis, University of Virginia
20. Sprigle S, Cheung KC, Brubaker CE (1990) Factors affecting seat contour characteristics. J Rehab Res Dev 27:127–134
21. Hagisawa S, Ferguson-Pell MW, Cardi M, Miller SD (1994) Assessment of skin blood content and oxygenation in spinal cord injured subjects during reactive hyperemia. J Rehab Res Dev 31:1–14
22. Ferguson-Pell MW, Hagisawa S (1995) An empirical technique to compensate for melanin when monitoring skin micro circulation use reflectance spectrophotometry. Med Eng Phys 17:104–110
23. Sprigle S, Linden M, Riordan B (2003) Analysis of localized erythema using clinical indicators and spectroscopy. Ostomy Wound Management 49:42–52
24. Silver-Thorn MB (2002) Investigation of lower-limb tissue perfusion during loading. J. Rehab Res Dev 39:597–608
25. Coleman LS, Dowd GSE, Bentley G (1986) Reproducibility of TcPO$_2$ measurements in normal volunteers. Clin Phys Physiol Meas 7:259–263
26. Dawson JB, Barker DJ, Ellis DJ, Grassam E, Cotterill JA, Fisher GV, Feather JW (1980) A theoretical and experimental study of light absorption and scattering by in vivo skin. Phys Med Biol 25:695–709
27. Hebden JC, Delpy DT (1997) Diagnostic imaging with light. Br J Radiol 70:S206–S214
28. Hebden JC Arridge SR Delpy DT (1997) Optical imaging in medicine. I. Experimental techniques. Phys Med Biol 42:825–840
29. Elwell J, Hebden JC (2004) http://www.medphys.ucl.ac.uk/research/borl/research/nir_topics/imaging_exp. htm

Magnetic Resonance Imaging and Spectroscopy of Pressure Ulcers

18

Gustav Strijkers, Jeanine Prompers, Klaas Nicolay

Introduction

In the previous chapters of this book, we have seen that pressure ulcers (decubitus ulcers) are extremely common in patients who are bed or chair bound, e.g. during hospitalization or because of spinal cord injuries. The ulcers can range from mild coloration of the skin to deep non-healing wounds, which extend into organs or bone. This complex pathology and aetiology of pressure ulcers makes a clinical evaluation by physical examination alone very difficult, if not impossible. Therefore, there is a great need for diagnostic methods to evaluate the depth and extent of pressure ulcers.

With their ability to measure structural, functional and metabolic parameters in healthy and diseased tissue, magnetic resonance imaging (MRI) and spectroscopy (MRS) offer a variety of fast and non-invasive tools that can be used not only for diagnosis and suitable planning of treatment, but also for a better understanding of the mechanisms underlying the formation of pressure ulcers.

In this chapter the current MR literature on pressure ulcers is discussed and new techniques that can be used in research and clinical diagnosis are proposed. The outline of the chapter is as follows. First the present role of MR techniques in pressure ulcer research is reviewed. Subsequently, a brief description of the basic principles of MR is given, followed by an explanation of a number of MR modalities and their (possible) applications in relation to the investigation of pressure ulcers. We conclude with a summary and perspective.

Present Role of MR

Magnetic resonance imaging has proven an important non-invasive experimental tool in the detection and characterization of pathologies in the musculoskeletal system (see e.g. [1–7]). The technique offers excellent soft tissue contrast and high anatomical resolution. Therefore, it is rather surprising that there are only a few systematic MRI studies of pressure ulcers in humans and animal models, especially because MRI can provide the clues for a fast and accurate diagnosis, which might prove crucial for efficient medical or surgical treatment.

Human clinical studies have been conducted mainly on debilitated patients with spinal cord injuries, who often develop chronic pressure ulcers (see other chapters of this volume). In a study by Hencey et al. [8], 37 male spinal cord injury patients who had current or recent sacral, ischial or peritrochanteric pressure ulcers were examined with MRI. It was concluded that MRI could play an important role in the clinical evaluation of decubitus ulcers. The technique was able to detect the extent of soft tissue changes, adjacent fluid collection and the involvement of bone.

In contrast, Rubayi et al. [9] reported a case study of six spinal cord injury patients with iliopsoas abscess evaluated by MRI, computed tomography (CT), conventional radiography, and radionuclide scanning. Iliopsoas abscesses were best diagnosed and treated using CT. From this study it was concluded that CT was superior to MRI and other radiographic methods.

More recently Huang et al. [10] evaluated the clinical accuracy of MRI was in the diagnosis of osteomyelitis in the pelvis/hips of 44 paralysed patients and the utility of MR mapping of the disease extent as a guide to the extent of surgical resection. It was found that MRI is able to diagnose the associated findings in spinal cord-injured patients and can also guide the surgeons as to the anatomic extent, allowing accurate and limited treatment.

Ruan et al. [11] also evaluated the use of MRI in making clinical decisions when assessing non-healing pressure ulcers and non-healing myocutaneous flaps for the presence of abscesses, osteomyelitis, sinus tracts and fluid collections. This was done in 12 patients as part of their pre- and postoperative diagnostic evaluation. A number of case studies illustrated the complicated treatment and evaluation. It was concluded that MRI could be used to identify and evaluate the pressure ulcers in the preoperative period.

To our knowledge, there are only a few histological animal model studies on pressure ulcers [12–15], and only one that combines histology and MRI [16]. In the latter work decubitus ulcers were induced in the tibialis anterior muscle and overlying skin in the right hind limb of the rat by compression from an indenter over the tibia. MR images were obtained in vivo 24 h after load application, and subsequently tissues were processed for ex vivo histological examination. The amount and extent of the damage determined with MRI and from histology were in good agreement. It was concluded that MRI, as it is non-destructive, is a promising alternative for histology in research on pressure ulcer aetiology and, especially, in follow-up studies to evaluate the development of muscle damage over time and in clinical studies.

The studies above, although limited in number, have clearly shown that MRI can be a useful tool for the clinical assessment and in the research of the aetiology of pressure ulcers. However, apart from the use of MRI, to provide basic contrast and mainly anatomical information, there are a number of MRI modalities available nowadays that have found no application in pressure ulcer research yet. Tagging MRI, diffusion-weighted MRI and perfusion MRI offer the possibility to measure local muscle fibre deformation, orientation and tissue perfusion, respectively. Magnetic resonance elastography measures the viscoelastic properties of muscle in relation to health and disease. Finally, with MRS the concentration of low-molecular-weight metabolites can be determined, which provides information on the biochemical status of tissues. The principles of these additional and alternative MR modalities and their potential value in pressure ulcer research will be discussed in the next sections of this chapter.

MR Techniques

Basic Principles and Practical Considerations

Nuclear magnetic resonance (abbreviated to MR in the biomedical literature) is a physical technique that is based on the fact that most atomic nuclei have a magnetic moment. When a large number of such nuclei are placed in a strong magnetic field, this leads to the generation of a net spin magnetization that can be detected with a radio-frequency receiver coil, after excitation by a short radio-frequency pulse. Many nuclei can be detected by MR, of which ^1H, ^{13}C, and ^{31}P are most relevant in biological tissues.

MR as applied in vivo has two basic modalities, MRI and MRS. MRI of biological systems is usually based on the measurement of the distribution of the hydrogen nuclei of water. The use of water as a probe molecule has many advantages: (1) the hydrogen nucleus has the highest sensitivity among biologically relevant nuclei; (2) water is present in high concentrations in most tissues; (3) the magnetic properties of water are sensitive to the local microstructure and composition of biological tissues as well as to environmental factors such as temperature and pH; (4) water displacement inherent to processes like diffusion, perfusion, flow, and movement can be quantified by specific MRI measurement sequences; and (5) the magnetic properties of the hydrogen nuclei in water can be modulated by interactions with paramagnetic entities, which are either endogenous to the tissue (e.g. deoxyhaemoglobin in the red cells of the blood) or can be injected as an exogenous contrast agent (examples include chelates of rare earth metal ions, or targeted nanoparticles containing paramagnetic centres). The above factors explain the rich spectrum of image contrast parameters for which MRI is so well known. As an imaging technology, MR has advanced considerably in the past 10 years, but it continues to evolve and new capabilities and applications will likely be developed (for introductory reading see [17–21]).

A MR system consists basically of the following components. A large magnet provides the static magnetic field. Radio-frequency coils transmit and receive the radio signals. Magnetic field gradient coils provide the spatial localization of the signal, and a computer is used to reconstruct the radio signal into the final image or spectrum. The MR examination of humans is usually carried out within the radiology department of a hospital. The patient is positioned on a narrow bed within the magnet and the MR technologist or radiologist performs the examination. An entire examination may take from 20 min to 1.5 h, depending on the type and amount of information required. The design of the MR system restricts the subjects to a horizontal lying position inside the bore of the magnet. This means that tissue deformation, relevant to pressure ulcer research, can be examined only in a lying position, not under realistic conditions in a sitting position, such as when a patient is confined to a wheelchair.

MR has no known negative effects on living tissue, but some potential hazards, related to metal objects entering the scan room, should be considered. Because of possible interference with the high magnetic and RF fields present, patients who have a heart pacemaker, surgical staples, aneurysm clips, or any other implanted metal device are not allowed to undergo a MR scan.

The MR examinations of animals are similar to those of humans, except that the animals are usually sedated to avoid movement during the scans. This also allows for longer scanning times, up to several hours. MR examinations on small laboratory animals are usually performed with specialized high-field animal scanners.

Basic Contrast

The proton density, and the T_1 and T_2 relaxation times provide the basic contrast in MR images. The proton density is the distribution of water in tissue, which gives the main anatomical contrast in the images. The brightness of pixels in the MR images also depends, however, on the chemical and physical environment of the protons, which can be described by T_1 and T_2. The spin-lattice or longitudinal relaxation time T_1 describes the exponential increase of the spin magnetization towards equilibrium when placed in a strong magnetic field or when disturbed by a radio-frequency pulse. The spin-spin or transverse relaxation time T_2 describes the exponential decrease of the spin magnetization in the transverse plane (perpendicular to the static magnetic field). This transverse magnetization, which is created by tipping the spin magnetization from longitudinal equilibrium by a radio-frequency pulse, creates the measured signal in MRI.

The intensity of the MR signal is given in first approximation by

$$I \propto N e^{-TE/T_2}(1 - e^{-TR/T_1}) \tag{1}$$

where N, T_1, and T_2 are the proton density, the spin-lattice relaxation time and the spin-spin relaxation time, respectively. TR is the radio-frequency pulse repetition time and TE is the echo time, or signal delay time. Contrast is obtained because different tissues have different proton densities and relaxation times [22–25]. Equation 1 shows that when TR is long and TE is short compared to T_1 and T_2, respectively, the contrast is mainly determined by the proton density, yielding a so-called proton density-weighted image. When TR is of the order of the spin-lattice relaxation time, contrast is obtained on the basis of differences in T_1, in which case the image is called a T_1-weighted image. When TE is of the order of the spin-spin relaxation time, contrast is obtained on the basis of differences in T_2, resulting in a so-called T_2-weighted image. Note that Eq. 1 holds only for a spin-echo imaging pulse sequence. For other imaging pulse sequences the intensity depends in a more complicated manner on N, T_1, and T_2 [20].

The spin-lattice relaxation time T_1 depends on the motion of water molecules in tissue and the interactions with surrounding macromolecules. The spin-spin relaxation time T_2 is in addition strongly affected by the slowly varying magnetic fields at the molecular level. A detailed discussion of the physical and chemical origin of the relaxation processes in living tissue is beyond the scope of this chapter. It is more useful to consider the relaxation times typically observed in musculoskeletal tissues and the effects of pressure ulcer pathology on these relaxation times. Table 18.1 shows typical relaxation times at 1.5 T for some relevant tissues.

The relevant pathologic conditions of pressure ulcers that affect muscle proton density and relaxation times are inflammation, haemorrhage, mass lesions, fibrosis, and fatty infiltration [1, 7]. Inflammation, oedema and haemorrhage usually lead to an increased proton density, caused by increased intracellular and extracellular free water. The T_1 and T_2 are increased because free water has longer relaxation times. Most mass lesions, such as solid neoplasms, abscesses and tumours, also are characterized by relaxation times that are prolonged relative to the surrounding tissues. Because both inflammatory processes and mass lesions lead to increased relaxation times, differentiation on the basis of relaxation times only is difficult. However, usually a clear distinction between the two can be made on the basis of morphology. Fibrous tissue formed by fibrosis does not provide much MR signal, due to low water content, and may be difficult to detect until a substantial amount of tissue has formed. Fat is characterized by a short T_1, and T_1-weighted MRI can therefore easily detect fatty infiltration.

Because of the well-documented effects of muscle pathology on the proton density and the relaxation times, contrast in proton density-weighted, T_1-weighted and T_2-weighted MRI provides a useful tool for the detection and diagnosis of pressure ulcers [8–11, 16]. This is illustrated in Fig. 18.1, showing transverse T_2-weighted MR images of the hind limbs of three rats

Table 18.1. Typical relaxation times for relevant human tissues at 1.5 T [22–25]		
Tissue	T_1 (ms)	T_2 (ms)
Muscle	1077	47
Adipose tissue	260	84
Nerve	740	77
Bone marrow	250	25

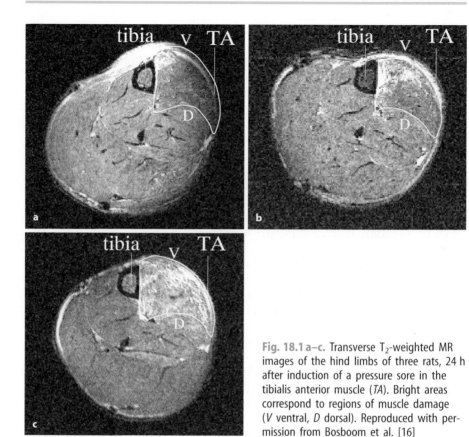

Fig. 18.1 a–c. Transverse T$_2$-weighted MR images of the hind limbs of three rats, 24 h after induction of a pressure sore in the tibialis anterior muscle (*TA*). Bright areas correspond to regions of muscle damage (*V* ventral, *D* dorsal). Reproduced with permission from Bosboom et al. [16]

24 h after induction of a pressure ulcer in the tibialis anterior muscle by compression [16]. Patchy regions with high signal intensity are observed in the muscle, probably caused by oedema due to inflammation. The amount of muscle damage assessed in vivo with MRI correlated well with the area of damage obtained from ex vivo histology.

Dynamic Deformation

In a number of recent studies it has been hypothesized that prolonged deformation of cells plays a major role in the onset of tissue damage [16, 26–31]. This hypothesis was tested on cultured cells [28, 31] and in a rat model in which the tibialis anterior muscle and overlying skin were compressed between an indenter and the tibia [16, 29, 30]. For the rat model, the amount and location of the pressure ulcers that developed were determined with histology and MRI (see Fig. 18.1), and the results were compared to finite-element calculations of shear strain distributions in the muscle during loading. Unfortunately, most calculations resulted in shear strain distributions not corresponding to the location and amount of muscle damage observed. The discrepancy was attributed mainly to insufficient knowledge about the exact deformations of the muscle induced by the indenter.

We propose an approach using MRI to locate the exact position of the indenter and the resulting amount of global deformation of the muscle. Figure 18.2 shows an ex vivo coronal MR image of the lower hind limb of a rat. In the image an indenter is visible, pressed into the tibialis anterior muscle. The indenter is visible because it is fabricated of a hollow Perspex tube, filled with regular water. The Perspex tube itself is not visible, but since the dimensions of the tube are known, the exact three-dimensional position of the end of the tube can easily be extrapolated from the position of the water in the tube. In this way the indenter can be pressed into the muscle in a precise and reproducible manner. The ex vivo MR image in Fig. 18.2 was recorded for demonstration purposes. The technique works in vivo as well.

With MR tagging it is possible to measure the three-dimensional tissue deformation also locally [32]. This technique uses a set of preparation radiofrequency pulses to produce a periodic modulation of the longitudinal magnetization prior to imaging. The resulting images show a characteristic striped or checkerboard pattern. Motion (deformation) between the time of preparation and imaging will show up as a displacement of the pattern. This technique is widely used to measure heart wall motion [33]. MR tagging can also be used to measure contraction and deformation of skeletal muscle. This is demonstrated in Fig. 18.3, which displays in vivo MR tagging images of a mouse hind leg at rest and during contraction by stimulation of the scia-

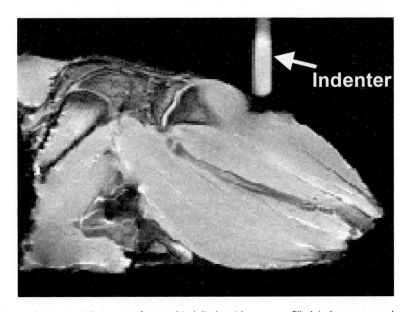

Fig. 18.2. Coronal ex vivo MR image of a rat hind limb with a water-filled indenter pressed into the tibialis anterior muscle. Courtesy of A. Stekelenburg and G. J. Strijkers, Eindhoven

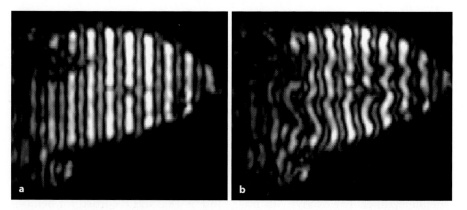

Fig. 18.3. Coronal in vivo MR tagging images of a mouse hind limb a at rest and b during contraction by stimulation of the sciatic nerve. Courtesy of A.M. Heemskerk, Eindhoven and M.R. Drost, Maastricht

tic nerve. By combining a set of slices at different positions and orientations, the three-dimensional local movements, deformation and stresses in the muscle can be determined. This technique can also be used in combination with the indenter shown in Fig. 18.2 to obtain accurate information about the exact deformation of the muscle under external pressure conditions.

Diffusion Weighting and Diffusion Tensor Imaging

The random motion (diffusion) of water molecules in living tissue can be measured with MR by using diffusion-weighted sequences, such as developed by Stejskal and Tanner [34]. Diffusion weighting can be achieved by introducing a set of pulsed magnetic field gradients, which subsequently dephase and rephase the proton spin magnetization. In tissue with diffusion, signal loss is observed, because moving spins are not completely rephased by the gradients.

Diffusion of water in biological tissue is composed of the random motion of water in the intra- and extracellular compartments as well as exchange processes. Diffusion-weighted imaging (DWI) can yield important information about the condition of healthy and pathological tissues [35]. DWI has been applied most extensively in the brain, in which it is highly sensitive to the detection of brain ischaemia in an early stage of development [36]. Necrotic tumour tissue can be differentiated from viable tissue by an increased diffusion-related signal loss [37–39]. Oedema, inflammation, and haemorrhage in soft tissue lead to increased free water content and therefore to strong diffusion attenuation of the signal in DWI [40]. It is expected that DWI might therefore prove useful in the detection and diagnosis of skeletal muscle pressure ulcers.

A high degree of orientation in tissue leads to anisotropy of the diffusion. This can be observed, for example, in white matter tracts in the brain [41–

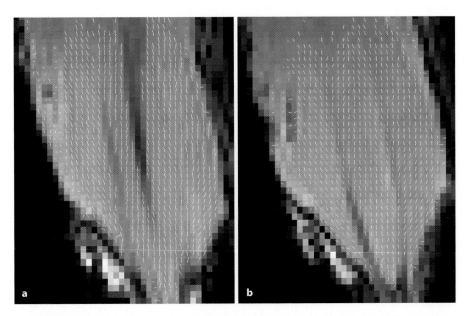

Fig. 18.4 a, b. Two slices of an ex-vivo diffusion tensor image of a mouse hind limb. The lines indicate the in-plane direction of preferential water diffusion, corresponding to the local muscle fibre orientation. The DTI data are plotted on top of a regular T_2-weighted MR image. Courtesy of A. M. Heemskerk and G. J. Strijkers, Eindhoven

44], but also in muscle [45–50]. Water diffusion along fibres is relatively fast, while diffusion perpendicular to the fibres is restricted. By measuring the directional dependence of the water diffusion and using the diffusion tensor concept for data analysis, the orientation of the fibres can be determined in three dimensions. This technique is called diffusion tensor imaging (DTI).

Figure 18.4 shows two slices of a diffusion tensor image of a mouse hind leg. The lines indicate the in-plane direction of easy water diffusion, corresponding to the local muscle fibre orientation. The DTI data are plotted on top of a regular T_2-weighted MR image. Muscle damage might lead to a localized decrease in the diffusion anisotropy. The muscle fibre orientation can provide input for mathematical finite-element models of skeletal muscle mechanics, relevant to pressure ulcer formation [16, 29, 30]. DTI can be combined with MR tagging to determine fibre orientation during contraction or deformation.

Perfusion

The aetiology of pressure ulcers is very complicated. One of the competing hypotheses suggests that local ischaemia of the tissue, caused by occlusion of the capillaries under pressure and subsequent reperfusion damage by oxygen free radicals, is an important trigger for the development of pressure ulcers (refs. [12, 13, 15, 51, 52] and Chap. 13 of this volume). Measurement of local perfusion and reperfusion of skeletal muscle could provide important clues concerning the development of pressure ulcers.

A number of techniques are available for measuring perfusion in skeletal muscle, such as strain-gauge plethysmography, the use of microspheres, radioactive tracer methods, thermodilution measurements and laser Doppler velocimetry [53–56]. None of these, however, is capable of providing the high temporal and spatial resolution desired when measuring in vivo muscle. MR, on the other hand, does offer a range of techniques to measure perfusion. Presently, most MR perfusion studies have been applied to the brain [57, 58], in which perfusion is higher and easier to measure than in skeletal muscle. Nevertheless, recent studies have demonstrated convincingly that perfusion measurements with high temporal and spatial resolution are possible in skeletal muscle too [59, 60].

Measurements of muscle perfusion with MR can be classified in two major techniques: the endogenous and the exogenous tracer methods. The first method uses endogenous water in blood as a contrast agent and is often called the arterial spin labelling (ASL) technique. ASL uses radio-frequency pulses to label the spin magnetization of arterial blood by inverting or saturating its magnetization. The labelled water molecules are delivered to the imaging slice by flow, followed by exchange with tissue protons. A control experiment is performed without labelling. The difference signal of control and labelled images, in which static tissue signals are identical, originates from blood that has perfused into the tissue only. Several ASL techniques have been designed, differing in how and at which position the blood is labelled [57, 58]. The drawback of ASL lies in its relatively low sensitivity and in the fact that quantification of the absolute perfusion is difficult and needs extensive mathematical modelling. The ASL technique is demonstrated in Fig. 18.5, showing perfusion images of the lower legs of four healthy volunteers. The images were recorded after the subjects had finished an exercise protocol in a plantar-flexion ergometer with weights of 10 lb (4.5 kg) and 20 lb (9.1 kg). Variations in perfusion rates with weight are clearly visible. Perfusion increases are associated with distinct muscle groups. Clear variations between different subjects can also be observed. The perfusion measurements were consistent with those obtained by traditional techniques. The results of this study show that perfusion measurements of skeletal muscle with the ASL technique are feasible.

The second perfusion MRI technique uses an exogenous paramagnetic contrast agent, such as gadolinium-DTPA. Following an intravenous injection of the contrast agent, the delivery of the agent to the tissue can be made visible with T_1-weighted fast MRI sequences. Recently this technique was successfully demonstrated in a rat model of hind-limb ischaemia [60]. After femoral artery ligation of one of the hind limbs, the remaining perfusion reserve was quantified using the Gd-DTPA uptake rate, obtained using a T_1-weighted fast imaging technique. Perfusion was also measured during hyperaemia, caused by stimulation of the sciatic nerves of both hind limbs. Figure 18.6 a shows the perfusion index for a cross section of the non-li-

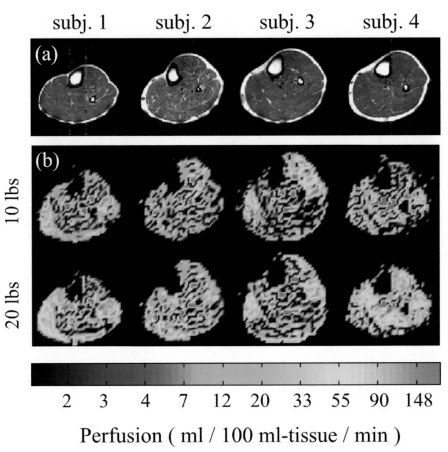

Fig. 18.5. a Anatomical axial MR images of the lower leg of four human subjects. **b** Perfusion images for both the 10-lb and the 20-lb exercise protocol. Courtesy of L.R. Frank et al. [59]: "Dynamic imaging of perfusion in human skeletal muscle during exercise with arterial spin labeling," Magn Reson Med 42, Copyright © 1999. Reprinted by permission of Wiley-Liss Inc., a subsidiary of John Wiley & Sons, Inc

gated and ligated hind limbs, at rest and after stimulation. The MR signal enhancement can be assumed to be proportional to the Gd-DTPA concentration, and the perfusion index was defined as the maximum Gd-DTPA uptake. The reduced perfusion index due to the ligation during hyperaemia is obvious. Very good agreement was observed between the MR perfusion data and microsphere blood flow measurements. In Fig. 18.6b the time course of the perfusion index during hyperaemia is shown from 1 h to 42 days after ligation, demonstrating that this technique can be applied reproducibly during a long period of time.

As shown, both endogenous and exogenous tracer methods have been successfully used to measure local perfusion in skeletal muscle. This opens the possibility of non-invasive measurement of perfusion changes in mus-

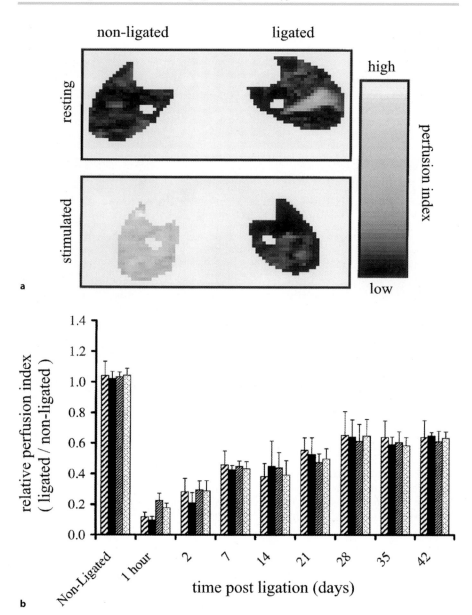

Fig. 18.6. a Examples of perfusion index maps from the hind limb muscles of a control rat and a rat with femoral artery ligation of one of the hind limbs, in resting condition and during stimulation-induced hyperaemia. The perfusion index was obtained with MR perfusion measurement using the contrast agent Gd-DTPA. **b** Time course of the perfusion index during hyperaemia after ligation. The *bars* indicate different muscle groups. From left to right: tibialis cranialis, tibialis caudalis plus flexor digitorum longus, gastrocnemius, and total muscle groups in the cross section. Courtesy of Y. Luo et al. [60]: "Evaluation of tissue perfusion in a rat model of hind-limb muscle ischaemia using dynamic contrast-enhanced magnetic resonance imaging," J Magn Reson Imaging 16, Copyright © 2002. Reprinted by permission of Wiley-Liss Inc., a subsidiary of John Wiley & Sons, Inc

cle during applied pressure and following reperfusion in relation to pressure ulcer formation. MR provides the possibility to measure acute changes in muscle perfusion on a short timescale. In addition, subtle changes in perfusion rates over extensive periods of time can be followed reproducibly. This might provide important new clues needed for unravelling the aetiology of pressure ulcers.

Magnetic Resonance Elastography

It is well known that a variety of disease processes lead to a change in the visco-elastic properties of tissue. A relatively new diagnostic method for detecting changes in the mechanical properties of tissue is magnetic resonance elastography (MRE) [61–64]. MRE can be applied to a variety of tissues. So far the technique mainly has been successful in the detection of tumours [65–68] (e.g. in the breast or brain), which are observable as stiff solid masses in the MRE images. Little is known about the elastic properties of muscle in vivo, and present MRE studies of muscle are therefore mainly focused on determining the mechanical properties of healthy muscle [69–72]. We anticipate that MRE can also be used to detect changes in muscle elasticity caused by decubitus ulcers in an early stage of development.

In brief, MRE works as follows: With MRE it is possible to directly visualize propagating acoustic strain waves in tissue. These waves are introduced into the tissue by excitation with a mechanical transducer. A velocity-sensitive phase-contrast MRI method is used to measure the small displacements when the waves propagate in the tissue. From these displacements, the velocity, wavelength and attenuation of the shear waves can be determined. Stiff material is characterized by a long wavelength and high wave velocity, elastic material by a short wavelength and low velocity. Figure 18.7 shows an example of MRE of the biceps brachii muscle of a healthy volunteer [69]. In this investigation MRE was applied to quantify the changes in stiffness of skeletal muscle under load. In Fig. 18.7a a schematic diagram of the experimental set-up is shown. The transducer, which excites the biceps tendon periodically, is placed on the skin. The volunteer holds a load of 4 kg. Figure 18.7b shows the conventional axial MR image of the arm, with the slice position of the coronal MRE wave image indicated by the rectangle. Figure 18.7c shows the MRE shear wave pattern at a single phase propagating in the coronal slice of the biceps. Combining wave images at different phases enables visualization of the propagating waves through the tissue.

For the characterization, modelling and diagnosis of pressure ulcers in skeletal muscle, MRE might be a very useful tool. Although no experimental evidence is available yet, we anticipate that oedematous ulcers will be visible as regions of changed elasticity [65]. MRE can provide the material parameters, needed for finite-element modelling of muscle deformation in relation to the formation of pressure ulcers (ref. [16] and Chap. 12 of this book).

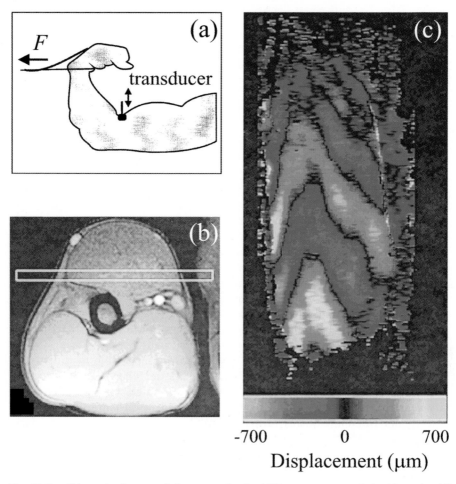

-700   0   700

Displacement (μm)

Fig. 18.7. a Schematic diagram of the set-up for the MRE measurements of the biceps brachii muscle under loading conditions. **b** Normal axial MR image of the arm. **c** MRE wave image at a single phase in the coronal slice indicated by the rectangle in **b**. Courtesy of M.A. Dresner et al. [69]: "Magnetic resonance elastography of skeletal muscle," J Magn Reson Imaging 13, Copyright © 2001. Reprinted by permission of Wiley-Liss Inc., a subsidiary of John Wiley & Sons, Inc

Magnetic Resonance Spectroscopy

In vivo ^{1}H and ^{31}P MRS might yield information of potential value in pressure ulcer research. ^{1}H spectroscopy provides a window on energy and fat metabolism, while ^{31}P MRS yields more specific biochemical information on tissue bioenergetics (for introductory reading see e.g. refs. [18, 21, 75]). Figure 18.8 shows examples of ^{1}H and ^{31}P NMR spectra from human skeletal muscle, using a magnetic field of 1.5 T.

The most sensitive nucleus for MRS is ^{1}H. Figure 8a shows a localized ^{1}H NMR spectrum of human skeletal muscle. During acquisition the high

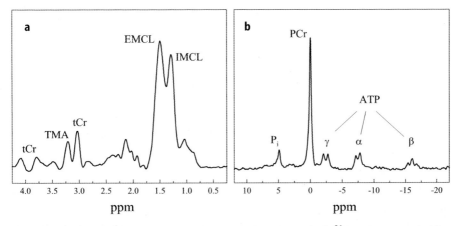

Fig. 18.8. a Localized ^{1}H NMR spectrum of human skeletal muscle. b ^{31}P NMR spectrum of human skeletal muscle. Courtesy of J. J. Prompers, Eindhoven

signal from free water is suppressed, to obtain a spectrum with the peaks of several metabolites that contain protons. From left to right the peaks correspond to methyl and methylene protons of creatine and phosphocreatine (total creatine = tCr), to protons in trimethylammonium groups (TMA), and to methyl and methylene protons of extra- and intramyocellular lipids (EMCL and IMCL). Creatine and phosphocreatine serve as a major energy buffer in muscle, and fatty acids are the main fuel for ATP synthesis. Lactate, an important marker for tissue ischaemia and hypoxia [75–78], cannot be observed in this spectrum because it is masked by the large lipid signals and occurs only in low levels in resting muscle. Two-dimensional NMR or spectral editing techniques are necessary to observe lactate in human skeletal muscle [78–81].

Figure 18.8 b shows a ^{31}P spectrum of human skeletal muscle. From left to right the peaks correspond to inorganic phosphate (Pi), phosphocreatine (PCr), and the three phosphate groups (a, β, γ) of ATP. The ^{31}P spectrum reflects the metabolic state of the tissue. Biologically relevant parameters, such as intracellular pH, free magnesium concentrations, and ADP concentrations, can be deduced.

MRS is much less sensitive than MRI because it measures metabolites that are present in millimolar concentrations, while tissue water that is utilized for MRI is present in bulk amounts. Consequently, MRS is usually restricted to measuring signal from a relatively large amount of tissue. For example, a rough estimate shows that a minimum volume of 30 cm^3 is needed to measure the ^{31}P ATP signal of skeletal muscle at 1.5 T with sufficiently high signal-to-noise ratio [81]. Volume selection can be achieved by applying single-voxel localization techniques or by using surface coils, which record the signals from a restricted area only. Multi-voxel localization and spectroscopic imaging techniques can be used to obtain spatially resolved metabolic information [21].

Summary and Future Perspective

As we have illustrated, there is a broad range of structural, functional, as well as metabolic parameters that can be measured non-invasively by MRI and MRS under in vivo conditions in humans and laboratory animals. This makes MR ideally suited for the detection and characterization of pressure ulcers. Most MRI and MRS techniques can be combined in a single experiment, which makes the information density of MR very high. T_1, T_2 and diffusion weighting provide the basic contrast, capable of detecting pressure ulcer pathology, e.g. oedema, inflammation and haemorrhage. Perfusion MR and MRS capture the nutrient flow and metabolic state of the tissue. Combinations of MR tagging, diffusion tensor imaging and MRE can provide information on geometry, fibre orientation, deformation behaviour and material parameters, indispensable for the mathematical modelling of the behaviour of muscle under pressure.

To conclude, MR is expected to gain importance and establish itself as an essential tool both in the clinical assessment of pressure ulcers and in research on pressure ulcer aetiology.

References

1. May DA, Disler DG, Jones EA, Balkissoon AA, Manaster AA (2000) Abnormal signal intensity in skeletal muscle at MR imaging: patterns, pearls, and pitfalls. Radiographics 20:S295–S315
2. Revelon G, Rahmouni A, Jazaerli N, Godeau B, Chosidow O, Authier J, Mathieu D, Roujeau JC, Vasile N (1999) Acute swelling of the limbs: magnetic resonance pictorial review of fascial and muscle signal changes Eur J Radiol 30:11–21
3. Nguyen B, Brandser E, Rubin DA (2000) Pains, strains, and fasciculations: lower extremity muscle disorders. Magn Reson Imaging Clin N Am 8:391–408
4. Reimers CD, M Finkenstaedt M (1997) Muscle imaging in inflammatory myopathies. Curr Opin Rheumatol 9:475–485
5. Beltran J (1995) MR imaging of soft-tissue infection. Magn Reson Imaging Clin N Am 3:743–751
6. Ruiz-Cabello J, Regadera J, Santisteban C, Grana M, Alejo RP, Echave I, Aviles P, Rodriguez I, Santos I, Gargallo D, Cortijo M (2002) Monitoring acute inflammatory processes in mouse muscle by MR imaging and spectroscopy: a comparison with pathological results. NMR Biomed 15:204–214
7. Berquist TH (ed) (2001) MRI of the musculoskeletal system. Lippincott Williams & Wilkins, Philadelphia
8. Hencey JY, Vermess M, van Geertruyden HH, Binard JE, Manchepalli S (1996) Magnetic resonance imaging examinations of gluteal decubitus ulcers in spinal cord injury patients. J Spinal Cord Med 19:5–8
9. Rubayi S, Soma C, Wang A (1993) Diagnosis and treatment of iliopsoas abscess in spinal cord injury patients. Arch Phys Med Rehabil 74:1186–1191
10. Huang AB, Schweitzer ME, Hume E, Batte WG (1998) Osteomyelitis of the pelvis/hips in paralyzed patients: accuracy and clinical utility of MRI. J Comput Assist Tomogr 22:437–443

11. Ruan M, Escobedo E, Harrison S, Goldstein B (1998) Magnetic resonance imaging of nonhealing pressure ulcers and myocutaneous flaps. Arch Phys Med Rehabil 79:1080–1088

12. Daniel RK, Priest DL, Wheatley DC (1981) Etiologic factors in pressure sores: an experimental model. Arch Phys Med Rehab 62:492–498

13. Salcido R, Donofrio JC, Fisher SB, LeGrand EK, Dickey K, Carney JM, Schosser R, Liang R (1994) Histopathology of pressure ulcers as a result of sequential computer-controlled pressure sessions in a fuzzy rat model. Adv Wound Care 7:23–24, 26, 28

14. Goldstein B, Sanders J (1998) Skin response to repetitive mechanical stress: a new experimental model in pig. Arch Phys Med Rehab 79:265–272

15. Peirce SM, Skalak TC, Rodeheaver GT (2000) Ischemia-reperfusion injury in chronic pressure ulcer formation: a skin model in the rat. Wound Repair Regen 8:68–76

16. Bosboom EMH, Bouten CVC, Oomens CWJ, Baaijens FPT, Nicolay K (2003) High-resolution MRI to assess skeletal muscle damage after prolonged transverse loading. J Appl Physiol 96:2235–2250

17. Callaghan PT (1991) Principles of nuclear magnetic resonance microscopy. Oxford University Press, Oxford

18. Gadian DG (1995) NMR and its applications to living systems. Oxford University Press, Oxford

19. Vlaardingerbroek MT, Den Boer JD (1999) Magnetic resonance imaging. Springer, Berlin Heidelberg New York

20. Haacke EM, Brown RW, Thompson MR, Venkatesan R (1999) Magnetic resonance imaging: physical principles and sequence design. Wiley, New York

21. De Graaf R (1998) In vivo NMR spectroscopy:principles and techniques. Wiley, Chichester

22. Venkatesan R, Lin W, Haacke EM (1998) Accurate determination of spin-density and T_1 in the presence of RF-field inhomogeneities and flip-angle miscalibration. Magn Reson Med 40:592–602

23. Breger RK, Yetkin FZ, Fischer ME, Papke RA, Haughton VM, Rimm AA, (1991) T_1 and T_2 in the cerebrum: correlation with age, gender, and demographic factors. Radiology 181:545–547

24. Breger RK, Rimm AA, Fischer ME, Papke RA, Haughton VM (1989) T_1 and T_2 measurements on a 1.5-T commercial MR imager. Radiology 171:273–276

25. Bottomley PA, Foster TH, Argersinger RE, Pfeifer LM (1984) A review of normal tissue hydrogen NMR relaxation times and relaxation mechanisms from 1–100 MHz: dependence on tissue type, NMR frequency, temperature, species, excision, and age. Med Phys 11:425–448

26. Ryan TJ (1990) Cellular responses to tissue distortion. In: Bader DL (ed) Pressure sores: clinical practice and scientific approach. Macmillan, London

27. Landsman AS, Meaney DF, Cargill RS, Macarak EJ, Thibault LE (1995) 1995 William J. Stickel Gold Award. High strain rate tissue deformation. A theory on the mechanical etiology of diabetic foot ulcerations. J Am Podiatr Med Assoc 85:519–527

28. Bouten CV, Knight MM, Lee DA, Bader DL (2001) Compressive deformation and damage of muscle cell subpopulations in a model system. Ann Biomed Eng 29:153–163

29. Bosboom EM, Hesselink MK, Oomens CW, Bouten CV, Drost MR, Baaijens FP (2001) Passive transverse mechanical properties of skeletal muscle under in vivo compression. J Biomech 34:1365–1368

30. Bosboom EM (2001) Deformation as a trigger for pressure sore related muscle damage. PhD thesis, Eindhoven University of Technology, ISBN 90-386-2962-1
31. Bouten CV, Breuls RG, Peeters EA, Oomens CW, Baaijens FP (2003) In vitro models to study compressive strain-induced muscle cell damage. Biorheology 40:383–388
32. Axel L,Dougherty L (1989) MR imaging of motion with spatial modulation of magnetization. Radiology 171:841–845
33. Reeder SB, Du YP, Lima JA, Bluemke DA (2001) Advanced cardiac MR imaging of ischemic heart disease. Radiographics 21:1047–1074
34. Stesjkal EO, Tanner JE (1965) Spin diffusion measurements: spin echoes in the presence of a time dependent field gradient. J Chem Phys 288–292
35. Le Bihan D, Breton E, Lallemand D, Grenier P, Cabanis E, Laval-Jeantet M (1986) MR imaging of intravoxel incoherent motions: application to diffusion and perfusion in neurologic disorders. Radiology 161:401–407
36. Hoehn M, Nicolay K, Franke C, van der Sanden B (2001) Application of magnetic resonance to animal models of cerebral ischemia. J Magn Reson Imaging 14:491–509
37. Maier CF, Paran Y, Bendel P, Rutt BK, Degani H (1997) Quantitative diffusion imaging in implanted human breast tumors. Magn Reson Med 37:576–581
38. Karczmar GS, River JN, Goldman Z, Li J, Weisenberg E, Lewis MZ, Liu K (1994) Magnetic resonance imaging of rodent tumors using radiofrequency gradient echoes Magn Reson Imaging 12:881–893
39. Lang P, Wendland MF, Saeed M, Gindele A, Rosenau W, Mathur A, Gooding CA, Genant HK (1998) Osteogenic sarcoma: noninvasive in vivo assessment of tumor necrosis with diffusion-weighted MR imaging. Radiology 206:227–235
40. Baur A, Reiser MF (2000) Diffusion-weighted imaging of the musculoskeletal system in humans. Skeletal Radiol 29:555–562
41. Le Bihan D, Mangin JF, Poupon C, Clark CA, Pappata S, Molko N, Chabriat H (2001) Diffusion tensor imaging: concepts and applications. J Magn Reson Imaging 13:534–546
42. Neil J, Miller J, Mukherjee P, Huppi PS (2002) Diffusion tensor imaging of normal and injured developing human brain – a technical review NMR Biomed 15:543–552
43. Sotak CH (2002) The role of diffusion tensor imaging in the evaluation of ischemic brain injury – a review. NMR Biomed 15:561–569
44. Lim KO, Helpern JA (2002) Neuropsychiatric applications of DTI – a review. NMR Biomed 15:587–593
45. van Doorn A, Bovendeerd PH, Nicolay K, Drost MR, Janssen JD (1996) Determination of muscle fibre orientation using diffusion-weighted MRI. Eur J Morphol 34:5–10
46. Van Donkelaar CC, Kretzers LJ, Bovendeerd PH, Lataster LM, Nicolay K, Janssen JD, Drost MR (1999) Diffusion tensor imaging in biomechanical studies of skeletal muscle function. J Anat 194 (Pt 1):79–88
47. Damon AM, Ding Z, Anderson AW, Freyer AS, Gore JC (2002) Validation of diffusion tensor MRI-based muscle fiber tracking. Magn Reson Med 48:97–104
48. Napadow VJ, Chen Q, Mai V, So PT, Gilbert RJ (2001) Quantitative analysis of three-dimensional-resolved fiber architecture in heterogeneous skeletal muscle tissue using nmr and optical imaging methods. Biophys J 80:2968–2975

49. Sinha U, L Yao L (2002) In vivo diffusion tensor imaging of human calf muscle. J Magn Reson Imaging 15:87–95
50. Bonny JM, Renou JP (2002) Water diffusion features as indicators of muscle structure ex vivo. Magn Reson Imaging 20:395–400
51. Kosiak M (1966) An effective method of preventing decubital ulcers. Arch Phys Med Rehabil 47:724–729
52. Dinsdale SM (1974) Decubitus ulcers: role of pressure and friction in causation. Arch Phys Med Rehabil 55:147–152
53. Guy RH, Tur E, Maibach HI (1985) Optical techniques for monitoring cutaneous microcirculation: recent applications. Int J Dermatol 24:88–94
54. Raynaud JS, Duteil S, Vaughan JT, Hennel F, Wary C, Leroy-Willig A, Carlier PG (2001) Determination of skeletal muscle perfusion using arterial spin labeling NMRI: validation by comparison with venous occlusion plethysmography. Magn Reson Med 46:305–311
55. P. Nuutila, Kalliokoski K (2000) Use of positron emission tomography in the assessment of skeletal muscle and tendon metabolism and perfusion. Scand J Med Sci Sports 10:346–350
56. Saltin B, Radegran G, Koskolou MD, Roach RC (1998) Skeletal muscle blood flow in humans and its regulation during exercise. Acta Physiol Scand 162:421–436
57. Barbier EL, Lamalle L, Decorps M (2001) Methodology of brain perfusion imaging. J Magn Reson Imaging 13:496–520
58. Calamante F, Thomas DL, Pell GS, Wiersma J, Turner R (1999) Measuring cerebral blood flow using magnetic resonance imaging techniques. J Cereb Blood Flow Metab 19:701–735
59. Frank LR, Wong EC, Haseler LJ, Buxton RB (1999) Dynamic imaging of perfusion in human skeletal muscle during exercise with arterial spin labeling. Magn Reson Med 42:258–267
60. Luo Y, Mohning KM, Hradil VP, Wessale JL, Segreti JA, Nuss ME, Wegner CD, Burke SE, Cox BF (2002) Evaluation of tissue perfusion in a rat model of hind-limb muscle ischemia using dynamic contrast-enhanced magnetic resonance imaging. J Magn Reson Imaging 16:277–283
61. Muthupillai R, Lomas DJ, Rossman PJ, Greenleaf JF, Manduca A, Ehman RL (1995) Magnetic resonance elastography by direct visualization of propagating acoustic strain waves. Science 269:1854–1857
62. Muthupillai R, Rossman PJ, Lomas DJ, Greenleaf JF, Riederer SJ, Ehman RL (1996) Magnetic resonance imaging of transverse acoustic strain waves. Magn Reson Med 36:266–274
63. Muthupillai R, Ehman RL (1996) Magnetic resonance elastography. Nat Med 2:601–603
64. Kruse SA, Smith JA, Lawrence AJ, Dresner MA, Manduca A, Greenleaf JF, Ehman RL (2000) Tissue characterization using magnetic resonance elastography: preliminary results. Phys Med Biol 45:1579–1590
65. Manduca A, Oliphant TE, Dresner MA, Mahowald JL, Kruse SA, Amromin E, Felmlee JP, Greenleaf JF, Ehman RL (2001) Magnetic resonance elastography: non-invasive mapping of tissue elasticity. Med Image Anal 5:237–254
66. McKnight AL, Kugel JL, Rossman PJ, Manduca A, Hartmann LC, Ehman RL (2002) MR elastography of breast cancer: preliminary results. Am J Roentgenol 178:1411–1417
67. Lorenzen J, Sinkus R, Lorenzen M, Dargatz M, Leussler C, Roschmann P, Adam G (2002) MR elastography of the breast: preliminary clinical results. Rofo Fortschr Geb Rontgenstr Neuen Bildgeb Verfahr 174:830–834

68. McCracken PJ, Manduca A, Felmlee JP, Ehman RL (2002) Mechanical transient-based MR elastography. Proc Intl Soc Mag Reson Med 10
69. Dresner MA, Rose GH, Rossman PJ, Muthupillai R, Manduca A, Ehman RL (2001) Magnetic resonance elastography of skeletal muscle. J Magn Reson Imaging 13:269–276
70. Jenkyn TR, Kaufman KR, An KN, Ehman RL (2002) Change in relaxed muscle stiffness due to joint positioning measured in vivo using magnetic resonance elastography. Proc Intl Soc Magn Reson Med 10
71. Sack I, Tolxdorff J, Bernarding T, Braun J (2002) Simulation of MR elastography wave images measured in the biceps brachii. Proc Intl Soc Magn Reson Med 10
72. Uffmann, Mateiescu S, Quick HH, Lado ME (2002) In vivo determination of biceps elasticity with MR elastography. Proc Intl Soc Magn Reson Med 10
73. Budinger TF, Benaron DA, Koretsky AP (1999) Imaging transgenic animals. Annu Rev Biomed Eng 1:611–648
74. Behar L, den Hollander JA, Stromski ME, Ogino T, Shulman RG, Petroff OA, Prichard JW (1983) High-resolution 1H nuclear magnetic resonance study of cerebral hypoxia in vivo. Proc Natl Acad Sci USA 80:4945–4948
75. Berkelbach, van der Sprenkel JW, Luyten PR, van Rijen PC, Tulleken CA, den Hollander JA (1988) Cerebral lactate detected by regional proton magnetic resonance spectroscopy in a patient with cerebral infarction. Stroke 19:1556–1560
76. Fenstermacher I, Narayana PA (1990) Serial proton magnetic resonance spectroscopy of ischemic brain injury in humans. Invest Radiol 25:1034–1039
77. Duijn JH, Matson GB, Maudsley AA, Hugg JW, Weiner MW (1992) Human brain infarction: proton MR spectroscopy. Radiology 183:711–718
78. Pan JW, Hamm JR, Hetherington HP, Rothman DL, Shulman RG (1991) Correlation of lactate and pH in human skeletal muscle after exercise by 1H NMR. Magn Reson Med 20:57–65
79. Shen D, Gregory CD, Dawson MJ (1996) Observation and quantitation of lactate in oxidative and glycolytic fibers of skeletal muscles. Magn Reson Med 36:30–38
80. Asllani I, Shankland E, Pratum T, Kushmerick M (1999), Anisotropic orientation of lactate in skeletal muscle observed by dipolar coupling in (1)H NMR spectroscopy. J Magn Reson 139:213–224
81. Chatham IC, Blackband SJ (2001) Nuclear magnetic resonance spectroscopy and imaging in animal research. ILAR J 42:189–208

Microelectrodes and Biocompatible Sensors for Skin pO$_2$ Measurements

19

Wen Wang, Pankaj Vadgama

Introduction

The potential of monitoring oxygen (O$_2$) levels on a continuous real-time basis gives the opportunity to both assess dynamic fluctuations and make a predictive assessment of O$_2$ trends in any particular localized environment [1]. Electrochemical and optical (fibre-optic) sensors provide a near ideal means of localized tissue monitoring other than totally non-invasive methods such as the near-infrared monitoring of the inter-converting Hb/HbO$_2$ chromophore pair pioneered by Jöbsis [2] and referred to in Chap. 17. In both electrochemical and optical sensors, a direct interfacial reaction takes place, which can be conveniently amplified and translated into a continuous electrical output using systems suitable for near-patient use. A key capability is that of virtually reagentless measurement in an optically opaque tissue matrix – ideal for subcutaneous measurement. With the advent of miniaturization techniques, including those adapted from the microelectronics industry, ethically acceptable, clinically invasive monitoring becomes feasible.

Application criteria include sensitivity, selectivity, stability, biocompatibility, reliability and overall safety. Undoubtedly, an important route to overcoming many of these problems was to retain sensors behind permselective membranes and appropriate encapsulants [3]. Interfacing with appropriate polymer membrane coverings has permitted the operation of many sensors independently of solution variables presented by the in vivo milieu.

Electrochemical Monitoring

The polarographic principle of electrochemical O$_2$ reduction at a noble metal working electrode polarized at approximately –0.65V vs. Ag/AgCl is well established. However, in the Clark electrode design [4], an O$_2$-permeable membrane separates an entire (two-electrode) electrochemical cell from the unmodified, undiluted biological matrix. This methodology has been the mainstay of implantable O$_2$ sensors. The membrane, typically made of PTFE, has a crucial role in restricting O$_2$ permeability sufficiently to limit evolved diffusion gradients to within the physical confines of the mem-

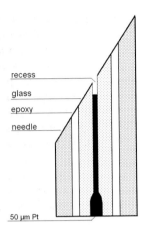

Fig. 19.1. Polarographic 'stab' electrode for tissue pO$_2$ monitoring (after [5])

recess

glass

epoxy

needle

50 µm Pt

brane material itself, so avoiding further impact of sample O$_2$ permeability variation due to sample matrix alteration – a particular consideration when devices are implanted within tissue.

For tissue monitoring such probes need to be of reduced diameter, and have tended to be fragile and difficult to construct. Van der Kleij and de Koning [5] constructed a needle electrode (Fig. 19.1) utilizing a platinum wire cathode of 5 µm diameter insulated in glass, and incorporated into a spinal needle of 0.5 mm bore. Here, to avoid a separate reference electrode, the stainless steel was used as the anode [6]. The key feature is that the working electrode is protected and O$_2$ diffusion gradients are internalized within the fluid column of the recess. This ensures that, as with a low-permeability covering membrane, the diffusion field extending into the tissue matrix is negligible. This means that the O$_2$ flux to the working electrode is independent of sample matrix and only reflects local PO$_2$. Schneiderman and Goldstick [8] examined the influence of recess dimensions and aspect ratios to determine the influence of externalized diffusion fields around the electrode tip. Undoubtedly, a recessed tip structure is able to stabilize O$_2$ measurements and to some extend protect the working electrode surface from biofouling. Indeed, Davies and Brink [8] had previously concluded that recessed-tip electrodes and intermittent voltage pulses to the working electrode were the only means of obtaining reliable pO$_2$ measurements in tissue.

Interest in tissue pO$_2$ has increased in view of the radiosensitization of O$_2$ and the value of relating O$_2$ tension to radiation dose. There was also the realization that steep O$_2$ gradients exist in tissue, and that it was necessary to understand the three-dimensional profile of pO$_2$, particularly in relation to the microcirculation. The additional advantage of using a microelectrode is the limit to the competition for O$_2$ consumption with cells in the immediate environment of the device. Silver [9] discussed the relevant issues and concluded that intermittent sweep potentials applied to the working electrodes reduced O$_2$ consumption and minimized equilibration time, thereby reducing artefactual influences on tissue and facilitating rapid clinical measurement. With the advent of microfabrication, miniaturized planar O_2 electrodes have been produced. In one example, Suzuki [10] produced a 350-µm-depth silicon structure which featured anisotropically etched V-grooves that contained electrolyte and whose surfaces included a cathode (working electrode) and an anode. This internal micro-reaction chamber for the polarographic reduction of O_2 was bounded by a gas-permeable membrane based on a negative photoresist. The membrane provided for electrochemical stability within the device, protected the sensing surface from biofouling and controlled O_2 flux. However, such a Clark-type electrode construction, whilst having advantages for bio-interfacing, does complicate microdevice construction and scale up of production. A commercially available medical system is that marketed by Eppendorf. This microelectrode comprises a recessed gold–platinum wire combination in an insulating glass needle, in turn housed within a 300-µm o.d. protective needle. The recessed gold surface is membrane protected, and so approximates to the desired structure for tissue measurements. Automated sub-millimetre advance and retraction within the tissue allows multiple location measurements, but with post-retraction measurement the problems of tissue compression are obviated. Tama-Dasu et al. [11] related the putative O_2 consumption of the electrode tip to simulated tissue measurements by differentially weighting O_2 at different 3-D locations in tissue. They concluded that, for limited measuring times, O_2 transport from more distant locations will be restricted; therefore, what the electrode provides is an "averaged" approximation of the time value of clinical validity, which is not appropriate for data input into more formal tissue-modelling procedures. By contrast, direct, free quantitative consumption of O_2 by a large electrode applied to the liver surface (Ag working electrode, diameter 3 mm) was used intentionally by Seifalian et al. [12] to measure perfusion-driven delivery of O_2 to the liver. The electrode had a highly permeable covering membrane. Such a construction could, perhaps, provide a measure of changes to the cutaneous circulation.

However, for non-invasive monitoring of the skin, the conventional approach has been that of the heated transcutaneous pO_2 electrode [13]. Here, heating permeabilizes the thick outer stratum corneum of skin to allow rapid O_2 diffusion. The route taken involves numerous biological barriers, but heating stabilizes, and also arterializes, the dermal capillary bed. Whilst accuracy is compromised in thicker adult skin relative to neonatal skin, where the electrode has seen most application, Stücker et al. [14] used such an electrode to measure O_2 consumption by the skin in patients with chronic venous skin lesions. They measured transcutaneous pO_2 reduction after arresting arterial O_2 supply. Using the pO_2 solubility coefficient for skin, they were then able to determine skin O_2 consumption differences between patients with and without venous ulceration. Evident lowering of transcutaneous pO_2 was judged to be a late-onset phenomenon.

A more distributive assessment of tissue O_2, short of a 3-D O_2 map is to create a pO_2 distribution profile. Using the Eppendorf short penetration/retraction procedure, Nozue et al. [15] undertook a thorough evaluation of pO$_2$ distribution in defined turnover volumes. There was semi-quantitative agreement between laboratories concerning the turnover hypoxic zones, and such a methodology could also enable more quantitative assessment of skin hypoxia.

Fibre-Optic O$_2$ Sensors

Optically based O$_2$ sensors almost all exploit the interference of O$_2$ on the quantum yield and/or lifetime of excited fluorescent or phosphorescent molecules. Specially formulated dyes with high-efficiency O$_2$ quenching have allowed for the fabrication of miniaturized fibre-optic probes able to monitor pO$_2$ over the medically important range [16]. The reversible, dynamic quenching occurs through the formation of an O$_2$ charge–transfer complex on collision of O$_2$ with the excited fluorophore which, in turn, leads to non-radiative transfer to the ground state. For the purposes of invasive, transcutaneous monitoring, it is optimal to attach the reagent to the fibre-optic tip. The fibre-optic probe of Peterson and Vurek [17] translated the principle of O$_2$-quenched fluorescence of a dye to a practical solution (Fig. 19.2). The advantage of this approach is that the electrode truly approaches equilibrium, and so does not consume O$_2$ as such, there is no dependence on external tissue flux, and so the device is independent of sample properties. Moreover, there is no external electrical interference. A simple probe can be used, without the need for a reference electrode. Flexibility of fibre-optics is certainly a disadvantage with respect to implantation, but if, for example, a narrow needle (Fig. 19.2) or indeed a retractable needle is used, then insertion is possible. The remaining device is a tissue-compliant, flexible probe that is less liable to induce pain, tissue irritation or ongoing trauma.

There is interest, now, in the development of microscale optical probes with tip diameters in the range of 10–30 µm. To further create compact systems, the O$_2$-quenched indicator requires activation by a light-emitting diode (LED) and a luminescent lifetime of greater than 1 µs [18]. Ruthenium (II) tris(dipyridye)-type organometallic complexes have proved attractive for this reason; they can have fluorescence lifetimes up to 5.0 µs,

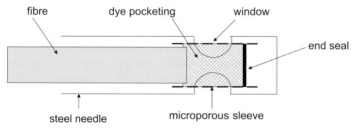

Fig. 19.2. Fibre-optic O$_2$ sensor based on dye fluorescence quenching exploitation of microporous membrane to retain perylene dibutyrate dye (after [49])

i.e. efficiently quenched by O$_2$, excitation wavelengths (approximately 460 nm) suited to blue LEDs and demonstrate large stokes shifts (emission maxima ~ 600 nm). Variants on the organometallic model include ruthenium and platinum phosphorescent complexes with porphyrins, which have proved attractive for microelectrodes because of strong phosphorescence, the ease of polymer matrix entrapment and high phosphorescence yields [19].

For microelectrode fabrication, the simple basic rules include [18]:

- An indicator of activity per unit area
- Mechanical integrity with strong adherence to the optical interface
- A higher degree of rigidity to the immobilizing matrices than for conventional, larger electrodes (viz. PMMA, sol gels).

With optimization of the retaining polymer matrix, it is possible to create multi-element arrays [20] not only for topological and spatial resolution, but to permit more sophisticated multivariate analysis for self-correction and measurement verification during use. Conversion to a practical structure was reported by Holst et al. [21], who formed multiple flame-tapered optode tips of 20–30 µm (Fig. 19.3) and retained indicator within a polystyrene matrix. They used reduced lifetime of the luminescence to determine O$_2$ quenching, thereby avoiding the effects of dye photobleaching, optical background, sample optical properties and the complicating effects of add-on optical insulation. The operational set-up utilized sinusoidal light excitation and the dye lifetime decay induced a phase delay in emitted light. Phase-angle shift allowed measurement of O$_2$ flux over the forearm skin surface from atmospheric air using a planar dye-loaded sensor foil [22]. In these studies, cuff inflation to occlude local circulation led to a drop in superficial skin pO$_2$ and therefore an increased air–skin pO$_2$ gradient, facilitating pO$_2$ uptake from the ambient air. Andrezejewski et al. [23] simplified the task of microsecond light decay processing by measuring signal amplitudes at two distinct frequencies for differentiated light modulation, readily followed by lock-in amplifiers instead of high-speed photodetectors.

For long-term monitoring, photobleaching is a concern, with evidence that, as well as expected decreases in emission intensity, decay time may also be affected. Hartmann et al. [24] monitored the contributory effects of singlet O$_2$ (produced by quenching) on photobleaching, and were able to mitigate these through co-incorporation of amine singlet O$_2$ scavengers.

The principle of fluorescence lifetime decay has been used for skin surface pO$_2$ imaging, on the basis that multiple electrode arrays cannot provide equivalent spatial resolution. Hartmann et al. [24] developed ruthenium (II) organometallic-based O$_2$ permeable films, and topographical lifetime images were obtained that related to spatial O$_2$ distribution on a submillimetre scale using a CCD camera. Transparent planar O$_2$ sensors for such imaging have been developed by Holst and Grunwald [25], who embedded ruthenium (II)-tris-4, 7-diphenyl-1, 10-phenanthroline with trimethylsilylpropanesulphonate as counter-ion in PVC coated over transpar-

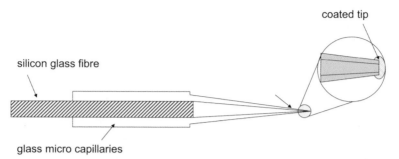

Fig. 19.3. O$_2$ microelectrode based on a tapered silicon glass fibre fixed in a glass microcapillary (after [21])

ent polyester. The advantage of the transparent construction is that pO$_2$ distribution can be correlated directly with structural images.

Future optical sensors will have greater stability and biocompatibility. However, improvements in optical characteristics such as excitation/emission maxima, air/nitrogen indicator stability, quantum yield and decay profile are likely with new indicators and better polymeric immobilization strategies [26].

Cutaneous Microcirculation

The cutaneous microcirculation has a unique anatomical arrangement that accommodates different often conflicting functions, namely, the supply of nutrients, clearance of waste products and control of heat exchange [27]. The arterial supply and venous drainage to the skin are located deep in the hypodermis. They give rise to arterioles and venules to form two important plexuses in the dermis: the deeper cutaneous plexus at the junction of the hypodermis and the dermis and the superficial sub-papillary plexus just beneath the dermal papillae [28]. The sub-papillary plexus supplies the upper layer of the dermis and gives rise to a capillary loop in each dermal papilla. In the epidermis, cells produced by mitosis in the germinal layer undergo different stages of maturation and move progressively to the outer layers. The cornified layer in the outermost region of the skin consists of flattened cell remnants that are constantly shed (Fig. 19.4).

The superficial layer of the skin is the region between the sub-papillary plexus and the surface of the skin. While there is recent evidence that O$_2$ entering the skin from the atmosphere may satisfy the O$_2$ requirements of the cells in these areas [29], there has been no investigation of counter-current-arranged capillary loops in the papilla and their significance to O$_2$ delivery to the epidermis [30, 31]. While there have been many studies on mechanisms of O$_2$ transport within tissues, including the skin (see reviews by Scheuplein and Blank [32]; Popel [33] and Pittman [34]), much of the experimental work on skin has been limited to estimates of mean tissue

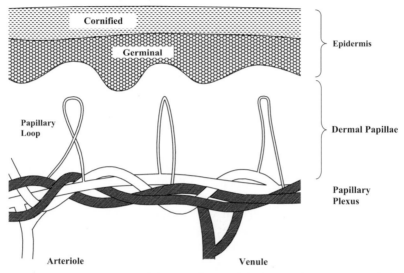

Fig. 19.4. Diagrammatic representation of the outer layers of the human skin, consisting of the dermal papillae and the epidermis. The papillary plexus gives rise to a single papillary loop in each dermal papilla. Cells in the epidermis undergo maturation from the germinal layer adjacent to the dermal papillae to the stratum corneum in the outermost layer, which is shed continuously

pO$_2$ from measurements of transcutaneous pO$_2$ or has used needle electrodes that were large relative to the dermal papillae [35–39]. There have been few attempts to relate the spatial distribution of pO2 to the arrangement of the cutaneous microcirculation using small, O$_2$-sensitive microelectrodes [1]. This study examined the distribution of pO$_2$ in the epidermis and dermal papillae in the skin of the finger nailfolds of healthy human subjects, when entry of O$_2$ from the atmosphere has been minimized by covering the skin surface with oil. Nailfolds were chosen for easy visualization of the microvascular architecture, since the cornified epithelium is thin and the most distal papillary loops lie almost parallel to the skin surface. The authors have also investigated changes in tissue pO$_2$ when the blood flow in adjacent capillaries is stopped and later re-started. In this chapter, we draw attention to this study in detail.

Microelectrodes for pO$_2$ Distribution in Superficial Layers of Human Skin

In studies using small microelectrodes, pO$_2$ measurements are limited to the superficial layers of the skin, since the penetration of deeper skin and underlying muscle requires much stronger, hence bigger, electrodes. O$_2$-sensitive microelectrodes were made using platinum–iridium wire, of 25 µm diameter, which was electrochemically etched to a slender profile with tip diameter less than 1 µm in saturated nitric acid solution. It was soldered to a conducting wire and was then fixed inside a 1.5-mm standard-walled glass pipette using the epoxy resin Araldite [40]. The glass pipette was mounted on a micropipette puller, which pulled the electrode to the desired tip size and profile and ensured that the glass sealed around the top of the wire. The tip of the electrode was bevelled using a micropipette grinder to enable easy tissue penetration. The surface of the metal electrodes was cleaned by sonication in distilled deionized water and was coated with Nafion perfluorinated ion exchange resin.

To investigate the effects of occluding the local microcirculation on the tissue pO$_2$, some electrodes were made with a special φ-shaped tip by repeated heating of the tip of the pulled electrode and fusing a small glass bead to the shaft approximately 200 μm above the tip. These microelectrodes behaved identically to conventional ones as they penetrated the tissue up to the depth at which the bulbous region of the glass shield came into contact with the skin surface. Further advance of the electrode compressed the underlying tissue, occluding the local microcirculation. This provided a convenient method for investigating the transient effects of microcirculatory arrest upon tissue pO$_2$.

It is not uncommon for electrodes of this size to break during experiments, often as a result of the unconscious movements of the finger. Penetration of skin and advance of electrodes in tissue were also occasionally responsible. Prior to the experiment, the stratum corneum was removed for easier electrode penetration using adhesive tape. The reference electrode (Ag/AgCl ECG electrode) was placed on the skin near the finger. The microelectrode was mounted on a 3-D remote hydraulic micromanipulator (Narishige, Japan) which, in turn, was mounted on a tri-axial coarse micromanipulator (Narishige, Japan). Both the working and the reference electrodes were connected to the potentiostat (CV37; BAS). Currents from the potentiostat at −0.75 V vs Ag/AgCl were recorded on a chart recorder.

Skin was illuminated using a cool light source. Paraffin oil was superfused over the finger to minimize transport of O$_2$ from the air and to reduce light reflections from the surface of the skin. A Wild M10 stereomicroscope (Leica) was used to visualize nailfold capillaries and flows in these capillaries. Although blood flow velocity was not estimated, the red blood cells were used as markers to indicate flow conditions, namely whether the blood flow had partially or fully stopped or was reinstated. The coarse micromanipulator was used to position an electrode just above the site of the measurement, while the remote hydraulic micromanipulator was used for the penetration of the skin and movement of the electrode within the tissue. In all measurements, the O$_2$ partial pressure of the air was considered to be 160 mmHg at sea level and at room temperature.

Spatial Variations of pO$_2$ in Superficial Layers of Skin

Mean values for the spatial variations of the pO$_2$ with depth in the outer skin are presented in Fig. 19.5. In Fig. 19.5a, mean pO$_2$ has been plotted for the superficial (5–10 µm), the middle (45–65 µm) and the deep (100–120 µm) regions in the dermal papillae of finger nailfolds. It is seen that the pO$_2$ increases with depth from the surface of the skin to the dermis. With paraffin oil applied, pO$_2$ was lowest at the surface of the skin. In the superficial region of the skin, pO$_2$ is approximately 8.0 ± 3.2 mmHg ($n = 6$). The value increases to 24.0 ± 6.4 mmHg ($n = 8$) in dermal papillae, and at the depth just above the sub-papillary plexus, pO$_2$ is approximately

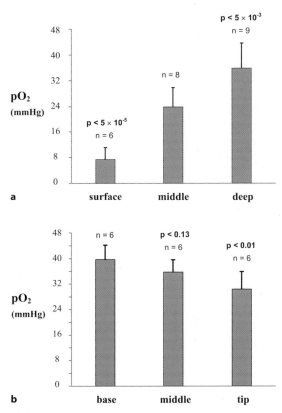

Fig. 19.5. Spatial variations of pO$_2$ in outer layers of nailfold skin. **a** Mean values for pO$_2$ at depths of 5–10 µm (*surface*), 45–65 µm (*middle*) and 100–120 µm (*deep*) in all areas of nailfold skin. The pO$_2$ at the surface and in the deep regions differ very significantly from those in the middle region ($p < 0.00005$ and $p < 0.005$ respectively). **b** Mean values for pO$_2$ with depth in tissue close to the axis of the capillary loops of the papillae. While pO$_2$ at the tip differs significantly from its value at the base ($p < 0.01$), the gradient is too small for significant differences to be detected between the pO$_2$ of the tissues around the middle of the capillary loops and the pO$_2$ at the tip and the base

35.2±8.0 mmHg ($n=9$). Analysis of variance (ANOVA) of the three sets of data showed highly statistically significant differences. Two-tailed Student's t-test yielded a p value of 0.005 or lower.

The pO₂ value was also measured along the axis of papillary loops. These measurements were carried out with the microelectrode tip at points in the tissue that were close to the most distal (and hence most horizontal) capillary loops of the nailfold. As shown in Fig. 19.5b, pO₂ generally decreased from the base to the tip of the papillary loop. At the base of the loop, pO₂ is approximately 40±4.8 mmHg ($n=6$), decreasing to 35.2±3.2 mmHg in the middle ($n=6$) and 30.4±5.2 mmHg near the tip of the loop ($n=6$). ANOVA of the three data sets confirmed statistically significant variations in the pO₂ along the axis of papillary loops. Student's t-test revealed that $p<0.01$ between data at the base and the tip of the papillary loop; however, the differences between values at the base and the middle of the papillary loop, and between those at the middle and the tip of the loop, were not statistically significant ($p>0.05$).

Temporal Variations in pO₂ Following Micro-Occlusion

Special ϕ-shaped electrodes were used to investigate the transient changes in skin pO₂ when the microcirculation is suddenly arrested and restored. In experiments where flow in the capillary and underlying sub-papillary plexus was either reduced or stopped, pO₂ in dermis decreased with the time in all cases by 16–24 mmHg. In several cases, there were initial short-lived increases in pO₂. These were most probably caused by interference from the slight movement of the electrode in the tissue. New steady values in pO₂ were reached within 30–60 s following alterations in capillary flow. The dynamic changes in pO₂ with time can be described by a single exponential decay function:

$$P = a \exp(-t/\tau) + b \tag{19.1}$$

where P is the value of pO₂ during the transient, τ is the time constant, a represents the difference between the initial and final values of pO₂ and b is the final value of pO₂.

After a period of microcirculatory arrest lasting between 1 min and 5 min, flow was restored. The increase in pO₂ can be described by a similar single exponential function:

$$P = a^* (-t/\tau^*) + b^* \tag{19.2}$$

where τ^* is the time constant for the exponential rise and a^* and b^* represent the range and the initial value of pO₂.

Time constants for the exponential decays (ischaemia) and rises (reperfusion) in pO₂ are shown in Fig. 19.6a. The mean time constant for the decay ($8.44±1.55$) was significantly higher than the corresponding value for

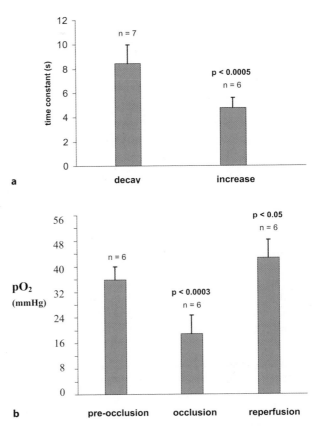

Fig. 19.6. Temporal characteristics in localized microvessel occlusion and reperfusion. **a** Time constants of mono-exponential decays of the pO_2 during microvessel occlusion differed significantly to those of exponential rises in reperfusion ($p < 0.0005$). **b** Mean values for pO_2 before, during and after local reduction in blood flow. After reduction in blood flow, mean pO_2 was significantly reduced ($p < 0.003$). After restoration of flow, pO_2 was increased to levels significantly above the initial control values ($p < 0.05$)

the increase (4.75 ± 0.82), a difference which was statistically significant ($p < 0.001$).

Figure 19.6b shows the steady values of the pO_2 following ischaemia after reperfusion and the values prior to arrest of the microcirculation (the control state). There was a significant decrease in the pO_2 following arrest of the local microcirculation. The pO_2 is reduced by an absolute value of 16 mmHg, representing a 45% decrease. When blood flow is restored pO_2 increases to 43.2 ± 6.4 mmHg, an approximately 125% increase over the ischaemic state value, which in turn is 23% greater than the control. Differences in pO_2 between ischaemia and control, and between ischaemia and reperfusion, were highly significant ($p < 0.001$). There was also significant difference between pO_2 values in control and in reperfusion ($p < 0.05$).

O$_2$ Supply to Skin

The study using small microelectrodes showed that when the skin of the human finger nailfold is covered with paraffin oil, the pO$_2$ in the tissue increases with depth from values close to zero at the surface to about 40–50 mmHg close to the sub-papillary plexus. These agree with previous experimental and theoretical estimates of pO$_2$ in this part of the skin [38, 41–43]. An increase in pO$_2$ with depth would be predicted if all O$_2$ is delivered to the papillary dermis and epidermis from the sub-papillary plexus. Under physiological conditions, however, O$_2$ can enter the outermost layers of the skin from the atmosphere, and recent measurements by Stücker et al. [29] have shown that this influx may be as much as 5.3 ml cm^{-2} min^{-1}, sufficient to meet the needs of the epidermis. Under these conditions the pO$_2$ profile with increasing depth beneath the skin surface might be expected to differ considerably from that reported by Wang et al. [1]. Although there is now strong evidence that O$_2$ can enter the skin from the atmosphere, the latter study demonstrates that when this is prevented, the O$_2$ supply to the epidermis and superficial dermis can be maintained by the papillary microcirculation [1]. There is also a suggestion that the papillary microcirculation is regulated to meet the O$_2$ requirements of the tissue at a very local level.

Effects of Localized Ischaemia–Reperfusion

Wang et al. [1] reported that when flow was stopped, pO$_2$ fell exponentially from a mean value of $\sim$38 mmHg to $\sim$21 mmHg with a mean time constant of just less than 8.5 s. In six of their seven experiments, the recording electrode was close to the sub-papillary plexus, as indicated by relatively high pre-occlusion values of the pO$_2$, i.e. in the range of 40 mmHg. When flow was stopped in vessels close to points near the base of the papillae, pO$_2$ fell to 20–24 mmHg, indicating that the supply of O$_2$ could be maintained, presumably by diffusion from surrounding vessels where microvascular flow was undisturbed. In one of their experiments, however, the electrode tip was at an intermediate depth in the tissue, where the arrest of local capillary flow brought pO$_2$ close to zero. This one observation strongly suggests that O$_2$ supply to the outer papillary dermis and epidermis is absolutely dependent on flow in the closest vessels.

The exponential decline in pO$_2$ when flow is stopped would be consistent with the discharge of O$_2$ from stores in the tissue. The most likely site of these O$_2$ stores is the haemoglobin of the red cells in the capillaries where flow has been arrested. The oxyhaemoglobin dissociation curve is approximately linear over the range of pO$_2$ between 15 mmHg and 40 mmHg, and the unloading of O$_2$ over this range might be expected to approximate to that of a single exponential function.

The rise of pO$_2$ to a new steady state as flow is restored is determined by the rate at which the pO$_2$ in capillaries is returned to their pre-occlusion values. This is primarily dependent on the blood flow velocity in the reperfused capillaries. If the tissue at the tip of the microelectrode is considered to be principally supplied by O_2 from a point along an adjacent capillary, the rate at which capillary pO_2 rises at this point will depend on how rapidly blood with a higher pO_2 reaches that point and how much the blood pO_2 falls between leaving the arteries and arriving at this point. Providing the O_2 consumption of the tissue remains constant, the extraction (i.e. the O_2 lost per unit volume of blood) should be largely dependent on the blood flow. If the post-occlusion flow is greater than in the pre-occlusion state, not only will the pO_2 rise rapidly, but it should rise above its initial level. The tissue pO_2 should then remain above its initial value for as long as the flow is elevated. This was observed in the experimental study. When blood flow is restored, tissue pO_2 rises to a value that is 23% higher than its pre-occlusion value. This is consistent with either a decrease in tissue O_2 consumption or a significant degree of reactive hyperaemia. Assuming that tissue O_2 consumption is the same as in the pre-occlusion state, the 23% increase in pO_2 is equivalent to an increase in O_2 saturation in the blood of the nearest capillaries from 70% to 85%. If the saturation of the arterial blood is 95%, the increase in blood flow equivalent to the rise in tissue pO_2 is of the order of 2.5-fold. This calculation indicates that reactive hyperaemia occurs with a high spatial resolution in skin, and this would be consistent with the very localized hyperaemic responses seen in some other tissues [44]. Although the rise in pO_2 accompanying reperfusion can be described approximately by a single exponential, the data were less regular than those describing the decline in pO_2 with vascular occlusion. This may represent fluctuations in blood flow velocity or red cell flux with the restoration in flow [45].

Future Prospects

The electrochemical and fibre-optic devices described in this chapter are best regarded as semi-implantable, minimally invasive devices. They have the potential to provide localized information on, at least, approximate pO_2 in pre-specified skin and skin ulcer microenvironments. There are two major developments likely to improve spatial discrimination and reliability. First, evolving microfabrication techniques will allow robust probe structures to be fabricated as arrays able to penetrate in and around the ulcer wound site, but with negligible local trauma. This 'atraumatic' insertion should minimize local tissue reaction with less tissue disruption. Devices will then become truly minimally invasive and yet have a high sensor/interrogation density, with features equivalent to a chemically reactive "Velcro". A further advantage will be a high level of sensor redundancy, allowing for greater confidence in the measurements. With appropriate additional microinjection capability along such arrays, it can be envisaged that pharmacologically active agents may be injected locally, e.g. vasodilators to monitor localized circulatory reactivity as a possible dynamic indicator of tissue integrity. The second key advance will come from materials science. Already, membrane technology has improved the stability and biocompatibility of biosensors. Further advances should help to further reduce the inevitable drift that O_2 sensors suffer due to surface fouling and contamination [46].

Other possible advances will exploit tissue-embedded optical nanoprobes coated with, for example, O_2-reactive dyes, so developing the recent concept of probes encapsulated by biologically localized embedding, so-called PEBBLE sensors [47]. Whist such micrometre-scale spheroids have allowed distributed sensing in vitro, the correct formulation may enable safe in vivo use; moreover, with near-infrared active dyes, interrogation of deeper skin layers becomes possible. The ultimate goal must be sensor-based feedback on a real-time basis so that local pO_2, a key surrogate of tissue metabolic status, can be used to optimize therapeutic regimens for pressure ulcers.

Acknowledgement. The authors thank Ms Monika Schoenleber for her help in preparing Figs. 19.1–19.3.

References

1. Wang W, Winlove CP, Michel CC (2003) Oxygen partial pressure in outer layers of skin of human finger nail folds. J Physiol 549 (3):855–863
2. Jöbsis FF (1977) Non invasive infrared monitoring of cerebral and myocardial oxygen insufficiency and circulatory parameters. Science 198:1264–1266
3. McDonnell MB, Vadgama P (1989) Membranes: separation principles and sensing. In: JDR Thomas (ed) Selective electrode reviews, vol 11. Pergamon Press, New York, pp 17–67
4. Clark LC (1956) Monitor and control of blood and tissue oxygen tension. Trans Am Soc Inter Organs 2:41–46
5. van der Kleij JA, de Koning J (1981) Tissue oxygen electrode for routine clinical application. In: Limmich HP (ed) Monitoring of vital parameters during extracorporeal circulation. Karger, Basel, p 95
6. Whalen WJ, Spande JI (1980) A hypodermic needle pO2 electrode. J Appl Physiol 48:186–187
7. Schneiderman G, Goldstick TK (1978) Oxygen electrode design criteria and performance characteristics recessed cathode. J Appl Physiol 45:145–154
8. Davies PW, Brink F (1942) Microelectrodes for measuring local oxygen tension. I. Animal tissues. Rev Sci Instrum 13:524–533
9. Silver IA (1986) In: Akhtar M, Lowe CR, Higgins IJ (eds) Biosensors. Proceedings of the Royal Society Discussion Meeting. The Royal Society, London
10. Suzuki H, Kojima N, Sugame A, Takei F, Ikegami K (1990) Disposable oxygen electrodes fabricated by semi conductor techniques and their application to biosensors. Sensors Actuators B1:528–532
11. Tama-Dasu I, Waites A, Dasu A, Denekamp J (2001) Theoretical simulation of oxygen tension measurement in tissues using a microelectrode. I. The response function of the electrode. Physiol Meas 22:713–725

12. Seifalian AM, Mallett S, Piasecki C, Rolles K, Davidson BR (2000) Non-invasive measurement of hepatic oxygenation by an oxygen electrode in human orthotopic liver transplantation. Med Eng Phys 22:371–377
13. Huich A, Huch R (1976) Transcutaneous, non-invasive monitoring of pO_2. Hosp Pract 6:43–52
14. Stücker M Falkenber M, Reuthor T, Altmeger P, Lübber DW (2000) Local oxygen content in the skin is increased in chronic venous incompetence. Microvascular Res 59:99–106
15. Nozue M, Lee F, Yuan F, Teicher B, Brizel DM, Dewhirst MW et al (1997). Interlaboratories variation of oxygen tension measurement by Eppendorf "Histograph" and comparison with hypoxic marker. J Surg Oncol 66:30–38
16. Wolfbeis OS (1991) Fiber optic chemical sensors and biosensors. CRC Press, Boca Raton, FL
17. Peterson JJ, Vurek GG (1984) Fibre-optic sensors for biomedical applications. Science 224:123
18. Kilmant I, Kühl M, Glud RN, Holst G (1997) Optical measurement of oxygen and temperature in microscale: strategies and biological applications. Sensors Actuators B38:29–37
19. Papkovsky DP, Olah J, Troyanovsky IV, Sadovsky NA, Rumyantseva VD, Mironov AF, Yaropolov AI, Savitsky AP (1991) Phosphorescent polymer films for optical oxygen sensors. Biosensors Bioelectron 7:199–206
20. Gauglitz G, Brecht A (1997) Recent developments in optical transducers for chemical and biochemical applications. Sensors Actuators B38:1–7
21. Holst G, Glud RN, Kühl M, Klimant I (1997) A micro-optode array for fine-scale measurement of oxygen distribution. Sensors Actuators B38:122–129
22. Holst GA, Köster T, Voges E, Lübbers DW (1995) Flox-on oxygen-flue-measuring system using a phase-modulation method to evaluate the oxygen-dependent fluorescence lifetime. Sensors Actuators B29:231–239
23. Andrzejewski D, Klimant I, Podrielska H (2002) Method of lifetime-based chemical sensing using the demodulation of the luminescence signal. Sensors Actuators B84:160–166
24. Hartmann P, Ziegler W, Holst G, Lübbers DW (1997) Oxygen flux fluorescence lifetime imaging. Sensors Actuators B38:110–115
25. Holst G, Grunwald B (2001) Luminescence lifetime imaging with transparent oxygen optodes. Sensors Actuators B74:78–90
26. Papkovsky BD (1995) New oxygen sensors and their application to biosensors. Sensors Actuators, B29:213–218
27. Wheater PR, Burkitt HG, Daniels VG (1979) Functional histology. Churchill Livingstone, New York, pp 116–127
28. Braverman IM (1997) The cutaneous microcirculation: ultrastructure and microanatomical organization. Microcirculation 4:329–340
29. Stücker M, Struk A, Altmeyer P, Herde M, Baumgärtl H, Lübbers DW (2002) The cutaneous uptake of atmospheric oxygen contributes significantly to the oxygen supply of human dermis and epidermis. J Physiol 538 (3):985–994
30. Wang W, Parker KH, Michel CC (1996) Theoretical studies of steady state transcapillary exchange in countercurrent systems. Microcirculation 3:301–311
31. Wang W (2000) A critical parameter for transcapillary exchange of small solutes in countercurrent systems. J Biomech 33:433–441
32. Scheuplein RJ, Blank IH (1971) Permeability of the skin. Physiol Rev 51 (4):702–747

33. Popel AS (1989) Theory of oxygen transport to tissue. Crit Rev Biomed Eng 17:257–321
34. Pittman R (1995) Influence of microvascular architecture on oxygen exchange in skeletal muscle. Microcirculation 2:1–18
35. Evans NTS, Naylor PFD (1966/7) Steady states of oxygen tension in human dermis. Respir Physiol 2:46–60
36. Spence VA, Walker WF (1976) Measurement of oxygen tension in human skin. Med Biol Eng 14:159–165
37. Lübbers DW (1987) Theory and development of trans-cutaneous oxygen pressure measurement. Int Anesthesiol Clin 25 (3):31–65
38. Jaszczak P (1991) Skin oxygen tension, skin oxygen consumption and skin blood flow measured by a tc-pO2 electrode. Acta Physiol Scand 143:53–57
39. Harrison D, Lübbers D, Baumgärtl H, Stoerb C, Rapp S, Altmeyer P, Stücker M (2002) Capillary blood flow and cutaneous uptake of oxygen from the atmosphere. In: Kessler MD, Mueller GJ (eds) Functional monitoring and drug tissue interaction. Proc SPIE 4623:195–205
40. Winlove CP, O'Hare D (1993) Electrochemical method in physiology. Curr Topics Electrochem 2:345–361
41. Grossmann U (1982) Simulation of combined transfer of oxygen and heat through the skin using a capillary-loop model. Math Biosci 61:205–236
42. Baumgärtl H, Ehrly AM, Saeger-Lorenz K, Lubbers DW (1987) Initial results of intracutaneous measurement of PO2 profiles. In: Ehrly AM, Hauss J, Huch R (eds) Clinical oxygen pressure measurement. Springer, Berlin Heidelberg New York, pp 121–128
43. Stücker M, Altmeyer P, Struk A, Hoffmann K, Schulze L, Rochling A, Lübbers DW (2000a) The transepidermal oxygen flux from the environment is in balance with the capillary oxygen supply. J Invest Dermatol 114:533–540
44. Burton KS, Johnson PC (1972) Reactive hyperemia in individual capillaries of skeletal muscle. Am J Physiol 223:517–524
45. Johnson PC, Wayland H (1967) Regulation of blood flow in single capillaries. Am J Physiol 212:1405–1415
46. Reddy SM, Vadgama P (1997) Membranes to improve amperometric sensor characteristics. In: Kress-Rogers E (ed) Handbook of biosensors and electronic noses: medicine, food, and the environment. CRC Press, Boca Raton, FL, pp 111–135
47. Xu H, Aylott JW, Kopelman R, Miller TJ, Philbert MA (2001) A real-time ratiometric method for the determination of molecular oxygen inside living cells using sol-gel based spherical optical nanosensors with applications to rat C6 glioma. Anal Chem 73:4124–4133
48. Stefansson E, Peterson JI, Wang YH (1989) Intraocular oxygen tension measured with a fibre-optic sensor in normal and diabetic drugs. Am J Physiol 256:H1127–H1133

New Tissue Repair Strategies

Debbie Bronneberg, Carlijn Bouten

20

Abbreviations

FGF	Fibroblast growth factor
EGF	Epidermal growth factor
GM-CSF	Granulocyte–macrophage colony-stimulating factor
IFN	Interferon-gamma
IGF	Insulin-like growth factor
IL	Interleukin
NGF	Nerve growth factor
PAF	Platelet-activating factor
PDEGF	Platelet-derived epidermal growth factor
PDGF	Platelet-derived growth factor
TNF	Tumour necrosis factor
TGF	Transforming growth factor
VEGF	Vascular endothelial growth factor

Introduction

Pressure ulcers are localized areas of tissue breakdown in skin and/or underlying tissue [1]. They are initiated by prolonged mechanical loads applied at the interface between skin and supporting surfaces and can be aggravated by a range of predisposing factors, such as the patient's nutritional status and disease. Although pressure ulcers can occur anywhere on the body, they often develop near joints and bony protrusions, e.g. in the trochanteric, ischial, heel, and sacral areas [2]. Patients as well as the clinical and nursing staff may not immediately be aware of these developing wounds, because they often occur in bedridden, paralysed, and elderly subjects undergoing treatments for other diseases. With progression, however, the wounds become painful and more difficult to treat and may considerably affect the patient's quality of life [3].

As is pointed out repeatedly in the first section of this book, the rates of occurrence of pressure ulcers are unacceptably high and represent a burden to the community in terms of health care and money. For instance, in the United States the incidence of pressure ulcers is estimated to be 5–10% among hospitalized patients [2, 4–9], 13% among nursing home patients

[2, 10], and up to 39% among those with spinal cord injuries [2, 11–12]. These high figures are mainly due to limited insights in pressure ulcer aetiology, and hence insufficient possibilities for pressure ulcer prevention, and have triggered substantial efforts to improve strategies for wound treatment and tissue repair.

By definition pressure ulcers are chronic wounds and, therefore, have an underlying physiological impairment that affects the wound-healing process [2]. Apart from reducing interface loads, extensive treatment of these wounds is essential to promote healing of existing ulcers and to prevent development of new ulcers. Today, a wide range of wound treatment strategies is applied with varying success ratios. These strategies include debridement of necrotic tissue and creation of a moist wound-healing environment (e.g. wound dressings). With ongoing developments in biotechnology and life sciences new treatment techniques are being developed, which mainly focus on improving wound healing via biochemical stimulation of the wound bed. The most promising new treatment techniques are discussed in this chapter, such as the exogenous application of growth factors, the application of living, engineered skin grafts, grown outside the body, and the application of gene therapy.

Acute and Chronic Wounds

Normal – or acute – wound healing proceeds through an orderly and timely sequence in which different phases can be distinguished: (1) haemostasis, (2) inflammation, (3) proliferation, and (4) maturation or remodelling [13]. No clear demarcation exists between the phases of wound healing, since tissue repair is a continuous process.

Tissue injury can cause both blood vessel damage and cell death [14]. The first phases of wound healing, therefore, focus on wound sealing, removal of debris and death tissue, and reduction of infection. Haemostasis, the arrest of bleeding, is achieved by vasoconstriction and clotting [13]. The formation of a clot serves as a temporary wound shield and provides a provisional matrix over which and through which cells can migrate during the repair process [15]. Importantly, the clot also serves as a reservoir of cytokines and growth factors that are released as activated platelets within the clot degranulate (e.g. PDGF, TGF-β1, TGF-β2, PDEGF, PAF, IGF-1, fibronectin, and serotin) [15–18]. These cytokines and growth factors play an important role in the subsequent stages of wound healing.

In the inflammatory phase, neutrophils and monocytes are attracted from the circulating blood to the wound site by a variety of chemotactic signals [15]. Neutrophils normally begin arriving at the wound site within minutes of injury. Their role is clearance of contaminating bacteria, as well as release of pro-inflammatory cytokines that probably serve as some of the earliest signals to activate local fibroblasts and keratinocytes [15, 19]. Unless a wound is grossly infected, the neutrophil infiltration ceases after a few days. Macrophages continue to accumulate at the wound site and are essential for effective wound healing [15, 20]. Their tasks include phagocytosis of any remaining pathogenic organisms and other cell and matrix debris. Once activated, macrophages release a battery of growth factors and cytokines at the wound site (e.g. FGF, EGF, VEGF, TNF-a, IL-1, and IFN-γ) [15–17]. These chemical messengers also stimulate the infiltration, proliferation, and migration of fibroblasts and keratinocytes [16, 18].

The proliferative phase comprises of (1) epithelization, (2) fibroplasia, and (3) angiogenesis. [13, 21, 22]. Within hours of injury the process of epithelization takes place, and keratinocytes proliferate and migrate from hair appendages and/or wound edges to cover the exposed tissue [13]. In order to cut a path through the fibrin clot or along the interface between the clot and the healthy dermis, the leading-edge keratinocytes have to dissolve the fibrin barrier ahead of them by means of fibrinolytic enzymes [15]. Once the denuded wound surface has been covered by a monolayer of keratinocytes, epidermal migration ceases and a new stratified epidermis with underlying basal lamina is established from the margins of the wound inward [15, 23]. Attracted by cytokines and growth factors, fibroblasts migrate into the wound site within several days of injury [16]. Once activated, the fibroblasts synthesize and deposit collagen and proteoglycans (i.e. fibroplasia), which ultimately bridge the edges of the wound and give it tensile strength. Like keratinocytes, fibroblasts also release proteases that dissolve the non-viable tissue and the fibrin barrier, which facilitates the remodelling of the matrix. This matrix serves as a scaffold for angiogenesis. Angiogenesis refers to the reconstitution of blood supply to the wound. The stimulus (angiogenic polypeptides such as bFGF, VEGF, TGF-a, IGF, and PDGF) for vessel formation and growth is provided by activated macrophages and keratinocytes [16, 24]. Blood vessels bud from intact vessels and the loops of these new capillaries give the matrix a red granular appearance (i.e. granulation tissue) [13].

The remodelling phase refers to changing patterns in the deposition and organization of matrix components during wound healing. Originally the collagen fibres, which are deposited by fibroblasts, are thin and randomly oriented [16, 17]. During the remodelling phase these collagen fibres become organized into thicker bundles and, aided by proteinases, are rearranged along the stress lines of the wound [13, 16, 17]. Remodelling may last up to a year and contributes to the development of tensile strength in the wound. However, the fibres do not completely revert to their original organization (basket-weave pattern), function, or strength [16, 17].

In pathological conditions such as non-healing pressure ulcers, the normal healing sequence is impaired and the ulcers are locked into a state of chronic inflammation [25]. Mast and Schultz [26, 27] and Tarnuzzer et al. [26, 28] have postulated that this healing impairment is due to the fact that in chronic wounds, repeated trauma, ischaemia, and infection increase the levels of pro-inflammatory cytokines (e.g. IL-1β and TNF-a), increase the level of matrix metalloproteinases (MMPs), decrease the presence of tissue inhibitors of metalloproteinases (TIMPs), and lower the level of growth factors. Cooper et al., using an enzyme-linked immunosorbent assay technique on retrieved wound fluids, showed that the levels of PDGF, bFGF, EGF and TGF-β were markedly decreased in chronic pressure ulcers compared with acute wounds [29, 30]. Recently, Diegelmann et al. demonstrated that an extensive neutrophil infiltration is responsible for the chronic inflammation characteristic of these non-healing pressure ulcers [25]. These neutrophils release significant amounts of MMPs (e.g. collagenase) that are responsible for the destruction of connective tissue matrix [25, 31, 32]. In addition, neutrophils release an enzyme called elastase that is capable of destroying important growth factors such as PDGF and TGF-α [25, 33]. Pressure ulcers further exhibit an environment containing excessive reactive oxygen species that can further damage the cells and the healing tissue [25, 34].

The Wound Healing Society's standards of care principles for pressure ulcers are pressure relief, moist wound environment, and debridement of necrotic tissue [35–36]. Stage II to IV pressure ulcers are often poorly responsive to standard treatment [37]. Because of the difficulty in treating this condition health care practitioners have often looked for an agent that will help to promote healing of these wounds. Advances in the treatment of these chronic wounds have relied heavily on concepts developed for acute wounds [38]. Wound-healing agents have traditionally included, for example, topical dressings, antimicrobial agents, disinfectants, wound cleaners, wound-debriding agents, and surgery (i.e. skin flaps) [37]. In the past few years, however, a new paradigm for the treatment of chronic wounds is emerging [38]. New therapeutic products are being developed that better address the pathogenic abnormalities of chronic wounds, such as the application of growth factors, tissue-engineered skin grafts, and gene therapy. However, healing of chronic wounds can only proceed once the inflammation is controlled [25]. To provoke an ideal response to these new therapeutics, it is important to properly prepare the wound bed first [25, 39, 40]. Therefore, "wound-bed preparation" should always be included in the standard protocol for the treatment of pressure ulcers, as well as aggressive nutritional supplementation of all malnourished or undernourished patients [2, 41, 42].

Wound-Bed Preparation

Recently, an extensive protocol for the successful treatment of pressure ulcers has been proposed [2]. An important step in this protocol is effective "wound-bed preparation". This treatment stage focuses on optimizing the wound bed of chronic wounds to facilitate the normal endogenous process of wound healing [38]. Wound-bed preparation is more than debridement alone. It is a very comprehensive approach aimed at reducing oedema and exudates, as well as on eliminating or reducing the bacterial burden and, importantly, correcting the abnormalities in chronic wounds that lead to impaired healing. Wound-bed preparation should be directed toward creating a moist wound-healing environment, while facilitating granulation tissue formation (i.e., new collagen formation and angiogenesis) and decreasing the bacterial count or load in the wound [2]. New treatments can be used additionally on these wounds to promote healing.

New Treatments

New wound-healing treatments aim at the biochemical stimulation of the wound bed to improve wound healing. Important new therapeutics in this category are reviewed below, such as (1) exogenous application of growth factors, (2) tissue-engineered skin grafts, and (3) gene therapy.

Growth Factors

Growth factors provide many of the cellular and molecular signals necessary for normal healing, but can be deficient in pressure ulcers [26, 30, 43]. Progress in the understanding of growth factors in wound healing and the ability to synthesize adequate quantities of these factors in their pure form, using recombinant DNA technologies, has led to clinical trials evaluating their use [44, 45]. Generally, the recombinant growth factors are delivered to the wound through the application of a gel or through subcutaneous injection around the wound edges [45].

Recombinant PDGF-BB is the only growth factor preparation currently approved for clinical use in diabetic foot ulcers [13, 46–48]. In 1992, the first randomized control study on the effect of recombinant PDGF-BB on pressure ulcers was published [49, 50]. This study demonstrated an increase in the rate of wound closure of stage III and IV pressure ulcers within 4 weeks of treatment with 1 $\mu g/cm^2$ PDGF-BB compared with the placebo control group and the groups treated with lower doses (0.01 $\mu g/cm^2$ and 0.1 $\mu g/cm^2$ PDGF-BB) [49]. In 1999, Rees et al. examined the effect of recombinant PDGF-BB (becaplermin gel) on chronic full-thickness pressure ulcers (stage IV) in a 16-week clinical trial [44, 51]. Healing was achieved in 23% of the group treated with becaplermin gel 100 $\mu g/g$, 19% of the group treated with 300 $\mu g/g$, 3% of the group treated with 100 $\mu g/g$ twice daily, and 0% of the placebo group. The negative dose–response effect, the fact that the rate of healing was considerable lower than rates reported with other standard treatments, and the finding that no ulcers healed in the placebo group make interpretations of this study problematic [44]. In another trial, Pierce et al. demonstrated that recombinant PDGF-BB failed to improve the rate of complete healing of pressure ulcers, although a 15% decrease in ulcer volume was observed in the treatment group [44, 52]. Taken together, these results indicate that the efficacy of recombinant PDGF-BB in the treatment of pressure ulcers is still somewhat unclear.

Other growth factors and cytokines, such as Il-1β, bFGF, GM-CSF, TGF-β3, and NGF have also been studied for the treatment of pressure ulcers. Robson et al. studied the safety and effect of topical treatment with recombinant IL-1β in the management of stage III and IV pressure ulcers in 26 patients [53]. The use of IL-1β in this study was safe, but the dose levels tested (0.01, 0.1 and 1 µg/cm^2) did not result in an improvement of the healing ratio. In another study, Robson et al. used recombinant bFGF to treat 50 patients with stage III and IV pressure ulcers in eight dosing regimes, and a trend toward faster healing was observed in six of the eight groups [44, 54]. Sequential use of recombinant growth factors has also been attempted in the treatment of pressure ulcers. In 2000, Robson et al. studied the effect of sequential GM-CSF and bFGF treatment on the healing of stage III and IV pressure ulcers [29]. A total of 61 patients were randomly assigned to receive GM-CSF for 35 days, bFGF for 35 days, sequential therapy of 10 days of GM-CSF followed by 25 days of bFGF, or placebo. The mean change in ulcer volume did not differ significantly among these four treatment groups. However, significantly more patients treated with any kind of cytokine achieved a greater than 85% decrease in ulcer volume than the placebo-controlled patients after 35 days. Furthermore, treatment with bFGF alone showed the best results in this study. In 2001, Hirshberg et al. studied the effect of recombinant TGF-β3 in the treatment of pressure ulcers [55]. The findings of this study indicate that the topical application of TGF-β3 is safe and is very effective at the earliest stages of therapy. At the termination of the study (16 weeks), however, no significant difference was observed in the healing rate among the three treatment groups (1 µg/cm^2 and 2.5 µg/cm^2 TGF-β3 and placebo control). In 2003, Landi et al. attempted to determine whether recombinant NGF is an effective treatment for patients with severe pressure ulcers [44, 56]. In this study, 18 patients with pressure ulcers of the foot were randomly assigned to receive topical NGF for 6 weeks and were compared with 18 patients that received a topical placebo. After 6 weeks of treatment the average reduction in ulcer area was significantly greater in the NGF treatment group than in the placebo control group. This finding indicates that topical treatment with NGF may be an effective therapy for patients with severe pressure ulcers. Recently, Thomas indicated that the data of this study might be somewhat limited due to the study design [44]. First, only pressure ulcers of the foot were studied, which does not limit the validity of the results but makes it difficult to extrapolate them to the treatment of pressure ulcers at other locations. Second, studies in which the healing rate of the control group is very poor should always be interpreted with caution, as part of the difference between the two treatment groups may be caused by failure of treatment in the placebo control group.

Since their introduction in wound healing, the prospects of topical recombinant growth factors as a new treatment for pressure ulcers were high, as preclinical studies showed very promising outcomes [38]. In contrast, the outcome of the clinical trials has been slightly disappointing. A number of explanations can be given for the limited success, and most probably all of them apply. First, it has been hypothesized that the dosage and mode of delivery of topically applied growth factors may have been wrong [29, 38, 57, 58]. Therefore, better insights into the effects and working pathways of growth factors in healing wounds are required. Second, topically applied growth factors could have been lost by the aggressive action of neutrophil-derived enzymes (proteases) such as elastase in pressure ulcers [25, 33]. In future, therefore, strategies need to be explored to down-regulate the neutrophil infiltration and also inhibit or neutralize the host of destructive proteases released from these powerful inflammatory cells [59, 60]. One way to tackle this problem is by effective "wound-bed preparation" before treatment with the growth factor being tested in the clinical trials.

Tissue-Engineered Skin Grafts

A current management option for non-healing pressure ulcers is surgical repair using autologous (i.e. obtained from the patient) skin flaps. Disadvantages of these skin flaps are the requirement for (large) skin biopsies and the additional donor-site wound complications, including delayed healing, scarring, pain and risk of infection [61, 62]. Tissue-engineered skin grafts can be ideal substitutes for these skin flaps. The term "tissue engineering" was adopted by the Washington National Science Foundation bioengineering panel meeting in 1987 [63, 64]. It refers to the application of the principles and methods of engineering and the life sciences toward the development of biological substitutes to restore, maintain, or improve function [64]. However, the essence of tissue engineering is the use of living cells together with natural or synthetic extracellular matrix components. Currently, skin products made of (1) only extracellular matrix materials, (2) mainly cells (e.g. keratinocytes and/or fibroblasts), or (3) a combination of cells and matrices have all been referred to as tissue-engineered skin. The development of tissue-engineered skin grafts has been triggered by advances in research that have focused on cell culture and the cryopreservation of living cells. A fundamental advance was made in 1975, when Rheinwald et al. successfully grew human epidermal keratinocytes for the first time in serial culture with fibroblasts [65].

The use of tissue-engineered skin grafts holds the promise of direct wound closure, while actively influencing and controlling the wound environment. The incorporation of cells in these grafts, which are able to secrete their own growth factors and other mediators of wound healing, might strongly improve the wound-healing process.

A wide range of tissue-engineered skin grafts is commercially available today, some of which are already used as therapeutic products for the treatment of patients with burns and chronic wounds (e.g. venous and diabetic ulcers). These skin grafts can be broadly categorized into *epidermal* grafts, *dermal* grafts, and *composite* grafts, depending on the type and number of cultured skin layers. Apart from the type of skin layer, these products mostly differ in respect of the source of the cells and extracellular matrix (i.e. autologous, obtained from the patient; allogenic, obtained from a human donor; xenogenic, obtained from an animal donor), culture conditions, shelf life, and costs. Autologous skin grafts, which require a small biopsy from the patient's skin, seem the most ideal skin grafts. However, only few autologous skin grafts are commercially available today, because they cannot meet the requirement of immediate "off-the-shelf" availability. In general it takes a couple of weeks to develop a skin graft, so autologous skin grafts cannot be used for direct wound treatment. Therefore, most skin grafts consist of allogenic and/or xenogenic donor material. Disadvantages of using non-autologous donor material are the risks of disease transmission and graft rejection. Therefore, several safety assessments are normally incorporated into the production process of these skin grafts [61]. First, the donor material needs to be screened for blood-borne pathogens and latent viruses. Second, the cell lines need to be fully characterized to minimize, for instance, possible oncogenic potential. Finally, the potential for rejection of non-autologous cells by the recipient's immune response, and the use of immunosuppression therapy, must be addressed early in the development process. The manufacturing and storage of the final product also requires careful consideration. These skin grafts need to be stored by cryopreservation or other techniques that maintain cell viability and efficacy.

An extensive overview of the most important commercially available tissue-engineered skin grafts is given in this section and is summarized in Tables 20.1–3. In general, the main disadvantages of these skin grafts are the high costs, the long culture time, the poor mechanical properties, the occurrence of scar contraction, and the scarcity of clinical data to support their tolerability and effectiveness. Furthermore, skin grafts that contain living cells usually have a limited shelf life. The US Food and Drug Administration (FDA) has approved some skin grafts for clinical use in wound healing. However, the role of these skin grafts in the treatment of pressure ulcers remains to be elucidated.

Epidermal Grafts

Epicel, developed by Genzyme Biosurgery, is one of the oldest autologous epidermal equivalents. It was first created in 1975, but has been commercially available only since 1988 [64, 66, 67]. For the generation of Epicel a small skin biopsy sample is required from which a cell suspension of epidermal keratinocytes can be obtained [67]. This cell suspension is seeded and cultured on lethally irradiated 3T3 mouse fibroblasts. At the moment the cultures reach confluence, the keratinocyte sheets are released with dispase and attached to a non-adherent gauze dressing [67, 68]. Epicel provides permanent wound coverage and has been used to treat burns [67, 69, 70], chronic leg ulcers [67, 71], and pressure ulcers [67, 72].

EpiDex, developed by Modex Thérapeutiques, is another autologous epidermal equivalent composed of a keratinocyte sheet [66]. This epidermal equivalent does not rely on skin biopsies, but is generated from the patient's hair. Precursor cells for epidermal keratinocytes can be easily obtained from plucked scalp hair follicles, and these cells retain a high proliferative capacity irrespective of the age of the donor.

The engineered keratinocyte sheets have always been fragile, hard to handle, and display unstable attachment without dermal substrate. Fidia Advanced Biopolymers is attempting to remove this disadvantage by providing a film of benzoylated hyaluronic acid as additional dermal equivalent (Laserskin) [73]. This film has periodic perforations through which the keratinocytes can migrate to reach the dermis of the host, and further the film is biodegradable. ConvaTec has also generated autologous keratinocyte sheets on porous films of hyaluronic acid (VivoDerm) [66]. This epidermal graft has mainly been used for burns and chronic wounds, such as venous ulcers [66, 74, 75].

In 1983 Pruniéras et al. rendered the culture of keratinocytes more physiological by raising the cultured keratinocytes to the air–liquid interface [76]. By doing so they obtained evidence of a more complete differentiation, as evaluated by morphological criteria. Under the electron microscope, several ultrastructural features reminiscent of those seen in situ could be identified, including tonofilaments, desmosomes, and cell-membrane thickening. The stratum corneum barrier function of the epidermal equivalent could be markedly improved by topical exposure to air.

Keratinocytes can be raised to the air–liquid interface by culturing them on dermal substrates or dermal equivalents. Episkin, developed by Episkin

Table 20.1. Epidermal grafts

Product name	Reference(s)	Company	Epidermal equivalent	Dermal equivalent
Epicel	[64, 66–72]	Genzyme Biosurgery	Autologous keratinocyte sheet	Non-adherent gauze dressing
EpiDex	[66]	Modex Thérapeutiques	Autologous keratinocyte sheet from hair follicle precursor cells	Not indicated
Laserskin	[73]	Fidia Advanced Biopolymers	Autologous keratinocyte sheet	A porous film of benzoylated hyaluronic acid
VivoDerm	[66, 74–75]	ConvaTec	Autologous keratinocyte sheet	A porous film of hyaluronic acid

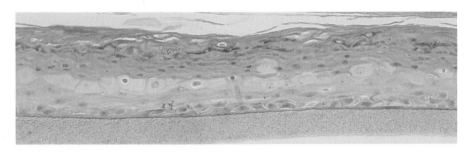

Fig. 20.1. A histological section of EpiDerm

SNC, is generated by seeding keratinocytes on a dermal substrate composed of a thin bovine collagen type I matrix surfaced with a film of human collagen type IV [77, 78]. MatTek Corporation also uses dermal substrates to expose the keratinocytes to air and generate epidermal grafts. EpiDerm is composed of human keratinocytes that are seeded on cell culture inserts coated with collagen. In Fig. 20.1 a histological image of EpiDerm is shown. SkinEthic, developed by Laboratoire SkinEthic, is also composed of human keratinocytes that are seeded on inert polycarbonate cell culture inserts. These three epidermal equivalents are, however, not employed to treat patients, but are mostly used as diagnostic products for topical irritation, corrosivity and other testing studies [73, 77–81]. The culturing of keratinocytes on dermal equivalents is discussed below in the section 'Composite Grafts'.

Dermal Grafts

Besides epidermal equivalents, dermal analogues are required to replace the dermis lost in chronic wounds and burns. Transcyte (formerly known as Dermagraft-TC), developed by Advanced Tissue Sciences (ATIS), was the first tissue-engineered dermal equivalent to receive approval by the FDA [64, 67, 73, 82]. For the generation of this graft, neonatal, allogenic fibroblasts are cultured and proliferate on nylon fibres that are embedded into a Silastic layer for 4–6 weeks [66]. After the synthesis of extracellular matrix components and growth factors, the fibroblasts are rendered nonviable by freezing. Transcyte was originally developed as a temporary covering for severe burns [73]. However, it is also used in the treatment of deep partial-thickness burns.

A modification of Transcyte is Dermagraft, which recently obtained approval by the FDA [73]. In contrast with Transcyte, this graft does not contain a Silastic layer and is a living dermal equivalent [64]. It can be obtained by culturing human allogenic fibroblasts from neonatal foreskin on a bio-absorbable polyglactin net in a sterile bag with circulating nutrients [64, 66]. These cells attach, multiply, and begin secreting growth factors. Investigation of Dermagraft has shown that it possesses considerable an-

Table 20.2. Dermal grafts

Product name	References	Company	Epidermal equivalent	Dermal equivalent
Transcyte	[64, 66, 67, 73, 82]	Advanced Tissue Sciences (ATIS)	A Silastic layer	Allogenic, neonatal, foreskin-derived fibroblasts cultured on a nylon scaffold and rendered non-viable after synthesis of extracellular matrix components and growth factors
Derma-graft	[64, 66, 73, 83–85]	Advanced Tissue Sciences (ATIS)	None	Allogenic, neonatal, foreskin-derived fibroblasts cultured on a bio-absorbable, polyglactin scaffold
Alloderm	[64, 66, 74, 86]	Life Cell Corporation	None	An acellular cadaveric dermis with an intact basement membrane
Xenoderm	[66, 74]	Life Cell Corporation	None	An acellular porcine dermis with an intact basement membrane
E-Z-Derm	[66, 67]	WoundCare	None	An acellular porcine dermis with cross-linked collagen
Oasis	[66, 67, 73]	Cook Biotech	None	A collagen matrix obtained from porcine small-intestinal submucosa
Integra	[64, 66, 67]	Integra Life Science Corporation	A bilaminated Silastic membrane	A matrix of bovine collagen and shark glycosaminoglycans

giogenic activity, which is enhanced by the cryopreservation process used to store the product [73, 83–85]. This graft is commercially available for use in diabetic foot ulcers [73]. The living fibroblast collagen matrix can be used alone or as a basis for a skin graft or an autologous skin flap [66].

Alloderm, developed by Life Cell Corporation, is made of salt-processed human cadaveric skin and comprises an acellular dermal matrix and an intact basement membrane complex, without an epidermis [64, 86]. This dermal substrate received FDA approval in 1992 [66]. Alloderm is decellularized, freeze-dried and biochemically stabilized [64]. This dermal graft has been used for the treatment of burns and dermal defects. Alloderm provides a template with natural dermal porosity for regeneration and allows the use of thinner additional grafts. Xenoderm is quite similar to Alloderm. This dermal substrate is developed by the same general process, but with material obtained from porcine skin [66, 74].

E-Z-Derm, developed by WoundCare, is a temporary skin substitute [66, 67]. This dermal substrate is an acellular porcine dermal matrix, in which the porcine collagen has been chemically cross-linked using an aldehyde. It is available as a perforated or a non-perforated dressing attached to a gauze liner that is discarded before application [67].

Oasis, developed by Cook Biotech, is made of material obtained from porcine small intestinal submucosa [66, 67, 73]. The serosa, smooth muscle, and submucosa are removed from this material [66]. The remaining collagenous, three-dimensional matrix serves as a reservoir for cytokines and cell-adhesion molecules, providing a scaffold for tissue growth after implantation. It has been proven that the structure and chemical composition of Oasis support tissue-specific remodelling [66, 67]. Oasis is supplied in hydrated (moist) or lyophilized (dry) sheets.

Integra, developed by the Integra Life Science Corporation, is composed of a bilaminated membrane consisting of a Silastic outer covering bonded to a collagen-based dermal equivalent, composed of bovine tendon collagen and shark glycosaminoglycans [64, 66, 67]. In 1996, Integra received FDA approval for use of Integra in burns. The main quality of this material are the pores induced in the matrix by a freeze-drying process that includes cross-linking [66]. At the moment the matrix becomes vascularized, the disposable Silastic layer is removed and can be replaced by a skin graft or combined to an autologous skin flap [66, 67].

Composite Grafts

Apligraf, developed by Organogenesis, is a bilayered skin equivalent that received FDA approval in 1998 [64, 66, 67]. This product is composed of both a dermal and an epidermal equivalent, containing living allogenic keratinocytes as well as fibroblasts. To generate Apligraf, human keratinocytes and human dermal fibroblasts are derived from neonatal foreskin and propagated in culture [64]. The dermal equivalent is composed of a mixture of bovine type I collagen and human fibroblasts. After 2 weeks of generating this mixture, a dense fibrous network of newly formed collagen and other matrix components is formed. A suspension of keratinocytes is placed on top of this mixture, to generate the overlying epidermal equivalent. Subsequently, these keratinocytes are exposed to an air–liquid interface to promote keratinocyte differentiation and the formation of a stratum corneum.

Apligraf resembles human skin histologically and can be thought of as 'smart' tissue. It has been shown to have the ability to self-regenerate when injured in vitro, and produces a number of growth factors and cytokines [64, 66]. It is hypothesized that the cells of this tissue-engineered skin can serve the environment into which they are placed, and take 'corrective action' by producing the appropriate soluble factors, IL-1, IL-3, IL-6, IL-8, TGF-α, TGF-β, and bFGF [64, 82]. In 2000, Brem et al. performed a clinical trial to test the efficacy of Apligraf in treating pressure ulcers [87]. In pressure ulcers of various durations, the application of Apligraf with the surgical principles used in a traditional skin graft (i.e. skin flap) is successful in producing healing. In patients with pressure ulcers, 13 of the 21 wounds healed in an average of 29 days. All wounds that did not heal in this series occurred in patients who had an additional stage IV ulcer or a wound with exposed bone. One possible limitation of this study is that it was a non-randomized study with no placebo group. However, it had been established earlier in separate prospective, randomized, placebo-controlled studies that Apligraf accelerates closure of two types of chronic wounds (i.e. venous and diabetic) [87–90]. The data presented in the study performed by Brem et al. indicate that when infection is controlled by debridement and other appropriate therapy, biological intervention with Apligraf provides a choice that assures lack of progression in pressure ulcers [87].

Orcel, developed by Ortec International, consists of allogenic fibroblasts and keratinocytes grown in vitro and seeded on the reverse side of a bilayered matrix of bovine collagen [66]. This bilayered skin equivalent has

Table 20.3. Composite grafts

Product name	References	Company	Epidermal equivalent	Dermal equivalent
Apligraf	[64, 66, 67, 87–90]	Organo-genesis	Allogenic, neonatal, foreskin-derived keratinocytes cultured on top of the dermal equivalent and exposed to air to promote keratinocyte differentiation and formation of a stratum corneum	Allogenic, neonatal, foreskin-derived fibroblasts cultured with bovine type I collagen to form a dense network of newly formed extracellular matrix components
Orcel	[66, 73]	Ortec International	Allogenic keratinocytes cultured on the non-porous upper side of the dermal equivalent	Allogenic fibroblast cultured in a porous cross-linked bovine collagen sponge matrix

also obtained FDA approval [73]. The collagen matrix of this skin equivalent consists of a cross-linked bovine collagen sponge with an overlay of pepsinized insoluble collagen [66]. The keratinocytes are seeded on the insoluble collagen and the fibroblasts are seeded on the underside of the porous sponge. Orcel has been used in the treatment of epidermolysis bullosa (EB). Ortec International has also submitted a pre-market approval application for the use of Orcel in treating skin graft donor sites and has performed successful clinical trials in diabetic and venous ulcers [73].

The abundance of engineered skin grafts indicates that substantial progress has already been made in the field of skin tissue engineering. Nevertheless, several drawbacks need to be overcome to generate grafts mimicking normal human skin with high accuracy, which might also be applicable for effective healing of pressure ulcers. In particular the mechanical properties and integrity of engineered skin grafts remain to be optimized, as these properties are essential for bearing the prolonged loads applied to the human body under predisposing conditions for pressure ulcer development. Therefore, current research in the field of skin tissue engineering focuses, for instance, on improving the skin barrier properties [91–93] and on improving the structural interaction of the epidermal and the dermal equivalent of composite grafts [94, 95].

Gene Therapy

The skin is an attractive target for gene therapy because it is easily accessible and shows great potential as an ectopic site for delivery of protein (e.g. growth factors and cytokines) in vivo [96]. The application of gene therapy to the field of wound healing is still in its infancy, but it may have potential. The purpose of gene therapy in this setting is either to promote wound healing or to reduce the healing complications that lead to scarring, keloid formation or chronic ulceration. Dependent on the type and the severity of the wound, different gene delivery strategies can be used to promote wound healing. The most appropriate treatment for large wounds, which are in need of skin replacements, is the use of genetically modified skin grafts. In this case, cells need to be cultured, genetically modified in vitro, and used to engineer a skin graft that can be transplanted in the denuded wound areas to facilitate in situ tissue regeneration. Cells can be genetically engineered to express a variety of molecules, including growth factors that induce cell growth/differentiation or cytokines that prevent immunological reaction to the implant. On the other hand, smaller wounds may be amenable to in vivo gene delivery using a variety of approaches including gene injection, gene gun, microseeding, and liposomal gene delivery. The results of preclinical studies of gene therapy for wound healing are promising, but numerous clinical trials have to be performed to determine the real effectiveness of this new treatment in healing chronic wounds, such as pressure ulcers.

The majority of gene therapy studies in wound healing used recombinant retroviruses to modify the epidermal keratinocytes of engineered skin grafts [96]. In 1998, Eming et al. showed that PDGF-A overexpression improved the performance of composite grafts when transplanted to full-thickness wounds on athymic mice [96, 97]. Seven days after transplantation, these grafts demonstrated reduced wound contraction and increased dermal cell density in comparison with unmodified control grafts. Earlier, it had been demonstrated by Eming et al. that transplantation of genetically modified epidermal grafts overexpressing PDGF-A increased the growth and vascularization of the underlying dermal tissue [96, 98]. These results demonstrate the feasibility of using genetically modified skin grafts overexpressing PDGF-A to modulate wound healing. In 2000, Supp et al. used a recombinant retrovirus to transfer the gene encoding for VEGF to epidermal keratinocytes of composite grafts [96, 99]. VEGF-modified and unmodified composite grafts were transplanted to full-thickness wounds on athymic mice, and elevated VEGF mRNA expression was detected in the modified grafts for at least 2 weeks after surgery. The VEGF-modified grafts further exhibited increased numbers of dermal blood vessels and decreased time to vascularization compared with the unmodified control grafts. Recently, Supp et al. demonstrated that the VEGF-modified grafts showed reduced contraction, which suggest more stable engraftment and better tissue development [96, 100]. Furthermore, an altered spatial distribution of blood vessels in the VEGF-modified grafts was demonstrated with more vessels in the upper epidermis, which is in close proximity to the modified epidermal cells. These results suggest that VEGF overexpression in genetically modified skin grafts can contribute to improved healing of full-thickness wounds.

Many technologies have also been developed for in vivo gene delivery to the skin [96]. The efficiency of these gene delivery methods for the treatment of (chronic) wounds has been determined in various preclinical studies. In 1999, Liechty et al. demonstrated that the application of a single dose of PDGF-B-encoding adenovirus on wounds in ischaemic rabbit ear, which have a 60% delay in healing, enhanced wound healing compared with placebo-treated control wounds, topical application of high concentrations of the PDGF-B protein, and placebo-treated non-ischaemic wounds [96, 101]. These results indicate that adenoviral-mediated gene transfer of PDGF-B overcomes the ischaemic defect in wound healing and, therefore, offers promise in the treatment of chronic non-healing wounds. A β-galactosidase-encoding adenovirus was also applied on wounds in the ischaemic rabbit ear [96, 102]. However, wound reepithelization was impaired in the β-galactosidase treated wounds compared with placebo-treated control wounds. This adverse effect is possibly a result of an acute inflammatory response to the adenoviral particles [96]. Therefore, selection of the proper transgene with appropriate biological activity in wound healing seems essential to avoid an adverse effect on the healing response. The gene gun or particle-mediated gene transfer is another gene delivery method that has been evaluated for wound healing [96]. Propelled from a ballistic device, gold microparticles conjugated with DNA penetrate cell membranes to transfect the cells of the wounded skin. It has been shown that the micro-projectile delivery of EGF, TGF-β and PDGF in the wound bed enhances wound healing rates and increases wound tensile strength [96, 103–105]. Microseeding is also being studied for gene delivery to wounded skin [96]. This method delivers DNA through a set of solid oscillating microneedles which are able to penetrate to various depths of the tissue. Eriksson et al. demonstrated that delivery of an EGF-encoding plasmid to partial thickness wounds in pigs via microseeding is more efficient than gene delivery by a single injection or even the gene gun [96, 106]. Besides physical methods, chemical methods of gene delivery have been employed for wound healing, such as liposomal gene delivery. Sun et al. showed that liposomal delivery of the FGF-1 gene in wounds of diabetic mice promoted wound healing in three administrations, compared with 15 administrations required to achieve a similar biological effect by the delivery of the protein [96, 107].

In addition to wound-healing technologies that introduce genes into target cells, antisense oligonucleotides (ODN) have been used to block unwanted gene functions [96]. This method allows the specific inhibition of the biosynthesis of a protein by adding to the cells a synthetic nucleotide complementary to a portion of the mRNA encoding for the protein [108]. The ODN penetrate into the cell and are thought to hybridize and block the recognition of the normal message [108, 109]. Choi et al. demonstrated that topical application of antisense ODN targeted to TGF-β1 mRNA reduced scarring compared with the control wound site on a mouse [96, 110]. This result indicates that antisense TGF-β1 ODN could be used for ameliorating scar formation during wound healing.

Future Perspectives

With the ongoing progress in biotechnology and life sciences a new paradigm for treating chronic wounds has emerged. New treatments are being developed that better address the pathogenic abnormalities of chronic wounds, such as topical application of growth factors, tissue-engineered skin grafts, and gene therapy. Despite their current shortcomings and limited clinical evaluation these new therapies have great potential for healing pressure ulcers. For widespread clinical application, however, conclusive studies regarding their long-term effects and cost-effectiveness need to be performed. In addition, ethical considerations apply when using, for instance, genetically modified or non-autologous cells as well as their products.

References

1. American Pressure Ulcer Advisory Panel (1998) Pressure ulcers prevalence, cost and risk assessment: consensus development conference statement. Decubitus 2:24–28
2. Brem H, Lyder CH (2004) Protocol for the successful treatment of pressure ulcers. Am J Surg 188 [Suppl 1A]:9–17
3. Bouten CVC, Oomens CWJ, Baaijens FPT, Bader DL (2003) The etiology of pressure ulcers: skin deep or muscle bound? Arch Phys Med Rehabil 84:616–619
4. Barrois B, Allaert FA, Colin DA (1995) A survey of pressure sore prevalence in hospitals in the greater Paris region. J Wound Care 4:234–236
5. Baumgarten M, Margolis D, Berlin JA, Strom BL, Garino J, Kagan SH, Kavesh W, Carson JL (2003) Risk factors for pressure ulcers among early hip fracture patients. Wound Repair Regen 11:96–103
6. Pearson A, Francis K, Hodgkinson B, Curry G (2000) Prevalence and treatment of pressure ulcers in northern New South Wales. Aust J Rural Health 8:103–110
7. Meehan M (1990) Multisite pressure ulcer prevalence survey. Decubitus 3:14–17
8. Bours GJ, Halfens RJ, Lubbers M, Haalboom JR (1999) The development of a national registration form to measure the prevalence of pressure ulcers in The Netherlands. Ostomy Wound Manage 45:28–33, 36–38, 40
9. Allman RM, Laprade CA, Noel LB, et al. (1986) Pressure sores among hospitalized patients. Ann Intern Med 105:337–342
10. Brandeis GH, Morris JN, Nash DJ, Lipsitz LA (1990) The epidemiology and natural history of pressure ulcers in elderly nursing home residents. JAMA 264:2905–2909
11. Walter JS, Sacks J, Othman R, et al. (2002) A database of self-reported secondary medical problems among VA spinal cord injury patients: its role in clinical care and management. J Rehabil Res Dev 39:53–61
12. Garber SL, Rintala DH (2003) Pressure ulcers in veterans with spinal cord injury: a retrospective study. J Rehabil Res Dev 40:433–441
13. Jeffcoate WJ, Price P, Harding KG (2004) Wound healing and treatments for people with diabetic foot ulcers. Diabetes Metab Res Rev 20:S78–S89
14. Calvin M (1998) Cutaneous wounds repair. Wounds 10:12–32
15. Martin P (1997) Wound healing – aiming at the perfect skin regeneration. Science 276:75–81
16. Hunt TK, Hopf H, Hussain Z (2000) Physiology of wound healing. Adv Skin Wound Care 13[Suppl 2]:6–11
17. Witte MB, Barbul A (1997) General principles of wound healing. Surg Clin North Am 77:509–528
18. Hunt TK, Zabel, DD (1995) Critical care of wounds and wounded patients. In: Ayres SM, Grenvik A, Holbrook PR, et al (eds) Textbook of critical care, 3rd edn. Saunders, Philadelphia, pp 1457–1486
19. Hubner G, Brauchle M, Smola H, Madlener M, Fassler R, Werner S (1996) Differential regulation of pro-inflammatory cytokines during wound healing in normal and glucocorticoid-treated mice. Cytokine 8:548–556
20. Leibovich SJ, Ross R (1975) The role of the macrophage in wound repair. A study with hydrocortisone and antimacrophage serum. Am J Pathol 78:71–100

21. Risau W (1997) Mechanisms of angiogenesis. Nature 386:671–674
22. Stephens P, Thomas DW (2002) The cellular proliferative phase of the wound repair process. J Wound Care 11:253–261
23. Gipson IK, Spurr-Michaud SJ, Tisdale AS (1988) Hemidesmosomes and anchoring fibril collagen appear synchronously during development and wound healing. Dev Biol 126:253–262
24. Feng JJ, Hussain MZ, Constant J, et al. (1998) Angiogenesis in wound healing. J Surg Pathol 3:1–8
25. Diegelmann RF, Evans MC (2004) Wound healing: an overview of acute, fibrotic and delayed healing. Front Biosci 9:283–289
26. Payne WG, Ochs DE, Meltzer DD, et al. (2001) Long-term outcome study of growth factor-treated pressure ulcers. Am J Surg 181:81–86
27. Mast BA, Schultz GS (1996) Interactions of cytokines, growth factors, and proteases in acute and chronic wounds. Wound Repair Regen 4:411–420
28. Tarnuzzer RW, Macauley SP, Mast BA, et al. (1997) Epidermal growth factor in wound healing: a model for the molecular pathogenesis of chronic wounds. In: Ziegler T, Pierce G, Herndon D, editors. Growth factors and wound healing. Springer, New York Berlin Heidelberg, pp 206–228
29. Robson MC, Hill DP, Smith PD, Wang X, Meyer-Siegler K, Ko F, VandeBerg JS, Payne WG, Ochs D, Robson LE (2000) Sequential cytokine therapy for pressure ulcers: clinical and mechanistic response. Ann Surg 231:600–611
30. Cooper DM, Yu EZ, Hennessey P, Ko F, Robson MC (1994) Determination of endogenous cytokines in chronic wounds. Ann Surg 219:688–691
31. Nwomeh BC, Liang HX, Diegelmann RF, Cohen IK, Yager DR (1998) Dynamics of the matrix metalloproteinases MMP-1 and MMP-8 in acute open human dermal wounds. Wound Repair Regen 6:127–134
32. Nwomeh BC, Liang HX, Cohen IK, Yager DR (1999) MMP-8 is the predominant collagenase in healing wounds and nonhealing ulcers. J Surg Res 81:189–195
33. Yager DR, Zhang LY, Liang HX, Diegelmann RF, Cohen IK (1996) Wound fluids from human pressure ulcers contain elevated matrix metalloproteinase levels and activity compared to surgical wound fluids. J Invest Dermatol 107:743–748
34. Wenk J, Foitzik A, Achterberg V, Sabiwalsky A, Dissemond J, Meewes C, Reitz A, Brenneisen P, Wlaschek M, Meyer-Ingold W, Scharffetter-Kochanek K (2001) Selective pick-up of increased iron by deferoxamine-coupled cellulose abrogates the iron-driven induction of matrix-degrading metalloproteinase 1 and lipid peroxidation in human dermal fibroblasts in vitro: a new dressing concept. J Invest Dermatol 116:833–839
35. Eaglstein WH, Falanga V (1997) Chronic wounds. Surg Clin North Am 77:689–700
36. Ehrlich HP, Diegelmann RF (1994) Responses from the wound healing clinical focus group at the Food and Drug Administration to the Government Relations Committee of the Wound Healing Society. Stars and Stripes Newsletter of the Wound Healing Society 4:5–12
37. Margolis DJ, Lewis VL (1995) A literature assessment of the use of miscellaneous topical agents, growth factors, and skin equivalents for the treatment of pressure ulcers. Dermatol Surg 21:145–148
38. Falanga V (2004) The chronic wound: impaired healing and solutions in the context of wound bed preparation. Blood Cells Mol Dis 32:88–94

39. Robson MC, Mustoe TA, Hunt TK (1998) The future of recombinant growth factors in wound healing. Am J Surg 176 [Suppl 2A]:80S–82S

40. Falanga V (1993) Growth factors and wound healing. Dermatol Clin 11:667–675

41. Lewis M, Pearson A, Ward C (2003) Pressure ulcer prevention and treatment: transforming research findings into consensus based clinical guidelines. Int J Nurs Pract 9:92–102

42. Strauss EA, Margolis DJ (1996) Malnutrition in patients with pressure ulcers: morbidity, mortality, and clinically practical assessments. Adv Wound Care 9:37–40

43. Bennett NT, Schultz GS (1993) Growth factors and wound healing: Part II. Role in normal and chronic wound healing. Am J Surg 166:74–81

44. Thomas DR (2003) The promise of topical growth factors in healing pressure ulcers. Ann Intern Med 139:694–695

45. Evans CA, Hagelstein SM, Ivins, NM (2000) Current challenges in wound care management: an overview. Br J Community Nurs 5:332, 334–336, 338–339

46. Steed DL (1995) Clinical evaluation of recombinant human platelet derived growth factor for the treatment of lower extremity diabetic ulcers. The diabetic ulcer study group. J Vasc Surg 21:71–78

47. Smiell JM, Wieman TJ, Steed DL, Perry BH, Sampson AR, Schwab BH (1999) Efficacy and safety of becaplermin (recombinant human platelet-derived growth factor-BB) in patients with nonhealing, lower extremity diabetic ulcers: a combined analysis of four randomized studies. Wound Repair Regen 7:335–346

48. Mulder GD (2001) Diabetic foot ulcers: old problems – new technologies. Nephrol Dial Transplant 16:695–698

49. Robson MC, Phillips LG, Thomason A, Robson LE, Pierce GF (1992) Platelet-derived growth factor BB for the treatment of chronic pressure ulcers. Lancet 339:23–25

50. Robson MC, Phillips LG, Thomason A, Altrock BW, Pence PC, Heggers JP, Johnston AF, McHugh TP, Anthony MS, Robson LE, et al. (1992) Recombinant human platelet-derived growth factor-BB for the treatment of chronic pressure ulcers. Ann Plast Surg 29:193–201

51. Rees RS, Robson MC, Smiell JM, Perry BH (1999) Becaplermin gel in the treatment of pressure ulcers: a phase II randomized, double-blind, placebo-controlled study. Wound Repair Regen 7:141–147

52. Pierce GF, Tarpley JE, Allman RM, Goode PS, Serdar CM, Morris B, Mustoe TA, Vandeberg J (1994) Tissue repair processes in healing chronic pressure ulcers treated with recombinant platelet-derived growth factor BB. Am J Pathol 145:1399–1410

53. Robson MC, Abdullah A, Burns, BF, Philips LG, Garrison L, Cowan W, Hill D, Vandeberg J, Robson LE, Scheeler S (1994) Safety and effect of topical recombinant human interleukin-1β in the management of pressure sores. Wound Repair Regen 2:177–181

54. Robson MC, Phillips LG, Lawrence WT, Bishop JB, Youngerman JS, Hayward PG, Broemeling LD, Heggers JP (1992) The safety and effect of topically applied recombinant basic fibroblast growth factor on the healing of chronic pressure sores. Ann Surg 216:401–406

55. Hirshberg J, Coleman J, Marchant B, Rees RS (2001) TGF-beta3 in the treatment of pressure ulcers: a preliminary report. Adv Skin Wound Care 14:91–95

56. Landi F, Aloe L, Russo A, Cesari M, Onder G, Bonini S, Carbonin PU, Bernabei R (2003) Topical treatment of pressure ulcers with nerve growth factor: a randomized clinical trial. Ann Intern Med 139:635–641

57. Robson MC (1991) Growth factors as wound healing agents. Curr Opin Biotechnol 2:863–867

58. Cross SE, Roberts MS (1999) Defining a model to predict the distribution of topically applied growth factors and other solutes in excisional full-thickness wounds. J Invest Dermatol 112:36–41

59. Diegelmann RF (2003) Excessive neutrophils characterize chronic pressure ulcers. Wound Repair Regen 11:490–495

60. Edwards JV, Yager DR, Cohen IK, Diegelmann RF, Montante S, Bertoniere N, Bopp AF (2001) Modified cotton gauze dressings that selectively absorb neutrophil elastase activity in solution. Wound Repair Regen 9:50–58

61. Jimenez PA, Jimenez SE (2004) Tissue and cellular approaches to wound repair. Am J Surg 187:56S–64S

62. Jones JE, Nelson EA (2000) Skin grafting for venous leg ulcers. Cochrane Database Syst Rev:CD001737

63. Nerem RM (1992) Tissue engineering in the USA. Med Biol Eng Comput 30:CE8–12

64. Lee KH (2000) Tissue-engineered human skin substitutes: development and clinical application. Yonsei Med J 41:774–779

65. Rheinwald JG, Green H (1975) Serial cultivation of strains of human epidermal keratinocytes: the formation of keratinizing colonies from single cells. Cell 6:331–343

66. Ramos-e-Silva M, Ribeiro de Castro MC (2002) New dressings, including tissue-engineered living skin. Clin Dermatol 20:715–723

67. Bello YM, Falabella AF, Eaglstein WH (2001) Tissue-engineered skin. Current status in wound healing. Am J Clin Dermatol 2:305–313

68. Green H, Kehinde O, Thomas J (1979) Growth of cultured human epidermal cells into multiple epithelia suitable for grafting. Proc Natl Acad Sci USA 76:5665–5668

69. O'Connor NE, Mulliken JB, Bank-Schlegel S, et al. (1981) Grafting of bruns with cultured epithelium prepared from autologous epidermal cells. Lancet I:75–78

70. Gallico GG 3rd, O'Connor NE, Compton CC, Kehinde O, Green H (1984) Permanent coverage of large burn wounds with autologous cultured human epithelium. N Engl J Med 311:448–451

71. Hefton JM, Caldwell D, Biozes DG, Balin AK, Carter DM (1986) Grafting of skin ulcers with cultured autologous epidermal cells. J Am Acad Dermatol 14:399–405

72. Phillips TJ, Pachas W (1994) Clinical trial of cultured autologous keratinocyte grafts in the treatment of long-standing pressure ulcers. Wounds 6:113–119

73. Mansbridge J (2002) Tissue-engineered skin substitutes. Expert Opin Biol Ther 2:25–34

74. Sefton MV, Woodhouse KA (1998) Tissue engineering. J Cutan Med Surg 3 [Suppl 1]:18–23

75. Phillips TJ (1999) Tissue-engineered skin: an alternative to split-thickness skin grafts? Arch Dermatol 135:977–978

76. Prunieras M, Regnier M, Woodley D (1983) Methods for cultivation of keratinocytes with an air-liquid interface. J Invest Dermatol 81 [Suppl 1]:28s–33s

77. Ponec M, Boelsma E, Weerheim A, Mulder A, Bouwstra J, Mommaas M (2000) Lipid and ultrastructural characterization of reconstructed skin models. Int J Pharm 203:211–225

78. Ponec M, Boelsma E, Gibbs S, Mommaas M (2002) Characterization of reconstructed skin models. Skin Pharmacol Appl Skin Physiol 15 [Suppl 1]:4–17

79. Coquette A, Berna N, Vandenbosch A, Rosdy M, De Wever B, Poumay Y (2003) Analysis of interleukin-1alpha (IL-1alpha) and interleukin-8 (IL-8) expression and release in in vitro reconstructed human epidermis for the prediction of in vivo skin irritation and/or sensitization. Toxicol In Vitro 17:311–321

80. Faller C, Bracher M (2002) Reconstructed skin kits: reproducibility of cutaneous irritancy testing. Skin Pharmacol Appl Skin Physiol 15 [Suppl 1]:74–91

81. Gibbs S, Vietsch H, Meier U, Ponec M (2002) Effect of skin barrier competence on SLS and water-induced IL-1alpha expression. Exp Dermatol 11:217–223

82. Eaglstein WH, Falanga V (1998) Tissue engineering for skin: an update. J Am Acad Dermatol 39:1007–1010

83. Mansbridge JN, Liu K, Pinney RE, Patch R, Ratcliffe A, Naughton GK (1999) Growth factors secreted by fibroblasts: role in healing diabetic foot ulcers. Diabetes Obes Metab 1:265–279

84. Pinney E, Liu K, Sheeman B, Mansbridge J (2000) J. Human three-dimensional fibroblast cultures express angiogenic activity. J Cell Physiol 183:74–82

85. Liu K, Yang Y, Mansbridge J (2000) Comparison of the stress response to cryopreservation in monolayer and three-dimensional human fibroblast cultures: stress proteins, MAP kinases, and growth factor gene expression. Tissue Eng 6:539–554

86. Phillips TJ (1998) New skin for old: developments in biological skin substitutes. Arch Dermatol 134:344–349

87. Brem H, Balledux J, Bloom T, Kerstein MD, Hollier L (2000) Healing of diabetic foot ulcers and pressure ulcers with human skin equivalent: a new paradigm in wound healing. Arch Surg 135:627–634

88. Falanga V, Sabolinski M (1999) A bilayered living skin construct (APLIGRAF) accelerates complete closure of hard-to-heal venous ulcers. Wound Repair Regen 7:201–207

89. Falanga V (1999) How to use Apligraf to treat venous ulcers. Skin Aging 25:30–36

90. Pham HT, Rosenblum BI, Lyons TE, et al. (1999) Evaluation of a human skin equivalent for the treatment of diabetic foot ulcers in a prospective, randomized, clinical trial. Wounds 11:79–86

91. Ponec M, Wauben-Penris PJ, Burger A, Kempenaar J, Bodde HE (1990) Nitroglycerin and sucrose permeability as quality markers for reconstructed human epidermis. Skin Pharmacol 3:126–135

92. Ponec M, Weerheim A, Kempenaar J, Mulder A, Gooris GS, Bouwstra J, Mommaas AM (1997) The formation of competent barrier lipids in reconstructed human epidermis requires the presence of vitamin C. J Invest Dermatol 109:348–355

93. Ponec M, Gibbs S, Pilgram G, Boelsma E, Koerten H, Bouwstra J, Mommaas M (2001) Barrier function in reconstructed epidermis and its resemblance to native human skin. Skin Pharmacol Appl Skin Physiol 14 [Suppl 1]:63–71

94. Medalie DA, Eming SA, Collins ME, Tompkins RG, Yarmush ML, Morgan JR (1997) Differences in dermal analogs influence subsequent pigmentation, epidermal differentiation, basement membrane, and rete ridge formation of transplanted composite skin grafts. Transplantation 64:454–465

95. Guo M, Grinnell F (1989) Basement membrane and human epidermal differentiation in vitro. J Invest Dermatol 93:372–378
96. Andreadis ST (2004) Gene transfer to epidermal stem cells: implications for tissue engineering. Expert Opin Biol Ther 4:783–800
97. Eming SA, Medalie DA, Tompkins RG, Yarmush ML, Morgan JR (1998) Genetically modified human keratinocytes overexpressing PDGF-A enhance the performance of a composite skin graft. Hum Gene Ther 9:529–539
98. Eming SA, Lee J, Snow RG, Tompkins RG, Yarmush ML, Morgan JR (1995) Genetically modified human epidermis overexpressing PDGF-A directs the development of a cellular and vascular connective tissue stroma when transplanted to athymic mice – implications for the use of genetically modified keratinocytes to modulate dermal regeneration. J Invest Dermatol 105:756–763
99. Supp DM, Supp AP, Bell SM, Boyce ST (2000) Enhanced vascularization of cultured skin substitutes genetically modified to overexpress vascular endothelial growth factor. J Invest Dermatol 114:5–13
100. Supp DM, Boyce ST (2002) Overexpression of vascular endothelial growth factor accelerates early vascularization and improves healing of genetically modified cultured skin substitutes. J Burn Care Rehabil 23:10–20
101. Liechty KW, Nesbit M, Herlyn M, Radu A, Adzick NS, Crombleholme TM (1999) Adenoviral-mediated overexpression of platelet-derived growth factor-B corrects ischemic impaired wound healing. J Invest Dermatol 113:375–383
102. Liechty KW, Sablich TJ, Adzick NS, Crombleholme TM (1999) Recombinant adenoviral mediated gene transfer in ischemic impaired wound healing. Wound Repair Regen 7:148–153
103. Andree C, Swain WF, Page CP, Macklin MD, Slama J, Hatzis D, Eriksson E (1994) In vivo transfer and expression of a human epidermal growth factor gene accelerates wound repair. Proc Natl Acad Sci USA 91:12188–12192
104. Benn SI, Whitsitt JS, Broadley KN, Nanney LB, Perkins D, He L, Patel M, Morgan JR, Swain WF, Davidson JM (1996) Particle-mediated gene transfer with transforming growth factor-beta1 cDNAs enhances wound repair in rat skin. J Clin Invest 98:2894–2902
105. Eming SA, Whitsitt JS, He L, Krieg T, Morgan JR, Davidson JM (1999) Particle-mediated gene transfer of PDGF isoforms promotes wound repair. J Invest Dermatol 112:297–302
106. Eriksson E, Yao F, Svensjo T, Winkler T, Slama J, Macklin MD, Andree C, McGregor M, Hinshaw V, Swain WF (1998) In vivo gene transfer to skin and wound by microseeding. J Surg Res 78:85–91
107. Sun L, Xu L, Chang H, Henry FA, Miller RM, Harmon JM, Nielsen TB (1997) Transfection with aFGF cDNA improves wound healing. J Invest Dermatol 108:313–318
108. Kim HM, Choi DH, Lee YM (1998) Inhibition of wound-induced expression of transforming growth factor-beta 1 mRNA by its antisense oligonucleotides. Pharmacol Res 37:289–293
109. Thierry AR, Rahman A, Dritschilo A (1992) Liposomal delivery as a new approach to transport antisense oligonucleotides. In Erickson R, Izant JG, editors. Gene regulation: biology of antisense RNA and DNA. Raven Press, New York, pp 147–161
110. Choi BM, Kwak HJ, Jun CD, Park SD, Kim KY, Kim HR, Chung HT (1996) Control of scarring in adult wounds using antisense transforming growth factor-beta 1 oligodeoxynucleotides. Immunol Cell Biol 74:144–150

Subject Index